APHASIA AND SENSORY-PERCEPTUAL DEFICITS IN ADULTS

Ralph M. Reitan, Ph.D.
Department of Psychology
University of Arizona
and
Neuropsychology Laboratory
1338 E. Edison Street
Tucson, Arizona 85719

APHASIA AND SENSORY-PERCEPTUAL DEFICITS IN ADULTS;

Published by:
Reitan Neuropsychology
Laboratories, Inc.
1338 E. Edison Street
Tucson, Arizona 85719

Contents

PREFACE . . . v

1. A SELECTIVE REVIEW OF TOPICS AND CONTRIBUTORS IN THE AREA OF APHASIA . . . 1
   - *Identification of Aphasic Deficits and Classification of Aphasic Disorders* . . . 2
   - *Correlation of Cerebral Localization and Aphasic Manifestations* . . . 5
   - *Tests and Methods for Examination for Aphasia* . . . 7

2. APHASIA, INTELLIGENCE, AND COGNITIVE IMPAIRMENT . . . 14
   - *Studies of the Nature of Aphasia* . . . 15

3. HISTORICAL AND CONCEPTUAL ASPECTS OF THE REITAN-INDIANA APHASIA SCREENING TEST AND THE REITAN-KLØVE SENSORY-PERCEPTUAL EXAMINATION . . . 21

4. INSTRUCTIONS FOR ADMINISTERING THE REITAN-INDIANA APHASIA SCREENING TEST AND THE REITAN-KLØVE SENSORY-PERCEPTUAL EXAMINATION . . . 26
   - *Aphasia Screening Test* . . . 26
   - *The Sensory-perceptual Examination* . . . 29
   - *Examination for Sensory-perceptual Disturbances* . . . 30

5. IDENTIFICATION OF DEFICITS ELICITED BY THE APHASIA SCREENING TEST AND THE SENSORY-PERCEPTUAL EXAMINATION . . . 32

6. BRAIN CORRELATES OF APHASIC AND SENSORY-PERCEPTUAL DEFICITS . . . 35
   - *Frequency of Occurrence of Aphasic Deficits* . . . 35
   - *Intercorrelations of Aphasic Symptoms* . . . 36

7. RESULTS FOR INDIVIDUAL PATIENTS . . . 46
   - *Intrinsic Brain Tumors* . . . 48
   - *Cerebral Vascular Disease* . . . 103
   - *Traumatic Brain Injuries, Parkinson's Disease, Multiple Sclerosis, Alzheimer's Disease, and Encephalitis* . . . 125
   - *Listing of Neurological Diagnoses for Individual Patients* . . . 166

8. CONCLUSIONS . . . 167

REFERENCES . . . 169

INDEX . . . 172

Preface

The principal purpose of this book is to provide examples of brain-related deficits on the Reitan-Indiana Aphasia Screening Test and the Reitan-Kløve Sensory-perceptual Examination. These procedures are being used by an increasing number of neuropsychologists and neurologists and it seemed important to provide a series of illustrations of the kinds of deficits in performance shown by persons with brain lesions. In addition, we have taken advantage of the opportunity to review the literature of aphasia briefly, to provide an organized survey of research findings based on our particular intruments, and to update and expand the instructions for administering these tests.

There are several points that are stated recurringly (perhaps repetitively) in this book, but the reason is that they are relevant in a number of contexts. First, while categories of aphasia have repeatedly been described in the literature, the deficits of individual subjects rarely neatly fit any of these categories. This book is about aphasic losses and related deficits that characterize individual human beings rather than ones that fit into categories. Secondly, we conceptualize dysphasic deficits as representing disorders of language functions (abnormalities), not as variations of normal language functions. We believe this position has distinct implications for the entire approach to evaluation of aphasia and differentiates our approach from the use of comprehensive aphasia tests that have been developed in recent years which emphasize a more general evaluation of both normal and impaired language usage. Finally, we postulate that it is necessary to use non-language as well as language tests to derive evidence that language deficits, found in clinical evaluation of individual persons, are unequivocally a result of cerebral damage. In addition, it is very helpful to include an inferential method that utilizes intra-individual comparisons to complement inter-individual bases of evaluating performance. In this volume we have systematically included a sensory-perceptual examination to extend the content of the data, to provide comparisons of the two sides of the body as a basis for drawing inferences regarding the two cerebral hemispheres (an intra-individual approach), and to relate this information to the evaluation of language disorders. Finally, we must emphasize the value of a comprehensive neuropsychological examination, including tests that go beyond those included in this volume, in order to understand brain-behavior relationships in the unit of value – the individual human being.

A number of persons have made contributions to this volume and the related procedures for examining aphasia and sensory-perceptual abilities. I should like to acknowledge the interest and cooperation of my colleagues in neuropsychology, neurology, neurosurgery and neuropathology, especially at the Indiana University Medical Center, for their joint study of the case material available to us. I am especially grateful to Robert F. Heimburger and Hallgrim Kløve for working with me in developing procedures for evaluation and insights into brain-behavior relationships. Ward C. Halstead, of course, was significant in each of these respects as well. Homer B.C. Reed, Sureyya Dikmen, Kathleen Fitzhugh-Bell, Donald G. Doehring and Loren Fitzhugh all contributed in analysis and evaluation of case material. William DeMyer, Mark Dyken, John Kalsbeck, and Wolfgang Zeman were of great help in evaluation of neurological and neuropathological findings. James C. Reed not only worked with me for years but also read the manuscript and offered many valuable critical suggestions.

Many persons have contributed specifically in preparation of the book. Judith Ann (Jan) Janesheski read the manuscript, updated and refined the instructions for the tests and prepared the index. Jim Hom and Janice Nici also read much of the manuscript and helped editorially. Vicki Gray prepared many of the figures and she, together with Janice Nici, Anne Bledsoe and Cathy Wicker, typed the manuscript. Sheldon Herring, Jim Hom, and Steve Mackie were of great help in organizing the material and preparing it for the printer. Katherine Vance and James LeRoy proofread the entire manuscript. Finally, we have studied many of these cases in our Workshops in Clinical Neuropsychology, and I thank the attendees for their valuable insights.

My particular approach to aphasia will be criticized by the aphasiologists and must remain my responsibility in addition to the shortcomings of this book. However, it is certainly rewarding, in its own right, to have received such excellent contributions from so many friends and collaborators.

Finally, the work of art on the cover depicts a representation of THE BRAIN done by a boy when he was 7 years of age; my son, Richard M Reitan.

I express my appreciation to them all.

Ralph M. Reitan

CHAPTER 1

A Selective Review of Topics and Contributors in the Area of Aphasia

The general discussion of aphasia customarily centers around (1) the nature and identification of aphasic deficits and (2) localization of these deficits in the brain. The purpose of this introductory chapter will be to provide a selective review of contributions to each of these concerns, together with a brief statement of current knowledge. It must also be noted, however, that localization of the lesion is not the only relevant characteristic in a biological sense. The type of lesion is distinctly relevant, the age at which the lesion was sustained has a great deal to do with aphasic manifestations, the duration of the lesion is of significance with respect to possible recovery, and the neurological character of the lesion (whether, for example, it is producing positive or negative types of symptoms) is another significant factor. The emphasis on localization, with relation to the nature of the deficit, has been given disproportionate significance in the writing of many persons concerned with aphasic manifestations. The case examples, given later in this volume, indicate quite clearly that, regardless of location of lesion, persons with slowly progressive or gradually resolving cerebral lesions demonstrate far less specific and severe deficits in the language area than is true for persons with recent insults, acute manifestations, and rapidly progressive lesions. The type and severity of aphasic deficits are associated with many variables that characterize the pathological dimensions of the lesion and, when the clinician becomes familiar with the brain-behavior correlates implied by specific deficits, rather detailed inferences can be drawn regarding the underlying pathology.

No attempt will be made to review historical considerations in the area of aphasia because Benton has published a number of such reviews, including a very recent one (Benton, 1964; 1965; 1976; 1977; 1981; and Benton and Joynt, 1960). These publications provide a detailed and valuable review of the historical aspects of aphasia, particularly as related to the more general area of human neuropsychology. In his most recent review Benton (1981) noted that aphasic disorders undoubtedly must have been observed even in the most primitive people who were able to speak. His review indicates that knowledge developed gradually, dating back to the time of the Hippocratic writings and continuing through modern times. Three to four hundred years ago case reports were published that noted impairment of language and verbal functions in persons who had suffered strokes, even to the point of citing dissociation of reading and writing abilities. Fairly detailed classification of the nature of aphasic disturbances was proposed early in the 19th century (Bouillaud, 1825). Since that time many significant problems in the area have been addressed and outstanding contributors have devoted major efforts toward their resolution. Benton reviews many of these problems and describes the work of persons such as Broca, Wernicke, Jackson, Marie, Henschen, Kleist, and Head. The serious student of aphasia should not only benefit from Benton's review, but should also gain more detailed knowledge of the approaches and contributions of these investigators.

Benton identifies the modern approach to aphasia as beginning with the detailed study of Weisenburg and McBride in 1935. These investigators developed a systematic method for evaluation of aphasic deficits and compared the language performances of aphasic and nonaphasic patients. Benton notes their results covered a broad spectrum and were not subject to a simple interpretation. Weinsenburg and McBride found that there were striking differences from one aphasic person to another, a conclusion that has systematically been repeated by investigators up to the present day. In fact Benton notes that "interindividual variability is an overriding feature of the performances of aphasic patients" (1981, page 17). In his historical review Benton goes on to review the work of many investigators, when contributions have been made, since the time of Weisenburg and McBride, noting that these contributions have centered around such topical considerations as cognitive factors in aphasia, the contribution of neurolinguistics to an understanding of aphasia, and the anatomical correlates of aphasic disorders.

While nearly every experienced investigator in the area cites the great interindividual variability among aphasic patients, references are also frequently made to the wide range and variety of specific kinds of aphasic disorders. The general characterization that is usually followed relates to categories of "fluent" and "non fluent" aphasic manifestations. Nevertheless, the reader should be aware that detailed categories of aphasia are frequently given concurrently with the statement that individual subjects do not fit these categories very well because of the uniqueness of their language deficits.

The approach in this volume will be to identify aphasic manifestations in individual subjects rather than to identify types of aphasia. Since the many types of aphasia that have been identified do not very well fit the manifestations of individual subjects, and if one is concerned with the individual human being as the unit of value, there would appear to be a need for identification of deficits shown by individual persons. In following this approach we will be less concerned with the conceptual classification of aphasic disturbances than with brain-related manifestations of language dysfunction in individual persons.

IDENTIFICATION OF APHASIC DEFICITS AND CLASSIFICATION OF APHASIC DISORDERS

In consideration of the requirement of identification and classification as fundamental elements of the scientific approach, it should scarcely be surprising that there has been a attempt to identify specific aphasic disorders and to organize and classify them into essentially non-overlapping groups. An attempt to accomplish these aims is obviously of advantage and promotes organization and understanding both of the types of deficits shown by individual patients and the types of aphasic disorders that may exist. However, in view of the great intra- and inter-individuality in expression of aphasic disorders, it is equally understandable that such efforts have at least engendered some disagreement and, at most, conflicting views and resulting controversy. In his monumental and fascinating work on aphasia, Head (1926) referred to the writing of John Hughlings Jackson who, more than 60 years earlier, had noted this problem and used it as a basis for caution. Jackson had observed the great intra-individual variability of response in persons with speech disorders due to cerebral damage. In fact, he felt that the individual subject frequently did not show the same deficits on successive examinations. This variability and uncertainty of obtaining the same results, even though the task did not vary, was viewed by Jackson as being quite characteristic of defective cerebral cortical activity. Many others have also reported that inconsistencies in performance across a broad range of functions, extending well beyond the language area, are quite commonly seen. Even the child in the classroom, who has sustained some kind of brain-related impairment, sometimes seems to be able to do a particular task quite well and at other times performs very poorly. This type of variability, even in terms of specific language responses, was viewed by Jackson as representing a serious problem in clinical examination of persons with aphasia and in the use of specific terms for identifying aphasic deficits. In his first clinical lecture in 1864, Jackson noted that some patients at one moment seemed to possess an ability and at a later moment to be entirely devoid of it. He wondered if terms such as "agraphia", "alexia" and "amnesia verbalis", and similar terms could be used if they could not be consistently applied to individual persons. Head noted that Jackson felt that the use of such terms communicated information that was "highly dangerous to the truth" by reason of their selective nature. Head extended this concern, raising a question as to whether a person might be suffering from agraphia when he was able to write certain things quite accurately but made significant errors on other tasks that had a similar degree of difficulty and familiarity. Head wondered whether a person had alexia when he was not able to read material that was given to him but who, at a later time, carried out the instructions quite accurately and apparently had understood them even though he initially was not able to read them aloud. Striking inconsistencies in performances of this type have been observed by everyone who has studied many persons with aphasic disorders, and these types of deficits occur particularly in persons with lesions that are acutely disruptive of brain functions. For example, one of the patients to be presented later in this volume showed very few specific aphasic disorders before surgical operation, even though he had a slowly growing intrinsic tumor in his left temporal-parietal area. After the operation, however, his aphasia was much more pronounced and he demonstrated striking inconsistencies in performances of the same tasks at different points in time. In fact, he was able to write words upon request quite legibly but, at a later point in time, when they were shown to him by the examiner, he had no idea what his own legible writing represented.

The problem of identification of specific aphasic deficits, and the application of terminology, may well be thought to be complicated by such inconsistencies in performance unless one adopts a view of aphasia as representing a set of specific abnormalities that are different from normal verbal communication. Anyone would agree that a person who was able to write words legibly but who could not read them at a later point in time, when they were perfectly clear to others, would have an abnormal type of language problem. Thus, if the patient shows evidence of distinct and definite abnormalities in the area of verbal communication, it would not be necessary to insist that he do so in every type of performance but that he do so in a clear cut and definite way at least some of the time. If, on the other hand, one views aphasic manifestations as representing varying degrees of deviations from normal expression, as contrasted with definite and distinct abnormality, one would have more of a problem in this regard. Inconsistencies in intra-individual responses, in such an instance, would in fact constitute a serious problem in measurement. If one were to attempt to evaluate language skills on a continuous scale, and judge the individual subject with respect to level of performance (how well the person did), the procedure would necessarily require a reasonable degree of consistency in performance. In other words, intra-individual unreliability of response can be viewed as a definitely abnormal manifestation, but it is not compatible with a requirement of scaling on a continuous distribution. To be perfectly explicit, where would one place an individual on a scale ranging from 0 to 100 with respect to reading, writing, and naming if the individual showed excellent performances at one moment and serious deficiencies the next? The point to be made here is that it is necessary to identify abnormalities seen in aphasic persons and pathognomonic deviations from normal language as contrasted with scaling of language abilities as with tests of verbal intelligence.

It should still be noted that Head was concerned about the use of selective terms of characterization of aphasic deficits. He noted that various terms, such as alexia and agraphia, were " . . . in fact purely grammatical designations." (1926, page 423). Nevertheless, Head did feel that there was no incompatibility between this concern and the use of systematic testing procedures to examine aphasic patients. He believed that formal testing procedures would often permit the examiner to show that pathological verbal responses of aphasic patients tended to assume certain distinctive forms even though the terms used for descriptive purposes might have certain limitations. Head said "no one who examined his patients with due care and an open mind would be able to discover an example of pure 'motor,' 'auditory,' or 'visual' aphasia." (1926, page 424). Head viewed brain functions that subserved language manifestations as representing a variable set of conditions that changed for the individual from one time to another. Thus, abnormal speech responses of the aphasic patient were presumed to be governed by conditions of the moment (permitting intra-individual variability from one time to another) and represented some type of interference with the mechanism necessary for perfect use of language. Since Head viewed aphasic deficits as representing abnormalities of speech and language, he did not feel that these abnormalities could accurately reveal the elements from which the normal use of language was composed, at least in any exact manner. Thus, he felt the study of aphasia could scarcely serve as a basis documenting elementary processes of normal language and that subdivision of language expression into categories as "motor" versus "sensory", and "auditory" or "visual" were not very meaningful. Thus, Head advocated the use of systematic tests to identify abnormal acts of speech in the widest sense but did not feel that the results of such examinations permitted identification of the analytical elements of the speech process or of language functions, either from a physiological or psychological point of view.

In spite of these many precautions, Head did identify certain clinical varieties of aphasia. He felt that *Verbal Aphasia* was characterized by difficulty in forming words for communicational purposes and that in this condition comprehension of the meaning of the words exceeded expressive ability. In Verbal Aphasia reading and writing might be adversely affected but arithmetical operations were done accurately except in severe cases. Head also identified *Syntactical Aphasia* as a disorder in which syntax suffers, balance and rhythm of verbal communication is deficient, and the patient has difficulty arranging words into coordinated phrases with oral communication possibly being in the form of jargon. *Nominal Aphasia* was characterized by impaired ability to use names, together with loss of comprehension of the meaning of words. Patients with Nominal Aphasia have extreme difficulty in reading, writing, and even in the understanding of single numbers or letters. Finally, Head proposed that *Semantic Aphasia* consists of rather generalized impairment in recognition of the full significance of words and phrases over and beyond their specific and direct verbal connotations. Such patients can read and write and understand words or short phrases, but show distinct deficits in comprehension of the general conception or meaning of the overall verbal communication. There have been many other classifications of aphasia, as will be noted in this chapter, but at this point we probably should comment that Sarno (1981) identifies a more specific criterion for Semantic Aphasia as including the substitution of a word or phrase for the intended (correct) expression even though the substitution is still in the same general meaning category. Sarno contrasts this criterion for Semantic Aphasia with the category of Verbal Paraphasia, in which the substitution is in another meaning category (such as boy for girl). Among the cases shown later in this volume, one will observe these various types of disorders that Head identifies. At the same time, the reader should have an opportunity, through study of these patients, to appreciate the precautions cited by Head with respect to use of specific terms of specific categories of classification. In other words, while these observations by Head are realistic, they do not necessarily constitute separate and non-overlapping categories of aphasic deficits. Certainly individual persons can be found who generally represent each of the categories, but the more apt generalization is that most patients represent overlapping aspects of these types of difficulties.

More recent volumes vary with regard to the extent that they use specific terms and identify different categories or classifications of aphasia. Brown (1972), in his volume on aphasia, apraxia, and agnosia, differentiates between these conditions noting that aphasia represents language disorders, apraxia is related to impairment in doing specific things (such as dressing), and agnosia involves failure to understand or appreciate non-verbal material. Differentiation of apraxia (expressive deficits) and agnosia (receptive deficits) from aphasia (verbal deficits) tends to ignore the fact that language disorders, as with any task that involves input, simple processing, and output, requires knowing (gnosis) and doing (praxis). In his book Brown goes on to include a final section that deals specifically with alexia in order to relate reading impairment to other aspects of aphasia as well as to differentiate between various types of alexia. More specifically, Brown indicates that aphasia refers simply to an acquired disorder of language manifested in speech, writing, or reading; agnosia refers to an acquired cortical sensory (apperceptive) or perceptual (associated) disorder, regardless of the modality concerned; and apraxia is associated with impairment of voluntary movement without obvious sensori-motor deficits. These definitions certainly do bring to mind Head's precaution that terms used for characterizing deficits may be purely grammatical designations. Nevertheless, these grammatical designations may have value in their communicational significance.

Brown's approach is to provide a detailed description of various types of aphasic manifestations and conditions. The work is of value in that he gives a brief historical introduction and clinical description of the nature of each deficit including a host of conditions such as anomia, semantic aphasia, Wernicke's aphasia, conduction aphasia, Broca's aphasia, word deafness, and related disorders that include sound agnosia, receptive amusia, pallilalia, paroxysmal speech disorders, and aphasic disturbances that are related to lesions of the thalamus. Brown goes on to identify a number of deficits in the category of apraxia, including ideational apraxia, ideo-motor apraxia, limb-kinetic apraxia, facial apraxia, truncal apraxia, dressing apraxia, and bimanual apraxia. Among deficits in the category of agnosia he cites apperceptive visual agnosia, associated visual agnosia, visual-spatial agnosia, prosopagnosia (inability to recognize faces), anosognosia (lack of awareness of disease or deficit) color agnosia, and autopagnosia (impairment in ability to identify body parts). Brown goes on with further classifications in the area of reading deficits, including agnosic alexia, agraphic alexia, aphasic alexia, and alexia in Broca's aphasia.

It would seem apparent that Brown's approach toward identification and classification of aphasic disorders stands in contrast to Head's approach in the sense that Brown offers a great number of classes whereas Head was much more conservative in this respect. Nevertheless, Brown's description of these various disorders is quite useful for those who wish to become familiar with types of disorders that are sometimes shown by individual persons and to review references to publications of various investigators who have been concerned with each of these topics. We should also note that the approach represented by Brown concentrates on types of deficits rather than on *patients* with these deficits. This type of approach is not at all uncommon, being the rule rather than the exception. However, the end result frequently is to concentrate on types of deficits as the units of importance rather than the particular deficits of the individual subject and their intra-individual relationships.

Serious students of aphasic disorders should be familiar with the significant contributions, over the years, of Hécaen and his collaborators (Hécaen & Albert, 1978; Hécaen, 1979). Hécaen has had a great deal of experience in examining individual patients with aphasia and other specific types of brain-related deficits. His investigative approach is definitely oriented toward elicitation of pathognomonic signs rather than normally distributed measurements. In this sense, his work generally falls more in the area of behavioral neurology than clinical neuropsychology. Nevertheless, he has gained a great deal of insight into the types of disorders that occur in aphasia. His chapter in Gazzaniga's *Handbook of Behavioral Neurobiology* provides an excellent and rather detailed review of the types of clinical manifestations of language disorders seen among aphasic patients. This review follows an approach that is similar in many respects to that used by Brown (1972), including many references to pertinent literature as well as to the historical development of various concepts. Hécaen and Albert (1978) have written an even more detailed book that provides a very valuable presentation of many aspects of human brain-behavior relationships. Although the authors point out that the book is not intended to be a comprehensive review of the literature, they have referred to many pertinent studies that will provide the student of aphasia with an excellent knowledge of contributions in the area. This book is devoted heavily to description of various types of disorders involved in dysphasia. While the authors have had a great deal of experience in examining individual subjects, the book is not oriented toward the specific kinds of deficits shown by patients but instead represents an abstraction of such data according to the conceptualizations of the authors. They do review the types of clinical manifestations shown by aphasic patients and, in addition, include detailed discussions of disorders of gestural behavior and disorders that involve sensory avenues including vision, audition, and somesthesis. Fairly extensive coverage is given to disorders of memory and the amnestic syndrome and a section is devoted to the types of disorders that have been reported to accompany frontal lobe lesions. A final chapter is concerned with recovery of function. While this book has a very strong orientation toward a pathognomonic sign approach, many of the references to the literature concern studies that have used more formal and extended testing procedures.

Damasio (1981) has written an interesting chapter in which he describes many of the manifestations of aphasia. He differentiates between aphasia and developmental language defects by noting that aphasia, in his judgment, is produced by acquired and recent cerebral lesions rather than congenital and longstanding genetic or environmentally induced pre- or perinatal cerebral disorders. This distinction requires that aphasic patients initially have developed adequate language abilities which then is followed by cerebral damage that results in a loss of these previously acquired skills. Developmental language defects, on the other hand, refer particularly to children in whom cerebral lesions may have produced developmental language deficits but whose language ability never has, and perhaps never will, reach a normal level. Since both aphasia and developmental language defects involve the use of language symbols for communicational purposes, this differentiation appears to be rather arbitrary insofar as it restricts the term "aphasia" to those persons who have already developed language abilities (as contrasted with persons with cerebral lesions that occurred early enough in life to preclude the opportunity of development of normal language functions). In this sense, the differentiation between the terms seems to refer rather exclusively to the time at which cerebral damage occurred, even though the damage was responsible, in each instance, for resulting language deficits. Since aphasia is customarily defined as impairment of language functions as a result of cerebral damage, it would seem quite possible to identify both early and later types of language disturbances as falling under the category of aphasia, even though the particular types of deficits may differ depending upon the stage of development at the time the brain lesion was sustained.

Damasio gives a useful description of the particular types of difficulties in the language area encountered by adult aphasics. He cites the general categories of fluent and nonfluent aphasic disorders and also follows the other traditional procedure of offering descriptions of many other types of aphasia including Wernicke's aphasia, Broca's aphasia, conduction aphasia, transcortical sensory aphasia, transcortical motor aphasia, global aphasia, anomic aphasia, alexia with agraphia, alexia without agraphia, pure word deafness, and atypical aphasia. In spite of the differentiation of these many types of aphasia, he cautions, as do many investigators, that the types of aphasia only approximate the deficit shown by individual patients, that "classifications are a necessary evil," and that a review of classification systems of aphasia can be a discouraging task. If such comments were, in fact, taken seriously one might wonder about the persistence of various authors in citing these terms and describing the manifestations that supposedly permit their use.

As is true in any area of scientific investigation, the more recent reports frequently represent elaboration of details. These details, obviously, may be of definite significance and certainly enrich knowledge in the area. Benson (1967) and Kertesz, Lask, and McCabe (1977) have studied patients with fluent and nonfluent aphasia and have found that nonfluent aphasia is more commonly associated with lesions in the anterior part of the language area whereas patients with fluent aphasia more commonly have posterior lesions. Heilman, Rothi, and Valenstein (1982) have added an additional finding to the effect that persons with more anterior lesions and nonfluent aphasia, as compared with persons having more posterior lesions and fluent aphasia, performed better when asked to engage in certain tasks as well as when asked to view on film certain pantomimed acts. Their results suggest that complex phenomena of apraxia, as associated with different types of aphasia and different lesion locations, may be further subdivided and delineated. It should be noted, however, that it is necessary to carefully compose selected groups of patients who meet specific criteria in order to demonstrate such phenomena and, while the information adds to knowledge in a very meaningful way, the results of such studies may not be applicable to heterogeneous groups of patients.

The literature in the field of aphasia has gone into many detailed studies that enrich knowledge in the area. Whitaker and Whitaker (1977) have been particularly instrumental in publishing such advances of knowledge in their three volumes entitled, *Studies in Neurolinguistics.* The first of these volumes presents interesting studies in the areas of neurolinguistic models of language and speech, subcortical language mechanisms, the role of phonology in linguistic communication, agrammatism, studies in syntax and semantics as related to aphasia, and transcortical motor aphasia. The second volume includes such specialized topics as jargonaphasia and jargonagraphia, the neurological basis of language as represented through gestures, and the relationship of "pure" alexia to aphasia. The third volume concentrates heavily on the important area of auditory comprehension deficits in aphasia and goes on to consider the nature of conduction aphasia, characteristics of acquired dyslexia, models of hemispheric function, and the possible significance of slow potentials as precedents of articulation. While it is important to investigate these areas of function, and relationships between variables, we may ask validly about the extent to which these advances in knowledge contribute to our significance of understanding of brain-behavior relationships for the individual human being.

CORRELATION OF CEREBRAL LOCALIZATION AND APHASIC MANIFESTATIONS

The many publications in this area date back more than a century and no attempt will be made to review this extensive literature. Instead, we will only direct the reader's attention to two recent summaries in the area and, in addition, to the studies of Penfield and Roberts (1959).

Damasio (1981) reviewed attempts that have been made in recent years to correlate types of aphasic deficits with localization results of computed tomography of the brain. She used the major categories of fluent and nonfluent aphasia for differentiation of types of aphasic deficits, and found that patients with fluent aphasia generally have lesions in the more posterior aspects of the language area of the left cerebral hemisphere whereas patients with nonfluent aphasia have lesions that tend to fall in the more anterior aspects. This finding, of course, agrees with many earlier reports. Even though this generalization holds fairly well, Damasio notes that "numerous exceptions exist." It must be added, of course, that these exceptions are represented by the complexity of brain-behavior relationships for individual subjects and that the individual patient frequently fails to show evidence of aphasic deficits that fall into a classical category. This problem of failure of correlation between results for individual subjects and the generalizations that exist in the literature probably will never be resolved until aphasiologists adopt an experimental approach that is aimed directly toward determining the limitations of prediction of lesion location on the basis of the manifestation of aphasic deficits made by the individual patient. This approach has been followed in the area of clinical neuropsychology (Reitan, 1962) in which neuropsychological test results, considered by themselves, were used for making predictions about individual patients. Such an approach, obviously represents the essence of individual diagnosis. Since individual diagnosis must necessarily be made in clinical evaluation of patients, it would seem that research approaches should come closer than they generally have in the past to simulating clinical procedures by testing the value of clinical categories (so frequently and repetitively described in the literature), with relation to their clinical utility. It is just not sufficient to offer clinical categorizations and continually cite the fact that "numerous exceptions exist" without attempting to determine, through individual prediction, just what types of exceptions seem to create the problems.

Marin, Schwartz, and Saffran (1979) present a detailed review of the parts of the brain that are specifically involved in the language process. These authors point out that two generalizations can safely be made. First, neural tissue involved in language is primarily neocortical. We should note that this generalization undoubtedly is true, even though some recent reports have suggested that subcortical centers, involving nuclei of the left thalamus, may be involved in language functions (Ojemann, 1975). The second generalization that can safely be made, according to these authors, is that this neural-cortical tissue is localized, for the most part, in the left cerebral hemisphere. This generalization also is hardly new. Additional attempts are made by these authors to identify the specific areas involved in language production or reception, citing the work of various authors. It should be noted, however, that they depend heavily upon the work of Conrad (1954). Conrad presented a detailed study in which he attempted to correlate the point of impact on the skull in head injury cases with the nature of resulting language deficits. In fact, he estimated the *midpoint* of the skull defect in persons with penetrating head injuries as a basis for presuming the point of cortical damage. The presumption in this regard was that the midpoint of penetration of the skull would correlate with focal cerebral involvement, a presumption that failed to take into consideration the fact that the lesion might be quite extensive, even possibly involving the other cerebral hemisphere as well as structures below the level of cerebral hemispheres. Nevertheless, this type of presumption is still taken seriously by a number of investigators, in spite of very good and longstanding evidence that damage in instances of penetrating head injury is scarcely limited to the point of penetration of the skull (Courville, 1942). It is difficult to understand why investigators continue to use such inadequate criteria for localization of cerebral damage. It probably is true, however, that the conclusion of these authors regarding the general location of the language area is relatively accurate. They conclude that language functions are principally represented in the left cerebral hemisphere, that the temporal lobe is involved almost entirely as well as the adjacent inferior aspects of the parietal lobe and the posterior-inferior part of the frontal lobe. This conclusion certainly would agree with our personal observations as well as the work of others (Mohr, 1978).

Marin, Schwartz, and Saffran (1979) recognized quite clearly the difficulty in precise identification of the area of damage in human beings with cerebral lesions. They pointed out, in fact, that cerebral lesions in human beings usually represent a biological accident of disease or injury that is not subject to precise control in terms of location or extent, is almost always irregular in its placement, and can rarely be reproduced. Thus, speculation rather than fact may be the end result in studies of correlations between language functions and localization of damage, especially considering the fact that the characteristics of cerebral damage may not be consistent between individual subjects. The authors note, however, that "in at least some proportion of cases the lesion rather specifically disrupts a particular aspect of language function" (1979, page 205), even though the language impairment may be variable from one subject to another and involve different elements and aspects of language functions. Thus, the problem is to correlate *two* sets of highly variable information (location of brain lesions and nature of language disorders) in aphasic patients. The authors suggest that it is possible to specify carefully and in detail the linguistic parameters of the language impairment even though it may not be possible, with as much precision, to identify the specific area of cerebral damage. Thus, they feel that the linguistic variables would have a logical priority in investigation and delineation of functional systems in the brain and that inquiries in this regard should be designed with respect to functional (language) units. In this sense, the authors suggest that language deficits in aphasic patients be identified as the independent variable rather than the brain lesion.

There is of course value in studying the various types of independent variables with relation to other measures, and this is hardly a new approach. For example, the relationships between the presence of aphasic deficits and loss on intellectual measures has been studied in patients in whom other variables were held constant, even though location of lesion was deliberately permitted to vary (Reitan, 1960). However, there is a real strategical problem in attempting to relate two variables when one of the two is not well defined or specified. Thus, if the location of the lesion is still presumed to correlate with the point of impact on the skull, and no further definition than this is achieved, one can hardly expect to advance knowledge of the relationships between sets of variables. Obviously, it is necessary to select cases in whom both variables to be correlated are relatively well known, rather than to perpetuate the grossly inaccurate criteria that are sometimes used in an uncritical manner.

The work of Penfield and Roberts (1959) still deserves special citation, particularly because of the fact that the independent variable (stimulation of specific areas of the cerebral cortex) was exactly identified. Of course, one must recognize the limitations of this variable and question its overall usefulness as a basis for generalization. However, these authors (the work on aphasia and language disorders was mainly contributed by Roberts) not only provided a brief, cogent historical review of aphasia, agnosia, and apraxia but also a statement regarding localization of functions within the language area. Their book presented findings on 569 patients who had been operated upon at the Montreal Neurological Institute for treatment of focal cerebral seizures. These patients had been evaluated for evidence of aphasia, before and after operation. Handedness had also been determined. The procedure was to apply electrical stimulation to points on the exposed cerebral cortex and to identify the kind of speech interference that occurred in the patient. (This was possible because the patient was under local anesthesia). Obviously a complete examination for aphasia could not be done under these conditions, but the standard procedure did involve conversation with the patient, asking the patient to give names of objects shown on pictures, having the patient count, having the patient write the names of objects shown on cards or in reply to questions, and having the patient write spontaneously. During the course of these activities the surgeon applied electrodes to the cerebral cortex at one point or another in the general area to be explored. When electrical stimulation interfered with the patient's performance, a notation was made of the point of application and the nature of the interference.

Several conclusions were reached. First, Roberts noted that dysphasia is quite rare with involvement of the right cerebral hemisphere alone, that interference with speech rarely occurred with right cerebral stimulation, and that the left cerebral hemisphere is usually dominant for speech regardless of handedness. Roberts also noted that recovery of speech and language functions, following damage to the left cerebral hemisphere, is not necessarily based on a presumption that the right cerebral hemisphere has "taken over" the language function. Roberts noted, for example, that even after a second or third operation on the left cerebral hemisphere, aphasic deficits tended to reappear. This was true particularly when the lesion was relatively small and did not involve all of the language area or a major part of the entire left cerebral hemisphere. This finding would suggest that remaining tissue in the language area might be of more critical significance in recovery of function, among adults, than the potential implicit in the function of tissue outside of the language area.

Roberts provided graphic information relating points of stimulation in the left cerebral hemisphere to interference with language activity. He included detailed maps that related points of stimulation to hesitation or slurring of speech, distortion and repetition of words and syllables, confusion of numbers in counting, inability to provide specific names of objects even though spontaneous speaking capability was preserved, misuse of a name even though prior responses had indicated that the patient was able to give the name correctly, and instances of misnaming of specific objects even though the use of synonyms for unrelated words was still possible. These examples of interference in language functions were not correlated with highly focal areas but rather were widely distributed in what might be considered the general speech area. As previously noted, this area includes principally the posterior-inferior part of the left frontal lobe, most of the left temporal lobe, and adjacent inferior aspects of the left parietal lobe.

It is necessary to observe that the tests used by Penfield and Roberts were principally dependent upon expressive aspects of language functions and did not constitute a complete examination for aphasia. Nevertheless, their results continue to be of important significance, including the observation that arrest or interference with speech was far less common with right than left cerebral stimulation.

TESTS AND METHODS FOR EXAMINATION FOR APHASIA

Both Spreen and Risser (1981) and Albert, Goodglass, Helm, Rubens, and Alexander (1981) have provided information with respect to general considerations in examining the aphasic patients and, in addition, Spreen and Risser (1981) have provided a valuable service in reviewing many of the instruments used for this purpose. Albert, et al., (1981) provide a fairly detailed description of the procedure for examination in use at the Boston VA Hospital Aphasia Center organized around the *Boston Diagnostic Aphasia Examination.* We should note that Darley and Spriestersbach (1978) also address these procedures, give a brief description of various tests for asphasia examinations, and note where these tests may be obtained.

The Brief Clinical Examination for Dysphasia

Spreen and Risser (1981) point out that the brief clinical examination is the primary method of assessing dysphasia and is the standard tool especially among neurologists and many speech clinicians. They cite the advantage of the clinical examination as offering flexibility, brevity, and suitability even for the severely impaired patient. In addition, a cursory clinical examination can be done at the bedside. While numerous versions of the clinical examination have been described in the literature, both Spreen and Risser (1981) and Albert, et al., (1981) note that a number of areas should be assessed. These include spontaneous and conversational speech; repetition of multisyllabic words, complex sentences, or verbal sequences; comprehension of spoken language; word finding or naming of common objects; reading; and writing. These areas of performance essentially cover the major abilities included in most examinations for aphasia. One might, then, wonder why a more formal and detailed examination would be necessary. A fundamental reason is to provide a systematic and organized assessment of language and related communicational skills within each of these areas and, in addition, to provide for the use of preselected stimulus materials with which the examiner can develop detailed familiarity. It is extremely important that the examiner know exactly the kinds of errors that are attributable to cerebral damage as contrasted with deficiencies in performance, shown by the individual subject, that are a result of other kinds of influences (such as limited educational opportunity and experience). As will be noted in many of the cases presented later in this volume, apparently minor deviations, in certain instances, carry a great deal of weight with respect to validity as indications of cerebral damage. Thus, the examiner must develop an appreciation of the particular kinds of errors that characterize cerebral damage and this requirement is greatly facilitated if the examiner is thoroughly familiar with the range of variation in performance shown by normal subjects as contrasted with the specific kinds of deficits that are frequently shown by subjects with cerebral lesions. As an illustration of this point, I was once told that writing abilities of Russian cosmonauts showed some deterioration in one of the rather early space flights. I was asked if it were possible to draw a judgment with regard to whether impaired cerebral functioning might be possible for this deterioration. I responded immediately that in many instances it is quite possible to detect impaired cerebral functioning through deterioration of writing abilities and I was shortly presented with a sample of the writing of the cosmonauts before and after fairly extended periods of time in space. It was perfectly apparent that the writing, after fairly extended periods of weightlessness, was much less disciplined and much more like a scrawl than the writing that had been done under normal conditions. However, it is equally apparent that the writing was in Russian, that I did not even know what it said, and that I had no competence whatsoever in deciding whether the change represented cerebral impairment or a more mechanical type of deficit relating to motor control.

Requirements for Tests of Dysphasia

Spreen and Risser (1981) note that three general requirements for aphasia tests are that they be standardized, reliable, and valid. These are the three general requirements used for most psychometric instruments and, in this sense, treat aphasia tests as belonging to the general class of psychometric instruments.

Under the heading of standardization these authors first note the requirement that test administration be standard and precisely the same from one subject to the next in order to produce comparable results. Secondly, they note another aspect of standardization that refers to the development of normative data against which the performance of an individual patient can be compared. They go on to cite factors such as age, gender, and socioeconomic status which may affect performance and indicate that separate norms must be established for such variables. They note that norms developed for normal subjects may not be adequate for evaluation of the aphasic subject. Nevertheless, they do not appear clearly to recognize that aphasia represents abnormalities in performance that, essentially, are not even included within the range of normal performances.

These authors state that the aphasia test should be reliable in the sense that similar results would be obtained on re-examination of the same subject under similar conditions. Reliability requires recognition of an interaction between the test itself and the patient or subject. In terms of this statement of reliability, any change in the test or the patient would diminish reliability as far as the procedure is concerned. As reported earlier in this volume, Head (1926) pointed out that it is common for the aphasic patient to demonstrate variable responses to the same stimulus material at different points in time. Thus, even though the stimulus material and procedure for administering the test were held constant, changes in the subject's responses would limit the identity (or similarity) of results obtained on separate occasions of testing, thereby reducing reliability. Given such circumstances as part of the situation to be expected among dysphasic persons, it would appear that the question of reliability, in a psychometric sense as applied to normal individuals, may need some modification with respect to evaluation of dysphasic persons.

Finally, the authors cite the requirement of validity. A test is valid if it measures what it is supposed to measure. In this sense the test should measure language deficits related to impairment of brain functions. To accomplish this aim, known correlations must be available between the test results obtained from individual patients and information regarding brain pathology. Relatively little detailed information of this kind is available for most of the tests that have been published. A later section in this monograph presents such results for our Aphasia Screening Test and Sensory-perceptual Examination.

Spreen and Risser (1981) go on with additional types of "psychometric" requirements that they feel relate specifically to aphasia and evaluation of brain damage. First, they note that the tests should cover a broad range of item difficulty, extending from easy to very difficult items. Obviously, if one considers aphasia to be an abnormality in performance, one would scarcely need the "very difficult" items. Such items would be useful to differentiate among persons with unimpaired abilities rather than persons with abnormalities of communicational skills in the language area as a result of cerebral damage. Secondly, Spreen and Risser (1981) note that it is necessary to use procedures that permit clarification of specific deficits. They cite instances in which the deficit may be on the sensory or input side, on the motor or output side, or may possibly represent a central kind of defect. Obviously, this is a very general requirement, necessary with any kind of examining procedure, even though it may be quite difficult to achieve in practice.

These authors also suggest that an aphasia examination should not overlap to any considerable extent with measures of general intelligence. They note that this is not a problem with "easy" items but that overlap occurs particularly with "difficult" items. The basic problem in this respect concerns the prior requirement cited by these authors to the effect that an aphasia examination should cover a broad range of item difficulty. If difficult items are included, one necessarily will create a procedure that overlaps with measurement of general intelligence. The basic problem in this respect concerns the fundamental conceptualization of aphasia. Inclusion of a broad range of items, in terms of difficulty-level, would require scaling of abilities that are normally distributed. The alternative approach presumes that aphasia represents the occurrence of abnormalities in the area of language communication. The testing requirement, stemming from this conceptualization, would be to include in an aphasia examination only items that were so easy and simple that anyone with a normal brain could be presumed to be able to perform them. If one adopts a conceptualization of aphasia as representing a brain-related abnormality in performance, there would appear to be little prospect of encountering confusion between aphasia and general intelligence except in mentally retarded persons who never had an opportunity to develop simple aspects of language communicational skills (perhaps as a result of minimal or absent educational experiences), or the young child who has not yet learned to use language symbols for communicational purposes.

Spreen and Risser (1981) also cite the usefulness of aphasia evaluation in assessing recovery of functions. Undoubtedly, recovery of functions is a very important aspect of assessment of the effects of brain damage. However, these authors state that to effect such an assessment it would be necessary to use rather different approaches than are customarily used in evaluating aphasia. They feel that learning trials would be necessary in order to assess the prospect for improvement shown by the patient and that the types of tests involved would be related to the requirements of measures in the learning area or the area of more general psychometric assessment. The authors indicate that they feel that such tests would be a major concern for test development in the future. While this recommendation may have distinct value, there already are extensive batteries for evaluating brain-behavior relationships that might well serve the purpose much more effectively than modifications of procedures to examine for aphasia.

Finally, Spreen and Risser (1981) note that one's conceptualization of the nature of aphasia undoubtedly will be a strong and necessary determinant of the kind of test constructed or used. They note that Benton (1967) has indicated that development of a model of language functioning is necessary as a preliminary step, much as a conceptualization of the nature of intelligence is necessary in order to develop an intelligence test. We must again note in this regard, however, that overview of aphasia relates to a *loss* in ability to express and understand basic aspects of language functioning rather than to a general model of language functioning (in agreement with Head, 1926). While language is undoubtedly extremely complicated, and the use of symbols for communicational purposes involves the entire area of linguistics, the essential nature of impairment of the aphasic subject concerns abilities in word finding, repetition, spontaneous speech, comprehension of language, reading and writing (and one might add arithmetical processes). In this sense an evaluation of aphasic symptoms ought principally to relate to simple manifestations of abilities in these areas, together with a method for identifying specific abnormalities or deviations from normal functioning, rather than to attempt a complete assessment of level or degree of competence in the entire area of verbal communicational skills.

Tests for Aphasia

In their excellent review of various approaches, methods, and tests used to evaluate patients, Spreen and Risser (1981) discuss various tests that have been developed to evaluate specific aspects of language functions such as auditory comprehension, expressive deficits, and word fluency, followed by a description of several short screening tests for aphasia. Next, communication profiles are reviewed and another section discusses the psycholinguistic evaluation of aphasic language. Finally, the authors describe a number of tests that they feel represent comprehensive examinations of the aphasic patient.

Among tests devised to examine specific aspects of language functions, Spreen and Risser first describe the *Token Test* that was designed by DeRenzi and Vignolo (1962). The materials for this test include 20 plastic or cardboard token stimuli of two sizes (large and small), two shapes (round and square), and five colors. These tokens are used as stimuli by which the subject is able to respond to verbal directions given by the examiner. These directions increase in difficulty from simple requests such as "show me a square" to more complex ones such as "pick up all squares except the yellow one." Obviously, this test is designed to evaluate the subject's ability to comprehend spoken language.

The *Reporter's Test* uses the same stimulus material as the *Token Test,* but in this instance the examiner engages in various acts (such as touching the large yellow square) and the subject is required to report what the examiner has done in a manner that would be sufficient to instruct a third participant to repeat the examiner's action (DeRenzi, 1980; DeRenzi and Ferrari, 1979). Customarily the *Reporter's Test* is given following administration of the *Token Test* so that the patient has already developed some familiarity with the stimuli and the testing procedures.

Another test for evaluation of auditory comprehension is called the *Auditory Comprehension Test for Sentences (ACTS)* (Shewan, 1980). In this test the examiner reads in consecutive order a series of 21 test items that represent sentences of various length, vocabulary difficulty, and syntactic complexity. The subject is required to listen to each sentence and to point to one of four visual displays to indicate which of the four is appropriate for the stated sentence.

Spreen and Risser describe two tests of word fluency which require the subject to say as many words as possible within a limited time period that begin with specified letters. Spreen and Benton (1977) have devised one of these tests as part of a more comprehensive examination which requires that the subject say as many words as possible which begin with the letters F, A, and S in a one minute time period. Another procedure of this kind was devised by Wertz (1979) that requires the subject to name words that begin with S, T, P, and C.

Spreen and Risser, in the description of short aphasia screening tests, identify the *Halstead-Wepman Aphasia Screening Test* (Halstead and Wepman, 1949). However, the authors confuse the test devised by Halstead and Wepman with the *Reitan-Indiana Aphasia Screening Test,* which is the instrument described in this manual.

Another screening test is the *Aphasia Language Performance Scales* (Keenan and Brassel, 1975) that consists of four 10-item scales in the area of listening, talking, reading, and writing. The items are arranged in approximate order of difficulty and a correct response (the type of response that might be expected from a normal adult) is given one point whereas a correct response that required prompting by the examiner is given only one-half point.

The *Sklar Aphasia Scale* (Sklar, 1973) is oriented toward evaluating receptive (input) and expressive (output) language capabilities. Four subtests are used that emphasize auditory decoding, visual decoding, oral encoding, and graphic encoding. Within each of these tests five areas of function are evaluated, each using five items. Each response is scored on a five-point scale which provides a score for each test as well as for the total performance.

Spreen and Risser describe two communication profiles, the *Functional Communication Profile* (Sarno, 1969) and *Communicative Abilities in Daily Living* (Holland, 1980). Rather than to provide a formal assessment of specific aspects of language impairment, these procedures attempt to assess language ability with relation to functional usefulness in everyday life. The *Functional Communication Profile* requires the examiner to rate 45 behaviors of the subject (e.g., the ability to indicate yes and no, to read newspaper headlines, to handle money) that are subdivided into categories of movement, speaking, understanding, reading, and miscellaneous activities (including such things as calculation and writing). A rather complicated system of scaling is required inasmuch as the examiner must estimate current ability as a proportion of what the subject's former ability may have been. Obviously, this type of rating system would require excellent clinical insight and experience. The *Communicative Abilities in Daily Living* consists of 68 items regarding the aphasic patient's functional communicative ability in situations that involve everyday activities. Each item is scored on a three-point scale (correct, adequate, or wrong). The items include various types of activities such as dealing with a receptionist, communicating with a doctor, driving, shopping, and making telephone calls. Since this test is heavily dependent on the patient's ability to understand verbal communication by the examiner, it is not surprising that Holland has reported that patients with Wernicke's aphasia performed less well than patients with Broca's aphasia. Interestingly, patients with global aphasia performed most poorly, suggesting that the overall degree of impairment may be reflected by the test results.

Undoubtedly communication profiles are of value in the assessment of individual patients with aphasia. It is important to know just how well the patient will be able to perform in practical kinds of situations that require language communication. On the other hand, evaluations of this kind undoubtedly measure general capabilities in addition to specific aspects of language use. Thus, a clear element of general intelligence, or impairment of brain functions that is not necessarily a part of language deficit, would enter into assessment. In this sense, communication profiles would reflect the influence of factors other than aphasia. As reported by Holland (1980) nonaphasics, as would be expected, perform better than aphasics, but noninstitutionalized persons perform better than institutionalized persons and younger persons better than older persons. If these measures are intended as procedures for assessing the general adaptive capability of brain-damaged or otherwise impaired individuals, it might be important to address such issues even more generally than these instruments do. In other words, if a comprehensive assessment of brain-behavior relationships is needed, a more complete battery should be used than one that centers on communicational aspects of language. It is apparent that these communication profiles attempt to assess language communicational skills that extend over a fairly broad and continuous range of abilities, in contrast to assessment of specific deficits or abnormalities in language performance.

Spreen and Risser briefly reviewed some of the very interesting and imaginative psycholinguistic approaches to evaluation of aphasic speech. These investigations require recording and analysis of conversational speech, although studies have also been done in experimental settings that permit analysis of types of errors produced by aphasic patients and of specific psycholinguistic characteristics. Wepman and his collaborators (1964) analyzed conversational speech of aphasic subjects along linguistic parameters that included grammatical form class usage, grammatical correctness, intelligibility, and word-finding problems. Howes (1964) has been particularly imaginative in his investigations of this kind. Differentiation was made of the speech production of fluent and nonfluent aphasic persons and analyzed according to rate of speaking, prosody, pronunciation, phrase length, effort, pauses, press of speech, perseveration, word choice, paraphasia, and verbal stereotypes. Particular characteristics of deficit, in turn, were related to the location of damage in the speech area. The results indicated that fluent language difficulties were more closely related to damage of the posterior parts of the language area whereas nonfluent disorders were more anterior in location. Spreen and Wachal (1973) have also performed comprehensive analyses of conversational speech of aphasics and normal speakers, analyzing various psycholinguistic aspects.

It must be noted that these psycholinguistic approaches to the evaluation of aphasia as compared with normal speech are of very definite interest and contribute significantly to an understanding of the nature of aphasic deficits. However, they have represented efforts in an interesting area of research rather than in the evaluation of individual patients and, while contributing to the understanding of aphasic deficits, have not been related pointedly to assessment of individual aphasic patients.

Spreen and Risser (1981) have described a number of comprehensive examinations for aphasia. These include *the Appraisal of Language Disturbance, the Boston Diagnostic Aphasia Examination, the Minnesota Test for Differential Diagnosis of Aphasia, the Multilingual Aphasia Examination, the Neurosensory Center Comprehensive Examination for Aphasia, the Porch Index of Communicative Ability, and the Western Aphasia Battery.* These tests have certain individualistic characteristics, but in general they include evaluation of oral expression, auditory comprehension, repetition, reading ability, and writing ability. They focus on diversity of performances and attempt to sample various tasks at different ability levels. As may be presumed in consideration of the fact that both easy and difficult tasks are usually included, these tests are oriented toward level of performance in the language area and, in this sense, may be considered somewhat comparable in many respects to the Verbal subtest of the Wechsler Scales. In other words, instead of using only items that are sufficiently easy so that they should be able to be performed by anyone with normal brain functions, the tests attempt to scale the adequacy of the individual subject with regard to verbal abilities. Such an approach is relevant with respect to the aphasic subject, because the aphasic subject obviously will do poorly in the area of language and verbal communication. On the other hand, an orientation toward aphasia as an abnormality in the use of language symbols for communicational purposes, as discussed above, tends to be lost. Identification of language deficits that are characteristic of cerebral lesions also tends to be underemphasized because the approach is a matter of one in which the individual's performance is placed on a continuous scale. We should note that these tests provide the opportunity for the individual aphasic subject to manifest his best capabilities, but the orientation is more directed toward performance on a psychometric type of instrument than toward a clinical examination for eliciting brain-related abnormalities of performance. Emerick (1971) developed the *Appraisal of Language Disturbance,* designing it as a method to examine input capabilities with relation to output capabilities and, in turn, to assess central processing requirements that intervene. The test is divided into three sections. The first of these evaluates eight input-output relationships such as an aural input to an oral output, aural input to a gestural response, visual input to a graphic response, etc. The second part of the test is concerned with central processes and requires the subject to engage in matching, sorting, and arranging tasks and responding to requests or demands. In addition, brief tests of the type frequently included in psychometric measures of intelligence are included such as a single object assembly test and a single verbal arithmetic problem. The *Peabody Picture Vocabulary Test* (Dunn, 1965), is also included in this section. The third section of this test is directed to evaluation of related factors such as tactile recognition, arithmetic, and questioning about paralysis or other physical abnormalities.

The Appraisal of Language Disturbance has been criticized (Spreen and Risser, 1981) because the test was not designed to identify types of aphasia. They note that Emerick has explicitly stated that it is more useful clinically to simply determine what the patient can and cannot do than to classify the aphasic manifestations in one category or another. From a clinical point of view, Emerick's position certainly can be supported, particularly considering the frequent statement by nearly all aphasiologists that the deficits manifested by individual patients rarely fall perfectly into any of the identified categories of aphasia.

The Boston Diagnostic Aphasia Examination was developed by Goodglass and Kaplan (1972). This test is divided into five language areas, each of which is evaluated by a number of subtests. The area of conversational and expository speech is based upon a sample of free conversation and a sample of narrative speech, with the analysis oriented toward verbal prosody, fluency, articulation, grammatical level, paraphasia, and word-finding difficulties. The second area, auditory comprehension, evaluates word recognition, body-part identification, ability to respond to commands, and responses of a yes or no nature to complex ideational material. Oral expression is evaluated through the use of 12 subtests that include naming, recitation, sequences of words, and repetition. The next area, understanding written language, is based upon four subtests that examine various aspects of reading comprehension. The final section of this test involves an evaluation of writing abilities.

The results of this examination provide a profile of strengths and weaknesses, based upon a standard-score conversion of results obtained in evaluation of 207 aphasic patients. There is, of course, a danger in using standard score conversions because of the necessary presumption that the normative group, on which the conversions were based, is entirely and adequately representative of the patients or samples seen by other examiners. Nevertheless, the procedure does permit a determination of the strengths and weaknesses of the individual subject in the various areas measured.

The Minnesota Test for Differential Diagnosis of Aphasia was developed by Schuell (1965, 1973) and provides a comprehensive examination of a wide variety of language behaviors at different levels of task difficulty. This test examines language and related abilities using a number of subtests, organized approximately according to level of difficulty, that fall in five major areas. These areas include auditory disturbances (nine subtests), visual and reading disturbances (nine subtests), speech and language disturbances (fifteen subtests), visual-motor and writing disturbances (ten subtests), and numerical relations and arithmetic processes (four subtests). This material is quite extensive in nature, but the procedure permits the examiner to estimate the level of difficulty at which one should begin and to discontinue testing when the patient fails 90% or more of the items. It should also be noted that the large number of subtests overlap with the type of material included in standard psychometric tests of intelligence rather than a test to identify aphasic deficits *per se*.

The Neurosensory Center Comprehensive Examination for Aphasia (NCCEA) was developed by Spreen and Benton (1977). This is a rather extensive test that evaluates language comprehension, language production, reading and writing. There are twenty subtests in the language area and four "control" subtests of visual and tactile functioning. The authors included non-language tests to provide information as to whether the deficits of the individual are specifically related to language or whether they might be due to another type of dysfunction. Further, the authors made the overall tests sufficiently complex that it would be possible to gain a rather precise measure of performance level. In addition to tests of verbal comprehension and word fluency, the subtests include measures of visual object naming, description of object use, tactile object naming for each hand, sentence repetition, sentence construction, object identification by name, oral reading of names and sentences, oral reading of names and sentences for meaning, object name writing, writing to dictation, copying sentences, and articulation. Scoring is based upon the number of correct responses. The scoring is arranged so that a profile of abilities for the individual subject may be determined.

The Porch Index of Communicative Ability (Porch, 1967, 1973) is another comprehensive method for assessing language functions in aphasic patients. The test is composed of eighteen subtests, four of which are verbal, eight gestural, and six graphic. Scores may be obtained for 180 individual items and these values may be transformed into an overall performance score, modality scores in the areas of verbal, gestural, and graphic communicative ability, and subtest scores for specific performances. The scoring system actually is quite complex. A given response to a test item is evaluated in five respects including accuracy, responsiveness, completeness, promptness, and efficiency. Sixteen categories have been developed that represent combinations of these five dimensions, resulting in a sixteen-point ranked scale from no response to a complex response. Porch stresses the need to have a well-trained examiner and the potential user is required to undertake a 40-hour workshop that emphasizes development of the scoring system and includes ten administrations of the test under the supervision of a previously trained and experienced clinician. Porch (1973) has provided percentile data against which the results for an individual patient can be ranked. This kind of information is useful for intraindividual comparisons as the patient recovers from aphasic deficits.

The Western Aphasia Battery, developed by Kertesz (1979, 1980), consists of four language subtests (spontaneous speech, comprehension, repetition, and naming) and three performance subtests, (reading and writing, praxis, and constructional abilities). The type of aphasia is determined by the pattern of performance of the individual on the four language subtests and an overall score may also be obtained, representing severity of deficit, called the Aphasia Quotient.

Although most of these testing procedures permit identification of specific deficits for individual patients, the general approach has been one of attempting to develop these tests along the lines of usual psychometric instruments which permit rating of the actual level of performance by the individual subject. In other words, the emphasis usually has not been on identification of specific deficits or abnormalities that characterize aphasia, but instead upon scaling the language performances of the individual and identifying areas of deficit that might permit classification of the subject with regard to the particular type of aphasia manifested. While such considerations may be important in providing a basis for determining the psychometric characteristics of the test, they tend to provide assessments of verbal and language abilities that would apply to the entire population rather than to aphasic patients specifically. The reader should note that the approach used in this volume, as applied to our *Aphasia Screening Test* and the *Sensory-perceptual Examination,* is oriented toward identifying brain-related *specific* disabilities. While it is undoubtedly important, in a clinical sense, to evaluate and rate the severity of disorder, it is not difficult to accomplish this purpose by means of an overall assessment of the patient's performances even if it is done subjectively. In fact, the severity and extent of aphasic disturbances is extremely variable among individual patients, as will be noted in the case interpretations included in this manual.

As noted above, many of these same tests are described by Darby and Spriestersbach (1978), and they also provide information regarding their publishers. In addition, these authors present a very thorough discussion of various dysarthrias, apraxia of speech, and their similarities and differences.

Finally, the reader must be referred to an excellent book recently published by a group of persons (Albert, Goodglass, Helm, Rubens, and Alexander, 1981) who have devoted the major focus of their professional lives to the area of aphasia. These authors are authoritative in their approach, are thoroughly experienced, and have presented a brief but balanced presentation of important topics in the area. In the preface the authors note that many professionals dealing with aphasic patients have complained that available books in the area tend to be theoretical, often representing selected approaches, and are not sufficiently directed toward the clinical manifestations of the patient. The available books that deal with aphasia provide information concerning labels, theoretical speculations, and categories of aphasic deficits, but individual patients with dysphasic symptoms often do not fit neatly into the available theoretical categories and clinical patterns of dysphasic symptoms rarely conform to the syndromes described in textbooks. This causes a particular problem for the beginner in the field, who may have learned the theories and labels, and now expects dysphasic patients to comply only to find that they do not. The authors point out that the need in the area is not for another book describing syndromes of dysphasia but instead a book that describes *"an 'approach' to the dysphasic patient."* (Italics theirs, page vii). The authors state that their purpose in writing this book would be to shift the emphasis from concern regarding the name of a dysphasic syndrome to a concern for the patient. Key questions would point toward the clinical manifestations of the patient's problems, the neurological disruptions underlying these problems, and the strengths of the patient that might be called upon for rehabilitation, and the therapeutic approaches that would be available.

It would seem from this stated purpose that these authors intended to write a book that would be directly applicable to evaluation and treatment of the individual aphasic patient. It must be noted, however, that while the book is clearly relevant to individual patients it is not *about* individual patients. This fact should not be taken as a major criticism of the book because it does an excellent job of presenting information for the person interested in a brief and authoritative review of aphasia. The authors describe the approach that should be followed in giving a brief, clinical (bedside) examination for dysphasia, but also provide a major section on the detailed and formal evaluation of aphasia. This section emphasizes the general nature of the examination, linguistic considerations, diagnostic aims, specific and non-specific indicators, and the various areas that should be evaluated (free conversation, auditory comprehension, productive speech, repetition, word retrieval, reading, writing, and the various dyspraxias). Nevertheless, it is necessary to report that the focus in this section is on the examination, and the factors underlying it, rather than the deficits shown by individual patients.

These authors also review the neuroanatomical and neurophysiological correlates of aphasia, citing briefly some of the historical considerations in this area and the contributions made by others. They provide a very cogent and informed conceptualization of the approach and problems in establishing brain-behavior correlates of aphasia. They discuss in detail the evidence for the areas of involvement relating to various types of dysphasia. However, they do *not* present a single description of the deficits of an individual subject nor the implications of such deficits with respect to localization of a lesion in a single brain.

The authors also present an excellent section on the major clinical manifestations of dysphasic syndromes, organized according to the manifestations shown in the various types and categories of aphasia (Broca's, Wernicke's, conduction, global, anomic, transcortical motor, transcortical sensory, mixed transcortical, dyslexias, dysgraphias, etc.). However, these descriptions represent the types and categories of aphasia rather than the aphasic manifestations shown by individual patients. Again, the focus is on deficits characterizing various types of aphasia rather than deficits shown by the individual patient.

The book includes an excellent major section on treatment of aphasia, but is organized principally according to treatment approaches to specific types of aphasic deficits (global aphasia, nonfluent aphasia, agrammatism, anomia, comprehension deficits, etc.). The authors also discuss factors and influences such as fatigue, perseveration, reinforcement and feedback, repetition, and sensory input. While they point out that these types of deficits are usually shown in a complex array by individual patients, the chapter is still organized according to types of deficits rather than the specific deficits shown by individual patients.

This book does take a step much closer to the kinds of difficulties shown by individual patients than is customarily true, and in this sense the stated aim of the authors is pertinent. Nevertheless, except for a single case example of treatment with "melodic intonation therapy," there is no presentation that is concerned with manifestations of the underlying disorder of a single patient. This criticism should not be intended to devalue the significant and excellent contribution of this book. It is important to learn about aphasia as well as aphasic patients.

CHAPTER 2

Aphasia, Intelligence, and Cognitive Impairment

My first contact with aphasic patients, and for that matter, patients with specific brain injuries, occurred in 1945 during World War II at the Mayo General Hospital at Galesburg, Illinois. My job at that time was to evaluate the deficits of soldiers who had sustained brain injuries and to try to make recommendations of steps that could be taken to facilitate the recovery process. I was completely fascinated with my observations of patients with organic language deficits. It seemed remarkable to me that these apparently intelligent persons were sometimes severely impaired in their ability to use even the most simple aspects of language for communicational purposes. I did not have any formal testing procedures available to me at that time, but I spent many hours with aphasic persons attempting to explore the kinds of difficulties that they had. In some instances the deficits seemed to be relatively mild and restricted in nature. For example, the patient might have only an occasional lapse, as far as I could tell, in using the name for a common object. In other instances severe and nearly total deficits would be present which caused a great deal of emotional stress and frustration for the subject. When this frustration built up to an extreme point, the person would be able finally to express words but they would be in the form of curse words and expletives. Following such an outburst, and after regaining a degree of emotional composure, the subject again would be unable to use language for effective communicational purposes.

While I had available no specific tests for evaluating aphasic symptoms, a number of other formal psychological tests that I was using permitted me to observe equally fascinating and highly specific deficits in persons who did not have apparent language problems. For example, in the case of a young man who had previously been a college student, and who I regarded as being quite intelligent and interesting to talk with, administration of the Block Design subtest of the Wechsler Mental Ability Scale provided an extreme surprise. This young man had been taking the Wechsler subtests seriously and doing quite well. However, when we reached the Block Design subtest, and the subject's task was to select the blocks and arrange them in such a way that the design would be reproduced, he began piling blocks on top of each other. At first I felt rather personally offended that he had decided to treat the task as if it wasn't worth taking seriously. However as I watched the performance I began gradually to realize that this apparently intelligent young man was completely confused and uanble to understand the nature of the task. He was completely unable to deal with the visual-spatial relationships that were required to perform the Block Design test and demonstrated a selective and specific manifestation of an extreme deficit in this area. I began to realize that striking losses of language functions might represent one of the consequences of cerebral damage but that other unexpected and highly specific kinds of losses might also be present. At that time I was aware that language impairment was frequently associated with cerebral lesions but had little notion of the significance of the right cerebral hemisphere for performance of tasks involving spatial relationships.

Additional observation of persons with aphasia were extremely impressive to me. I recall a young man with serious damage to his left cerebral hemisphere who, at the time I first met him, was grossly and severely impaired in the use of language. He was scarcely able to give his name or other information that represented basic aspects of his identity and past life. I recall a feeling of great compassion for this man, considering how important verbal communication is in so many aspects of everyday living. I had an opportunity to get to know this man and observe him closely over about a three month period. During that time he showed a remarkable recovery of language functions, even though we had no specific program of language and were not able to give him any formal help. Nevertheless, he was in constant contact with other persons on the ward and in the hospital more generally, continually faced with the necessity of attempting to engage in verbal communication to the best of his ability, and made progress that was to me almost unbelievable at that time. In fact, at the time of his discharge, about three months after my first observations of him, I was not able to detect any significant language loss that manifested itself in our casual contacts. It is entirely probable that I would have been able to identify language difficulties at this time with formal testing procedures, but I had no such instruments available. There was no doubt, however, that this young man had shown an absolutely remarkable recovery considering the severity of his initial deficits. I did not realize at that time that recovery of this type was possible in persons with biologically stabilized conditions of brain damage, whereas much less recovery, or even progressive deterioration of language functions, may be associated with progressive types of brain disease or more generalized involvement of the cerebral cortex.

These observations in 1945 did not teach me a great deal about the nature of aphasia but they did provide some insight into the specificity of language deficits that might occur even in persons who otherwise seemed quite intelligent. I also learned about some of the frustrations that accompany limitation of the ability to use language for communicational purposes after brain damage has occurred and observed the possibilities of recovery of language functions in individual persons (as documented by Wepman in more detail, 1951). Perhaps the most important thing that I learned from these observations was the importance of language functions and verbal communication as a manifestation of the brain. This, in turn, resulted in a continuing interest in the nature of language-brain relationships.

STUDIES OF THE NATURE OF APHASIA

In an historical perspective, the principal question regarding the nature of aphasia concerned the extent to which aphasia was a manifestation of general impairment of intellectual functions as contrasted with an exclusive involvement of speech, language or words without relationships to other aspects of intelligence. This problem has been debated in the literature since it was first considered by Hughlings Jackson in the 1860's (Jackson's Selected Writings, 1932). Jackson cautioned against the assumption that aphasic patients' intellectual impairment was as great as would appear from their language difficulties. In other words, he felt that there was a dissociation between language capabilities and other aspects of intelligence and that aphasic manifestations might be quite severe without involvement of other areas of intelligence. Head (1926, 1951) noted Jackson's postulates in this respect and felt, on the basis of his own observations, that general intelligence and memory were not primarily affected. He conceived aphasia as a disorder of symbolic formulation and expression which was represented primarily as a language deficit. While mechanisms for verbal expression might be considered as a necessary aspect of general intelligence, only in this respect could the aphasic person be considered deficient in general intelligence. Kennedy and Wolf (1936) were quite explicit in postulating that intellectual impairment, as such, bears no relationship at all to aphasia. These authors said:

> We believe that there is a distinction between intellectual defect and aphasia, that thought is possible without speech or words, that defective speech can exist as something apart from intelligence, ideation, attention, memory, and powers of association. There are many examples to demonstrate the truth of this statement.

These investigators did not mean to imply that aphasia and intellectual impairment were entirely incompatible but merely that they were separate types of manifestations. They pointed out that intellectual impairment could accompany aphasia and that, in fact, they often occur together. They said:

> Although thought processes are affected in aphasics, especially with large lesions, it is no more fitting to regard "mind" and speech as one than it is to expect every moron to be aphasic.

Marie (1906), however, had represented a rather different position. He pointed out that aphasia invariably consists of a defect in general intelligence plus a special language disorder. He felt that speech was closely tied to intelligence and that failure to use language for effective communicational purposes necessarily represented some degree of impairment of intelligence. Goldstein (1948), in his extensive consideration of organic language disturbances, was somewhat more explicit in emphasizing that intellectual deficit frequently was found in aphasic patients. Goldstein felt that impairment in the ability to assume the abstract attitude was a fundamental characteristic of intellectual loss in persons with cerebral lesions and that word finding difficulties, or amnestic aphasia, was integrally related to this loss in abstraction. However, he also distinguished between the "instrumentalities of speech" and abstraction abilities. In instances of paraphasia he believed that these "instrumentalities of speech" were impaired even though there might be no significant loss to the subject in his understanding of the meaning of words or in his capacity for abstraction. Thus, Goldstein felt that certain types of aphasic manifestations were more related to word usage and other aphasic symptoms were representative of fundamental intellectual losses. Nevertheless, he emphasized the impairment of abstraction ability in subjects with amnestic or nominal aphasia, pointing out that they were unable to give the name of objects even shortly after the correct name had been applied and a deliberate attempt made to relate the object and the word for it. He said that this kind of deficit was not primarily a memory loss but instead it was one expression of impairment of the abstract attitude. He felt that the aphasic subject could not find the proper word because he was not able to assume the attitude in which the proper words would normally appear. Even when, in some cases, he was able to find the word that belonged to an object, Goldstein said that these words were not normal for the aphasic subject and had lost meaning. The extent to which the impairment of the abstract attitude might, in Goldstein's judgment, be an *essential* feature of aphasia is difficult to assess from his writings. It is well known that Goldstein (1942) believed that impairment of the abstract attitude was one of the major consequences of brain injury in essentially every instance, regardless of the presence or absence of aphasia.

In 1935 Weisenburg and McBride noted that the relationship between aphasia and intelligence was a highly significant factor in attempting to gain an understanding of aphasia. They said, "The old question of the extent to which aphasia involves a "defect of intelligence" is of course an integral part of the whole discussion of the nature of aphasia." Their own conclusions were similar to those expressed by Head. They said:

> Much naturally depends upon the definition of intelligence, but it is clear that aphasia does not involve a "general intellectual defect", such as Marie postulated, in addition to the special defect of language. As the majority of authors since Broca have maintained, the clear-cut aphasic patient does not show a general diminution in intelligence. His intelligence suffers in particular ways . . . Marie was wrong in maintaining that aphasia was in any way a general defect of intelligence, but was right in his belief that other types of mental functioning beyond the language might be affected . . . The extent to which intelligence may be said to be affected varies from case to case; but for aphasic patients as a group it is evident, first, that intelligence suffers insofar as the language processes disturbed are necessary to the carrying out of intelligent behavior and, second, insofar as non-verbal activities are handicapped by changes in mental functioning which extend beyond language processes and are not dependent upon them.

While the above references have been principally to the neurological literature, the relationships between language and thinking have been studied in many scientific disciplines. No attempt will be made here to review the detailed consideration given to this topic by philosophers and even poets, as well as in the earliest recorded writings. An excellent review of the background of the problem has been presented by Meyers (1948) and related to the continuing historical interest in language and thinking as one of the persistent problems that has concerned man in his attempt to understand himself. In the history of psychology, John B. Watson, who generally has been regarded as the father of behaviorism, proposed the most intrinsic of relationships between language and thinking to the effect that thinking is merely subvocal speech (1924). There is little doubt that present-day psychologists view language and verbal communication as a tremendously important, perhaps *the* most important, aspect of human behavior. Watson undoubtedly has had a tremendous influence in promoting this view of language. Nevertheless, it is probable that few psychologists would accept the implication that thinking is nothing more than subvocal speech because such a statement implies that thinking is impossible without speech. Even so, one frequently encounters statements such as that made by Kimble (1956) in his general psychology textbook to the effect that, "Language is inseparably bound up with thinking and other symbolic behavior." Munn (1951), in a psychology textbook that was widely used, said, ". . . we must admit that the symbols which represent most of our world are language symbols (verbal, gestural, or written) and that most of our thinking appears to be an internal manipulation of such symbols."

Wepman (1951) studied 68 aphasic brain-injured subjects and estimated intelligence levels prior to the injury for comparison with measured results after brain damage. Because these were soldiers in World War II, he was able to obtain scores on the *Army General Classification Test* and convert them to IQ equivalents. He compared these results with IQ's measured with the *Wechsler-Bellevue Scale of Adult Intelligence* that were obtained in each instance at least six months after the injury. Wepman found the pre-injury intelligence quotient estimate to be 98.5 and the post-injury quotient for these same subjects to be 70.4, a decrease of 28 points. In fact, a mean of 70.4 represents a strikingly deficient level of general intelligence, falling generally within the lower 2% of the population. If Wepman's results are accurate, one would necessarily conclude that general intelligence is significantly and seriously impaired in aphasic subjects, whether or not aphasia and intellectual deficits are basically the same.

Meyers (1947) has pointed out that the occurrence of aphasia offers ". . . a singular opportunity to inquire into the language-thought relationship." If aphasic subjects show definite evidence of losses on both language and non-language tests, compared to brain-damaged subjects without aphasia, it would appear that the presence of aphasia has serious consequences for general intellectual capabilities. In fact, as recognized by Meyers, the significance of language for intelligence and thought (considered to be so critical by some psychologists and philosophers and almost uniquely representative of the human state) might be tested. Weisenburg and McBride(1935) stated the question when they said:

> The extent to which intelligence may be said to be affected is a moot point. Some investigators have held that intelligence suffers because speech is disturbed because of the intellectual disorder.

In spite of the general interest in developing an understanding of the nature of aphasia, there have been few controlled experimental investigations of the problem. Meyers (1947, 1948) administered a nonverbal abstraction type of problem to dysphasic subjects and non-dysphasic controls. He did not find that the dysphasic subjects had any special disadvantage with respect to their performances. Nevertheless, he was conservative in his generalizations from this study because he had used small sample sizes and had not used a variety of problem-solving procedures. I have investigated this problem in several studies (Reitan, 1953; 1954; 1954b; and 1960). My first opportunity for formal psychological testing of aphasic subjects occurred years ago when I was using the *Rorschach Test* and the *Wechsler Mental Ability Scale.* The *Rorschach Test,* at that time, had been proposed as a specific psychological technique for evaluating, among various personality characteristics, the effects of cerebral damage (Piotrowski, 1937; Klopfer and Kelley, 1942; and Beck, 1944 and 1945). In fact, Piotrowski (1937) had published specific diagnostic criteria of "signs" that supposedly reflected the effects of cerebral disease or damage on the *Rorschach Test.* There were other tests available at that time for evaluation of the effects of cerebral damage, but they were relatively few in number. In one study I compared three groups each containing 18 subjects. One group had cerebral traumatic lesions and showed evidence of definite aphasia, a second group was comparable in age, education, and vocabulary level and had sustained traumatic brain lesions but showed *no* evidence of aphasia, and a third group of control subjects had no current or past evidence of cerebral disease or damage. In examination of vocabulary level a deliberate attempt was made to avoid penalizing the aphasic subjects because of verbal fluency. In other words, the examiner made every effort to determine whether each subject, aphasic or not, knew the meaning of the words and even took the liberty, in individual instances, of departing from standardized administration procedure to the point of suggesting multiple alternatives of definition. We found that this procedure appeared to be quite plausible inasmuch as the aphasic patients consistently rejected, in decided terms, alternatives that they considered to be incorrect.

We had expected that the *Rorschach Test* would show definite deficits for the aphasic subjects as compared with the non-aphasic brain-injured comparison group, particularly because the Rorschach technique is strictly a visual-verbal procedure. Although the subjects are required to observe ink-blots visually, the entire response mechanism depends upon verbal communication. To our surprise, results of the study showed that the two brain-damaged groups were essentially similar in their performances on the test. However, both brain-damaged groups differed from the control group especially with relation to manifestation of "signs" of brain injury that had been previously proposed by Piotrowski (1937).

I interpreted these results as being in essential agreement with the postulations of Jackson, Weisenburg and McBride, Kennedy and Wolf and others who have held that the language dysfunction in aphasia is not directly associated with losses in basic intellectual functions resulting from brain injury, at least as indicated by ability to form associations to the Rorschach ink blots. Failure to find any substantial differences between the aphasic and non-aphasic brain-injured subjects lended no support to the postulates of Marie and others who felt that aphasia represented a fundamental loss of intelligence. Wepman's findings of striking loss of intelligence following brain injury was not substantiated with regard to specific effects of aphasia since brain-injured subjects without aphasia also showed comparable types of losses. More specifically, the severe deficit that Wepman found in comparing *Army General Classification Test* results with findings on the *Wechsler-Bellevue Scale* were not supported, but this might very possibly have been influenced by the use of different instruments. Goldstein's identification of impairment of the abstract attitude and loss in "instrumentalities of speech" as a basis for aphasia did not receive support from the results because both brain-damaged groups were essentially similar. It would seem likely that the deficits of the brain-damaged groups, in comparison to the controls, might be due at least in part to impaired abstraction abilities, but the findings did not point toward a special association between abstraction impairment and aphasic manifestations.

In terms of consideration of face validity, it would seem surprising that aphasic subjects performed essentially as well as non-aphasic brain-injured subjects on a task that requires strictly verbal responses. As Reitan (1954) pointed out in another publication, a careful scrutiny of the *Rorschach Test* protocols of the aphasic patients revealed a possible basis for this finding. The verbal responses for many of the aphasic subjects actually demonstrated significant and even serious difficulties in the use of language for communicational purposes. In some instances, for example, the subject was not able to name the object of which he was reminded, but would solve the problem by pointing to an appropriate part of his body or some object in the room. Thus, in one way or another, the subject would be able to communicate his association. In other instances subjects would use an incorrect word, recognize it as incorrect, and after some hesitation and word-finding effort would be able to communicate the correct word. Occasionally rather indirect descriptions of the associational process would occur. For example, in one instance a subject said, "These look like . . . oh, . . . I can't think of it . . . animals . . . last Sunday (which was Easter Sunday) they used them for decorations . . . you know." While this information was recorded, the examiner waited until after the examination to question the patient further and determine that the subject had, indeed, been reminded of a rabbit. In some instances the subject would use an incorrect word but give additional information through pointing. As an example, one subject said, "I could get a thyroid . . . a . . . you know what I mean . . . (points to chest) picture, in here." Later, when the subject was questioned it became clear that "thorax" was the word that the subject had been seeking. These kinds of responses strongly suggested that aphasic difficulties are rather specific in nature, representing a significant element of the types of impairment that are associated with cerebral damage, but not necessarily limiting the adequacy of neuropsychological functioning over and beyond the specific language difficulties and other more general effects of brain damage.

In one sense, the results of these investigations would raise a question regarding the total validity of psychometric measures of intelligence which are conceptualized as linear functions that are normally distributed. It seems unlikely that the components of intelligence can be individually identified and that human intelligence, as a whole, can be represented merely by an additive process based on the supposed individual components. If we postulate that measurement of intelligence should be rooted in an understanding of basic biological principles, it may be advantageous to refer briefly to certain fundamental assumptions in this area. E.B. Wilson (1925) noted that individual elements of the living cell could scarcely be added together to effect a composite understanding. He said, ". . . we cannot hope to comprehend the activities of the living cell by analysis merely of its chemical composition . . ." He pointed out that even the cell, as the individual structural unit, requires recognition of the fact that it represents an *organic* system in which there is a complex structure and organization. Sinnott (1950) carried this thought further saying:

> Others, however, . . . realized that it is not the *character* of the constituents of a living thing but the relations between them which are most significant. An organism is an *organized* system, each part or quality so related to the rest that in its growth the individual marches on through a series of specific steps to a specific end or culmination, maintaining throughout its course a delicately balanced state of form and function which tends to restore itself if it is altered. This is the most important thing about it. (p. 20.)

In this frame of reference, it may not be surprising that the human organism, even when having suffered brain injury and accompanying basic disruption of language communicational processes, still somehow manages to produce a degree of intelligent behavior even through the verbal mechanism.

As noted above, I also had used the *Wechsler Mental Ability Scale* to evaluate aphasic and non-aphasic brain-injured soldiers. The results in this experiment were somewhat different, showing that the aphasic subjects had lower scores on each of the Verbal subtests than did either the non-aphasic brain-injured subjects or the controls. Interpretation of these results, however, should consider the cultural background against which the types of tests that compose the Wechsler Scale have been developed. As noted above, contributions from nearly every field of thought have emphasized the importance of speech and language with relation to intellectual function, and it is not surprising that a test of intelligence, such as that composed by Wechsler, has attempted to represent language functions quite specifically. Schelling, for example, has said, "Without language it is impossible to conceive philosophical, nay, even any human consciousness." Bain commented, "Thinking is restrained speaking and acting," and Ribot said, "A thought is a word or an act in a nascent state . . . a commencement of muscular activity." John Stewart Mill carried this notion a little further: "Reasoning, the principal subject of logic, takes place usually by means of words, and in all complicated cases can take place in no other way." Leibneiz said, "It troubles me greatly to find that I can never acknowledge, discover, or prove any truth except by using in my mind words or other signs . . . If these characters were absent, we should never think or reason distinctly." Even Wordsworth said, "The word is not the dress of thought, but its very incarnation." Considering this type of emphasis on the importance of language and verbal communication, it is not surprising that our value system, in terms of behavioral correlates of brain function, has emphasized the special significance of an area in the left cerebral hemisphere, in contrast to other areas of the cerebral cortex, even though it represents only a delimited portion of the entire cerebral cortex (Penfield and Roberts, 1958). Perhaps it is not even surprising that the various investigators of human split-brain preparations, as judged from their scientific procedures and reports, scarcely knew how to address the right cerebral hemisphere when language was not a specifically appropriate medium. Further, it is probably not surprising that the type of intellectual function that seems, on the basis of much experimental evidence, to be most generally distributed throughout the cerebral cortex (abstraction, reasoning, and logical analysis), has been relatively neglected both in our attempts to understand the higher-level effects of cerebral damage as well as in our attempts to train the brains of children in the educational system. However, in administering the *Wechsler Mental Ability Scale,* a procedure that has in many respects developed from our value of language and verbal communicational skills, we did find evidence of impairment on the Verbal subtests among the aphasic subjects. One might wonder why a deficit appeared in this context when it had not appeared on the *Rorschach Test.* Specific experiments to answer this question have not been performed, but it is likely that the Wechsler Verbal subtests do not give the subject much leeway or option for expressing his response in such a form that he can obtain credit. For example, if the subject is asked to name the capital of Italy it is necessary that he come up with a single correct word and the types of associational processes, described above in response to the Rorschach ink-blots, would be of little avail. On this basis one might actually ask the question as to whether Verbal tests that are as inflexible as many of those included by Wechsler in his Scale actually do represent meaningful verbal intelligence. It is clear that on such measures aphasic subjects do have certain difficulties. It should be noted that in comparison of the Performance subtests the aphasic and non-aphasic brain-injured subjects did not show evidence of differences in results. The aphasics, in fact, had somewhat higher scores on four of the five measures even though these did not reach levels of statistical significance.

It is worth noting that if one selects specific deficits from the *Reitan-Indiana Aphasia Screening Test* as a basis for composing groups of subjects, the results relate differentially to Verbal and Performance Intelligence Quotients as measured by the *Wechsler-Bellevue Scale.* This hypothesis was confirmed even in a group of mentally retarded subjects by Davis and Reitan (1967). Eighty mentally retarded residents of the Fort Wayne State Hospital and Training Center were rated on certain performances based on the Aphasia Screening Test and the Reitan-Kløve Sensory-perceptual Examination. A classification system for each subject was developed with regard to whether he fell in the upper 50% or the lower 50% of the sample on variables related to left hemisphere function as contrasted with a variable that is more closely related to the status of the right cerebral hemisphere. The left cerebral "indicators" represented simple items from the aphasia test involving reading ability, right-left orientation, arithmetic ability, and finger localization. The right cerebral indicator was based on the subject's ability to copy the shape of a Greek cross. When the subjects were classified into appropriate groups with respect to their performances on these measures, the results showed a significant relationship to level of Verbal and Performance IQ values. The subjects who performed in the upper 50% on the left hemisphere measures had better Verbal IQ values and those who performed better in their ability to copy the spatial configuration of the Greek cross had better Performance IQ's. It does appear from these findings that specific deficits, as represented by the Aphasia Screening Test, do relate in an orderly and meaningful way to results obtained on the Wechsler Scale and this, in turn, suggests that the Wechsler Scale is composed of examining procedures that are somewhat more specific in nature than those required by the Rorschach Test. All of these results, up to this point, have been consistent in suggesting that aphasia represents a fairly specific kind of disorder that involves verbal and language symbols for communicational purposes whereas brain damage, without evidence of aphasia, may constitute a broad range of additional kinds of deficits. The types of losses in brain-damaged aphasic patients may include this broad range of deficits and, in addition, the more selective and specific types of verbal and language impairment that constitute aphasia. Again, considering the fact that the language area represents only a limited portion of the cerebral cortex (Penfield and Roberts, 1958), these findings tend to place the importance of language and verbal communicational skills in an overall behavioral context that would appear to be more appropriate and delimited than would be suggested by the historical and cultural references noted above.

The final study in this series (Reitan, 1960) attempted to reach a definitive answer regarding the nature of aphasia by using an extensive series of neuropsychological measures to compare aphasic, non-aphasic, and control subjects. Three individual groups of 32 subjects were composed of patients with brain lesions and dysphasia, brain lesions but without dysphasia, and a control group of patients hospitalized for various reasons but with no anamnestic or clinical evidence of cerebral disease or damage. The groups were matched in triads according to gender, age, and education. In addition, the brain damaged subjects were matched with regard to the type of brain lesion present. In order to compose these groups it was necessary to review detailed medical records and results of the aphasia examination on a total of 1500 patients who had already been given the complete and extensive set of neuropsychological tests. In addition, in order to put the question of the effect of aphasia to a stern test, the persons with aphasic difficulties were deliberately composed of those who had significant and serious deficits. Tests given included all of the variables developed by Halstead (1947); Parts A and B of the Trail Making Test (Reitan, 1955 and 1958); and the eleven subtests of the *Wechsler-Bellevue Scale.* This battery of tests included a number of measures that were dependent upon either receptive or expressive aspects of language communication and a number of tests in which language communication was necessary only for giving instructions. It should be noted, however, that instructions were repeated and elaborated as necessary to be sure that every subject knew exactly the nature of the task and what was required of him.

Comparisons of these groups yielded results that were quite definitive. Both brain-damaged groups had lower mean scores on every measure than did the controls. Thus, there was a general effect of brain damage that was apparent throughout the tests administered. In comparing the aphasic and non-aphasic brain-damaged groups, however, the results demonstrated significant differences only on measures that explicitly required the use of language functions (receptive, expressive, or both). In each of these instances the aphasic subjects earned lower mean scores. In every other instance, regardless of the complexity of the task or any presumptions that might be made with regard to implicit verbalization, the aphasic subjects showed no significant losses. One would have postulated, as I did, that implicit verbal reasoning on the Category Test (which is a complex test of logical analysis, concept formation, and abstraction) would have been a valuable aid in solving the task and that the aphasic group would thus perform more poorly. However, the results did not turn out to support any such postulate. In fact, the aphasic and non-aphasic groups obtained practically identical scores on the Category Test, both of which were significantly poorer than the controls.

The long-standing discussion and argument about the nature of aphasia with relation to intelligence appears to have received a consistent answer from the results of the various experiments. Performances that require explicit language use do, as might be expected, show evidence of impairment among dysphasic subjects. However, problem-solving and other adaptive abilities related to intelligence do not appear to suffer special impairment among dysphasic subjects as compared with non-dysphasic brain-damaged subjects unless there is a specific language component involved in the task. These findings suggest that language impairment is a relatively independent deficit associated with cerebral damage rather than a direct manifestation of defective intellectual or thought functions. Further, the findings tend to delimit the significance of verbal and language communicational skills with regard to the higher-level aspects of brain functions in human beings. It is important to recognize that other types of abilities are also of great importance, even in consideration of the extent to which human beings have developed such an awesome language competence. The interpretation of these findings should not downgrade the importance of language and verbal communicational skills, but should serve to suggest that they represent only part of the tremendous higher-level achievements of the human brain. A practical consequence of this finding, of course, is that an aphasia examination cannot be expected to represent all aspects of brain function. Even though such a test limits itself to rather simple kinds of behavioral performances, it would be important to include types of tasks that were related more generally to the cerebral hemispheres, including the right cerebral hemisphere, such as we have done in our Aphasia Screening Test. An approach oriented toward specific kinds of deficits, as is true in our Aphasia Screening Test and is also true, for example, in many of the tests developed by Luria, tends to underestimate if not even fail to measure many of the general characteristics of brain functions as well as the more specialized function of the right cerebral hemisphere. Only in the context of more extensive evaluations and research studies does it become possible to recognize both the strength and limitations implicit in any examining procedure.

CHAPTER 3

Historical and Conceptual Aspects of the Reitan-Indiana Aphasia Screening Test and the Reitan-Kløve Sensory-perceptual Examination

The *Aphasia Screening Test* is an adaptation of the *Halstead-Wepman Aphasia Screening Test.* Doctor Halstead had something of an interest in the area of aphasia when he was developing various standardized experiments and tests for evaluating brain functions in his laboratory at the University of Chicago. He had started the first full-time laboratory in the world for investigation of the behavioral correlates of brain functions in human beings and had developed a number of very interesting examining procedures which have turned out to have great value. However, he had not shown a great deal of interest in verbal or language tests. In 1946, when I began working in his laboratory as a graduate student, I had already observed brain-injured soldiers at the Mayo General Hospital and, as noted earlier in this manual, had developed a special interest in aphasic difficulties as well as sensory-perceptual deficits. Thus, I noticed with interest that Dr. Halstead had a number of 3 × 5 inch cards on which various stimulus items had been noted. These cards, in fact, constituted an examination for simple aspects of verbal communication (aphasia). They were not used routinely for examination of subjects and, in fact, no data had been collected with them in any systematic or standardized manner. Joseph Wepman, who returned to the University of Chicago in the late 1940's, had studied aphasic deficits in brain-injured soldiers which resulted in his book, *Recovery from Aphasia* (1951), and had stopped to visit with Dr. Halstead. Dr. Halstead showed Dr. Wepman the cards that he had developed for possible examination of aphasic difficulties and a plan developed between them to put together a formal test for aphasia. This plan resulted in the publication of the Halstead-Wepman Aphasia Screening Test (1949). It must be noted, however, that neither of these men had made any extensive use of the test prior to its publication.

I began using the *Halstead-Wepman Aphasia Screening Test* routinely after my move to the Indiana University Medical Center in 1951. I found that many of the items in the test were relatively useless for one reason or another. For example, the item that required the examiner to whistle or hum "Yankee Doodle" seemed to produce a broad range of responses from subjects that was not very helpful in the overall assessment. As another example, few people had difficulty identifying the larger or the smaller among three circles. The first of these items was intended to demonstrate musical agnosia when it occurred and the item involving the circles was intended to represent a size agnosia. However, in fact, neither of these procedures seemed to be very discriminating nor representative of patients with cerebral lesions. In total, I found that some of the items in the test were very useful but others were essentially a waste of time in the examination procedure. Thus, it was apparent to me that a revision of the test was necessary.

At about this time one of the residents in neurology, Dr. Charles Bonsett, had developed a rather strong interest in aphasic manifestations of patients with cerebral lesions. However, he found that it was quite disadvantageous to have to carry around the *Halstead-Wepman Aphasia Screening Test* because it was about 12 inches by 12 inches. Dr. Bonsett wondered if the test could not be organized on a flip-card basis so that he could carry it conveniently in his black bag. I proceeded to develop a version of the test in this form and Dr. Halstead had it printed in about 1954. However, this version still included all of the items of the *Halstead-Wepman Aphasia Screening Test* and I felt that some items should be omitted whereas additional items should be included. Thus, about two years later I developed a final version of the test, using a flip-card format. This version of the test, which presently is known as the *Reitan-Indiana Aphasia Screening Test,* is the one which has been used for collection of essentially all of our research data.

The purpose of the Aphasia Screening Test is relatively simple and straightforward. My interest was in composing a set of simple procedures that would cover the major areas of language and verbal expression (oral speech, recognition of letters, recognition of numbers, simple arithmetic, simple spelling, simple reading, simple writing, perception of auditory verbal communications, enunciatory skills, and right-left orientation). In addition, it seemed useful (as Halstead had also felt) to include evaluation of ability in copying simple spatial configurations (square, cross, triangle, and key). The test was not intended to represent an in-depth evaluation of abilities. Instead, just the opposite was intended. The purpose was to examine simple performances that presumably could be done correctly by nearly anyone with a basic grade school education. In this sense the test was never designed to provide measurements of abilities that would be represented by a normal probability distribution. Instead, the distribution was intended to be dichotomous with the great majority of persons being able to perform all items adequately. When a deficit in performance occurred we wanted that deficit to be sufficiently clear that we would be able to identify it as an abnormal response. While this is not entirely possible with every subject's performance on every item, the tasks involved usually do not strain the competence of normal subjects. An approach of this kind represents the customary procedure in developing an aphasia test as contrasted to the measurement of scaled performances, representing actual ability levels, as used in most psychological tests.

The above discussion clarifies the fact that an aphasia test customarily uses what has been referred to as the "sign" approach. I recognized on the basis of my early observation of brain-injured soldiers that some persons, even including those with generally good abilities, would sometimes show signs of distinct abnormalities in performances that were an indication of cerebral damage. Even at this early point in my study of brain-injured persons it seemed to me that there would be an advantage, in evaluating the behavioral correlates of brain functions, explicitly to incorporate a sign approach into a battery of tests for neuropsychological measurements. I have discussed in another text at some length the several approaches to neuropsychological measurement that deliberately have been built into the *Halstead-Reitan Neuropsychological Test Battery* (Reitan, 1974). These approaches complement each other and form the basis for a complete neuropsychological evaluation.

Obviously, it is necessary to evaluate adequacy of level of performance on a number of measures that fall in a normal probability distribution. In this sense, one learns whether the subject's general abilities are average, above average, or below average. However, neuropsychological assessment obviously cannot depend upon a level of performance approach alone. Many persons are below average (presumably about 50%) even though they have not sustained any significant damage or impairment of brain functions. Other persons are well above average in many respects even though they have sustained some cerebral damage. Thus, in terms of individual assessment it is perfectly clear that a level of performance approach can hardly be sufficient by itself.

Research studies have shown that patterns and relationships among higher-level functions may sometimes reveal information regarding the differential degree of integrity of various areas of the cerebral cortex. This approach represents a modification of the level-of-performance approach. For example, a person with a right cerebral lesion may have a significantly lower Performance IQ than Verbal IQ. In other instances persons may have relatively respectable IQ values, indicating that their abilities in the past have been relatively good, but peform quite poorly on the Halstead Impairment Index, revealing evidence of impairment on measures that are more immediately related to the biological condition of the brain. A variety of hypotheses have been developed, showing at least a degree of validity, that represent patterns and relationships among higher-level measurements.

A third approach, deliberately built into the *Halstead-Reitan Neuropsychological Test Battery* compares identical or very similar performances on the two sides of the body. The presumption, in this case, is that homologous areas of the two cerebral hemispheres may be compared by evaluating contralateral performances, taking handedness into account when relevant. This approach, based on right-left comparisons, has also turned out to be very valuable in neuropsychological assessment of brain functions.

Finally, a "sign" approach is also quite important even though, in many instances, brain-damaged persons may be able to perform the task satisfactorily. The "sign" approach obviously has its particular value when positive findings occur. Since relatively simple tasks are used, little information is gained when positive findings are not present.

The *Aphasia Screening Test* and the *Sensory-perceptual Examination,* as described in this volume, represent the principal aspects of the "sign" approach in the Halstead-Reitan Battery. It should be clear, however, that many persons, even with lesions that are sometimes associated with positive results, show negative findings in that they can perform the critical task satisfactorily. Reference to Table 12 should make this clear. For example, although no subjects with right cerebral lesions showed evidence of naming deficits (dysnomia), and only 1% of the controls was judged to have this kind of problem, 53% of the subjects with left cerebral lesions demonstrated this difficulty on the Aphasia test. In other words, 47% of the subjects with left cerebral lesions showed *no* difficulties in the simple naming problems used in the *Aphasia Screening Test.* Thus, when positive findings occur they may have very distinct and definite significance, but it is necessary to recognize that when normal performances are present the possibility of a cerebral lesion is not ruled out. Thus, the strength of the "sign" approach is based upon the presumption of positive findings and the weakness of the "sign" approach is reflected in negative findings. This situation is fundamental and inescapable in the use of a sign approach. If the "sign" is defined in a manner that is sufficiently stringent to relate positive findings to the criterion condition in question (such as left cerebral damage), it must be defined so stringently that some persons with left cerebral damage will not demonstrate the difficulty. If the "sign" is defined more loosely it is likely that it will no longer be a specific sign for *any* particular condition. If one recognizes the weaknesses implicit in the "sign" approach, (the limited information implicit in satisfactory performances), it becomes possible to use this approach quite effectively in conjunction with other procedures. Used by itself, however, the "sign" approach is certain to generate a large number of false-negative conclusions. This limitation of the "sign" approach is not restricted to evaluation of aphasia but creates the same types of problems in many other areas of evaluation. This approach is the principal basis underlying the physical neurological examination as well as for clinical interpretations of electroencephalography, and it is not surprising that in each of these procedures a considerable proportion of negative results occur even in persons with cerebral disease and damage. An important contribution could be made to the value of the physical neurological examination and EEG by systematic research regarding the use of complementary inferential methods such as has been done in interpretation of the *Halstead-Reitan Neuropsychological Test Battery.*

The above considerations have one clear implication. If one uses the Aphasia Screening Test alone, one must expect to find many instances of essentially normal performances on particular variables or tasks even when the criterion condition is present. In fact, recognition of this situation should alert the neuropsychologist to a clear realization that use of the "sign" approach, by itself, cannot represent a complete neuropsychological assessment. In this sense we strongly recommend that the Aphasia Screening Test be used in conjunction with a more complete and comprehensive evaluation of brain-behavior relationships.

Another distinct limitation of the Aphasia Screening Test is that it is necessary for the examiner to be able to recognize abnormalities of performance as contrasted with performances that may be somewhat deficient but still within the range of normal variation. Abnormal performances are indicative of cerebral damage whereas mildly deficient performances may not indicate anything more than that the subject has limited skill, possibly due to environmental factors such as a poor education. There is probably no substitute for neuropsychological experience in developing the ability to identify brain-related deficiencies as contrasted with relatively inadequate performances that stem from other types of factors. As one example, it is not unusual for a person with a limited educational background to spell SQUARE as S-Q-U-A-R. Omission of the E at the end of the word is fairly common among persons with limited educational training and is not a factor that necessarily indicates cerebral damage. However, spelling deficiencies in which the subject is not able to use letters properly to represent the sound of the word are often manifestations of left cerebral damage. While the case illustrations presented later are intended to provide the reader with experience in developing ability in identifying cerebral "signs", it is clear that any such skill is a function of one's total degree of experience. We cannot overstate the importance to the neuropsychologist, therefore, of developing experience in learning to recognize the kinds of abnormalities elicited by the Aphasia Screening Test as a result of cerebral damage.

Finally, there has been a growing tendency among many psychologists, even in published investigations, to *score* the deficits in performance that occur on the Aphasia Screening Test. Sometimes the scoring consists only of counting the number of deficits and sometimes the deficits are scaled with relation to their severity. As noted above, the Aphasia Screening Test was never intended to present a scaled performance of adequacy of abilities. In fact, just the opposite was intended in that the items and requirements were supposed to be so simple in nature that any person with a normal brain and minimally adequate education would be able to do them satisfactorily. Thus, as repeatedly noted, the important aspect of the test is to elicit *abnormalities* of performance that are compatible with cerebral damage and are not within the range of normal abilities. In this sense we wish to discourage the tendency to score the performances. A much better job of scoring performances can be done by developing testing and scaling procedures such as those used by Wechsler. There are two different inferential methods herein involved – one that is concerned with eliciting abnormalities in performance and another that is concerned with level of performance. In this sense, we must emphasize that the "sign" approach complements and supplements a level-of-performance approach. For example, some persons with cerebral lesions may earn a relatively normal score on the Arithmetic subtest of the Wechsler Scale but, when confronted with the problem of 85 − 25 = , will add instead of subtract. There is no way to "score" this type of error, but it does not occur in persons without cerebral damage and is about four times as frequent in cases with left cerebral lesions as with right cerebral damage. It must be recognized that there is a difference in the approach represented by identification of an abnormal performance or a pathological performance as contrasted with a scaled type of representation of the subject's abilities.

As noted above, in some instances investigators identify and count the number of positive signs. While this is not necessarily a gross deviation from the intended use of the test, one "sign" is probably not directly comparable in significance to another. In addition, it is quite important, in individual evaluation, to note the types of deficit rather than merely to count them.

In summary, there is no substitute for gaining experience in interpretation of results obtained on the Aphasia Screening Test if one wishes to use the results for understanding of brain-behavior relationships of the individual subject, especially in the context of a more complete neuropsychological examination.

The *Sensory-perceptual Examination* tests a number of simple functions in the areas of vision, audition, and tactile perception. The areas of the cerebral cortex that subserve these sensory avenues are quite well known, at least in a general sense. Thus, deficits in one or another of these sensory modalities have at least regional localizing significance. For example, disorders of tactile perception probably relate principally to impairment of the parietal areas; deficits in the area of auditory perception relate principally to the temporal lobes; and deficits in the visual area may relate to more posterior or occipital involvement. One must keep in mind that the neural pathways serving these sensory functions have a rather extensive distribution and the lesion responsible for the deficit may involve the pathway rather than the cerebral cortical projection area. For example, lesions of the geniculostriate pathways can be responsible for visual perceptual disturbances. It should also be noted that deficits on this examination, including visual perceptual difficulties, relate principally to the posterior parts of the cerebral hemispheres (as contrasted with the frontal lobes).

As previously noted, the sensory-perceptual tests do not provide a complete basis for neuropsychological examination of the individual subject. Impairment of motor functions, for example, as included in the *Halstead-Reitan Neuropsychological Test Battery,* should be considered in conjunction with sensory-perceptual deficits because the more posterior parts of the frontal areas (particularly Brodmann's area 4) represent motor functions. Obviously, both motor and sensory-perceptual abilities are in the category of lower aspects of brain functions and additional tests are needed to examine the higher-level functions (language, visuo-spatial problem-solving skills, and abstraction and reasoning abilities). Even though evaluation of sensory-perceptual skills does not constitute a complete neuropsychological evaluation, the results can be very helpful in identifying persons with impaired brain functions.

The *Reitan-Kløve Sensory-perceptual Examination* is based on methodological procedures which involve the "sign" approach and intraindividual comparisons of performances on the two sides of the body. The "sign" approach has been discussed and evaluated with regard to its strengths and weaknesses in the previous section. The basic requirement for its application is that the test requires only such simple performances that nearly anyone with a normal brain and the ability to cooperate in taking the tests should be able to perform satisfactorily. Thus, the tasks involved in the Sensory-perceptual Examination are basically simple and we expect any normal adult to be able to perform them with practically no mistakes or errors. As with any application of the "sign" approach, a number of false negatives can be expected. In other words, a number of people with cerebral damage will fail to show positive evidence on the test. Thus, the value of the procedure, in terms of individual interpretation, stems particularly from instances in which positive findings (errors or mistakes) are found. An occasional mistake might possibly be due to lack of close attention on the part of the subject, but any considerable number of errors probably has significance with respect to impaired brain functions. Thus, the occurrence of errors characterizes persons with cerebral damage or impaired brain functions.

The second approach involved in the Sensory-perceptual Examination is concerned with comparisons of performances on the two sides of the individual's body. Deficits on the right side implicate the left cerebral hemisphere and deficits on the left side point toward right cerebral damage. We should note that allowance for lateral dominance (handedness) is not of much significance with respect to interpretation of the results on the Sensory-perceptual Examination. We have found evidence that suggests possibly a slightly better performance for the preferred hand, but this tendency was of such a mild nature that it can hardly be applied to the results of individual subjects. Thus, we expect the performances to be essentially the same on both sides, regardless of the subject's handedness. The basic procedure in using this approach is to compare the performances on the two sides of the body. If deficits on the left side are predominant, the results would suggest that the right cerebral hemisphere of the individual was more impaired than the left. Conversely, particular evidence of impairment on the right side of the body would implicate the left cerebral hemisphere. Instances in which deficits were prominent on both sides, even though not necessarily perfectly equal, would tend to point toward generalized or bilateral cerebral damage.

We should note that the Sensory-perceptual Examination uses two techniques within the framework of right-left comparisons. In evaluating tactile finger localization (finger agnosia) and finger-tip number writing perception, the procedures involve a direct comparison of the independent functional capability of each cerebral hemisphere. If the patient makes a number of mistakes on the left hand, as compared with right-handed performances, the results would point toward right cerebral damage (right versus left comparisons), but each cerebral hemisphere is tested independently. (The fact that we always proceed with testing of the right hand first, regardless of the handedness of the subject, does not seem to affect the results to any significant extent).

With measures of simultaneous sensory stimulation, a somewhat different procedure is involved even though it still compares performances on the two sides of the body as a basis for evaluation of the functional status of the two cerebral hemispheres. In these tests, information is delivered simultaneously to each cerebral hemisphere and the cerebral hemispheres are tested in terms of their functional relationships rather than being tested independently. The testing procedure first tests each cerebral hemisphere independently (unilateral stimulation), but the critical test concerns perception of a stimuli delivered to both sides of the body at the same time (double simultaneous stimulation). Usually even a damaged cerebral hemisphere is able to respond correctly to unilateral stimulation, although in some instances correct perception even of unilateral stimulation is precluded by the severity of cerebral damage, and this information in its own right is definitely of value for lateralization of cerebral damage. With double simulateneous stimulation, however, the question concerns the comparative status of the two cerebral hemispheres, evaluating the perceptual capability of the impaired hemisphere when in competition with the unimpaired hemisphere. To be more specific, the subject might be able quite satisfactorily to identify a light touch to either his right or left hand when the touch is given on one side alone. However, when both hands are unexpectedly stimulated simultaneously, the patient with a damaged right cerebral hemisphere might report the stimulus only to the right hand. In other words, the stimulus to the left hand, following pathways into the damaged right cerebral hemisphere, could be perceived under conditions of unilateral stimulation but not perceived when in competition with a stimulus from the other hand coming to the opposite cerebral hemisphere. Thus, the test for bilateral simultaneous sensory stimulation in effect puts the two cerebral hemispheres into competitive function at the same time and the damaged cerebral hemisphere, under these conditions, sometimes fails to register a perception of the stimulus.

With respect to tactile stimulation, in most instances a stimulus to the face is more readily perceived by the brain than a stimulus to the hand. Thus, while no abnormal results may be obtained in bilateral stimulation of the hands, it is not uncommon to find imperception of the stimulus to the hand when given in competition with a stimulus to the contralateral face. The greater sensitivity of the face as compared with the hand may possibly be due to a larger cortical representation of the face than the hand. In fact, in some instances of severe generalized deterioration of cerebral functions, one finds that either hand, regardless of side, tends to be impaired in its tactile perception when a stimulus is given simultaneously to either side of the face. The practical consideration is that the face is somewhat more sensitive than the hand and that face-hand comparisons tend to yield positive findings more frequently than hand-hand comparisons.

We should note that the Sensory-perceptual Examination is somewhat different than the Aphasia Examination in terms of methodological aspects of approach. As noted above, the Sensory-perceptual Examination is based on the "sign" approach and right-left comparisons. The Aphasia Examination is based principally on the "sign" approach and does not involve comparisons of performances on the two sides of the body. It is possible, however, when using the Aphasia Examination to draw intra-individual comparative conclusions regarding adequacy of performances on various types of tasks. For example, it is always useful to compare the patient's abilities in drawing simple spatial configurations with evidence of abilities in dealing with simple language functions. Results in such a comparison may give a basis for drawing inferences regarding the status of the right and left cerebral hemispheres. The neuropsychologist's evaluation in this regard represents a modification of evaluation of patterns and relationships of the subject's capabilities, but since it is based on the "sign" approach it cannot hope to be especially sensitive. Thus, it is important to note that the Sensory-perceptual Examination represents a major addition methodologically to the Aphasia test because of its direct comparisons of the two sides of the body. Exactly the same tasks are involved, and the same points of sensory stimulation are used on the two sides of the body. Thus, the subject has an equal chance for performance on either side. When deficits occur on one side rather than the other for the individual subject, they almost inescapably have significance with respect to nervous system impairment rather than having other implications.

The use of right-left comparisons represents a very powerful method when positive results are obtained because of the intra-individual nature of the comparisons, the identity of procedures with respect to both sides of the body, and the anatomical organization of the nervous system. Thus, the Sensory-perceptual Examination provides a powerful approach in identification of brain disorders, especially when used in conjunction with other methods of evaluation. For this reason, we felt that this examining procedure and results obtained with it were especially important to include with the Aphasia Examination. In a practical sense, one examination complements the other to a tremendous extent. In fact, the whole area of aphasia may well have been clarified, especially in differentiating specific losses of language skills as contrasted with failure to develop language skills, if sensory-perceptual deficits had routinely been included as a source of additional evidence within which to evaluate language deficits.

CHAPTER 4

Instructions for Administering the Reitan-Indiana Aphasia Screening Test and the Reitan-Kløve Sensory-perceptual Examination

(The author gratefully acknowledges the important contributions to this section that were made by Judith Ann (Jan) Janesheski. Ms. Janesheski has had more experience than any other person in training individuals to administer this test and the rest of the Halstead-Reitan Neuropsychological Test Battery.)

APHASIA SCREENING TEST

The instructions for administration of the Aphasia Screening Test and the Sensory-perceptual Examination are included in the text rather than in an appendix in order to emphasize the importance to the reader of specific and detailed knowledge of the content and procedures involved before reviewing case material. In addition, detailed knowledge of the testing procedures is necessary to understand the meaning and limitations of research results. Thus, we urge the reader to study the methods of administration of the tests at this point.

The Aphasia Screening Test is rather simple to administer but it is important that the examiner follow the instructions explicitly. Because of the nature and purpose of the test (an investigation of possible abnormal performances) we do not hesitate to repeat items or to amplify instructions in an attempt to elicit the patient's best performances. The examiner should be careful to avoid giving actual help with any item, but we do want the subject to be sure to understand exactly what is required in each instance. Sometimes it is difficult to communicate the instructions because a subject demonstrates a receptive language abnormality and impaired ability to understand the instructions (auditory-verbal dysgnosia). Such difficulties should be noted and considered as part of the test results.

Very brief instructions for each item are given on the back of the flip-card that can be seen by the examiner at the same time the corresponding stimulus, on the front of the card, is seen by the subject. These very brief instructions are intended only as a cue to the examiner rather than as a substitute for the actual instructions used in administering the test. In practice it is recommended that the examiner follow the recording form rather than to depend on the brief instructions on the back of the stimulus cards. (The cross-hatched instructions are for items that have no visual stimulus for the subject.) The most likely type of deficit associated with a defective performance on each item is also noted on the back of the stimulus card. We must observe, however, that the deficit may be either receptive or expressive, or possibly a combination of both. An individual subject may not be able to name an object because of an expressive naming difficulty (dysnomia) or, alternatively, because of a deficit such as visual form dysgnosia. There is no absolute manner in which to resolve a question of whether the deficit is expressive or receptive. Even the most simple type of response requires input, central processing, and output in order for the cycle to be completed. Sometimes the limitation of the subject is on the input or receptive side (dysgnosia) and in other instances on the output or expressive side (dyspraxia). The particular responses of the subject may make the nature of the difficulty (receptive or expressive) quite clear. In other instances it is important to consider recurring difficulties, on separate items of the test, to gain additional insight. A judgment regarding a preponderance of expressive or receptive aphasic problems can often be gained confidently by a review of similar types of difficulties on various items of the test.

Before beginning with instructions for administering the test itself, we should review some general information with regard to the procedure that should be followed. First, as with all of our neuropsychological testing procedures (in contrast, for example, with some of the recommendations given by Wechsler for his test), the examiner should make every effort to elicit the best performance of which the subject is capable. We are interested in learning how well the subject's brain is able to perform. Thus, the instructions should be given in such a manner that the subject understands that a formal test is being administered and that she/he is expected to do as well as possible. With many brain-damaged persons this approach may cause a certain amount of stress. The examiner should be aware, however, that the neuropsychological testing is intended to stress the subject's brain in order to find out what it can and cannot do. When the subject has difficulty on any particular task, the deficient performance may, in fact, take the subject quite by surprise. He may not know that he has this kind of problem and may have been entirely unaware of it. This is true even in some instances of patients with definite aphasia. In casual, everyday situations the patient may think that he has some type of problem with verbal communication, but uses various devices such as circumlocution to avoid the problem. In a formal testing situation, however, the patient must do what the test calls for and follow the examiner's instructions. The specificity of the required response often reveals specific deficits. If the subject obviously feels stressed, it is permissible to give her/him some general support and verbal comfort, but it is not permissible for the examiner to give the subject specific information regarding how to do the individual tasks nor to do the tasks for the subject.

The examiner should be alert to the fact that she/he should provide every subject the best possible opportunity to perform correctly *on his first attempt.* While additional trials may be given for the same item, additional trials do permit a degree of positive practice-effect which often is difficult to evaluate. Thus, the examiner should be sure that the subject does not perform in a careless manner on the first trial. If the subject has difficulty on tasks such as drawing the square, cross, or triangle, standard practice requires that at least one additional trial be given in order to determine whether the subject is able to show improvement or, as occurs in some cases, whether he has continued or even more serious difficulties. The examiner may give three or more trials if there seems to be variability in the performance, although this rarely is necessary.

When the subject has difficulty on an item, it is important that she/he be given an opportunity to correct this difficulty if possible. In other words, quite neutral requests should be made such as, "Would you try that again?" or "Are you sure that is right?" More specific verbal suggestions may be given later, but only after the subject has had an opportunity to correct her/his own error. The fact that an error occurred initially is not "excused" by a correct performance on the second trial. Since the tasks on the Aphasia examination are quite simple in nature, most persons who make a serious attempt to do well are able to perform quite adequately. In other words, if the subject was able to perform correctly on the second trial, he should not have made the mistake in the first place! Frequently a *correct* response on the second trial merely documents the evidence of brain dysfunction that was manifested on the first trial, considering the fact that simple material is used and presuming careful and deliberate testing techniques are used by the examiner.

It is important that the examiner record the actual responses of the subject for each individual item on which deficits occur. If the responses are without error, we customarily leave the appropriate space on the recording form blank. However, if there is hesitation, apparent confusion, or some difficulty in responding, this should be noted even though the response is correct. Self-corrections, whether spontaneous or prompted, should also be noted. Sometimes a verbatim response is difficult to record, but the examiner should make an attempt to do this so that full details are available for interpretation. For example, when the subject is asked to repeat METHODIST EPISCOPAL, it is not satisfactory for the examiner merely to write down that the subject had difficulty. The examiner should listen very carefully to the exact sounds said by the subject and write the subject's response phonetically. Secondly, it is important that the examiner influence the subject to make an actual attempt to perform each task. The examiner should not accept responses such as, "I don't know", since such responses do not yield any significant information. Since this test depends upon the "sign" approach, it is important to determine whether or not the subject demonstrates a *sign* of brain damage. In addition, unless the subject makes an actual attempt on each task, the examiner in effect has deleted some of the items from the test. Under such circumstances it may be difficut to interpret the results and determine, in terms of the overall pattern of responses, whether the deficit is expressive, receptive, or both. In reaching a judgment regarding this problem it is often important for the examiner to have made notes regarding the subject's ability to understand the instructions. If the subject is continually confused with regard to the instructions, this constitutes an important indication of auditory receptive difficulties in the language area.

It is important that the subject *not* be permitted to cross out performances or erase. Persons who have difficulty frequently want to delete the incorrect performance. Obviously, this may destroy the evidence of cerebral disease or damage.

Finally, we should state quite explicitly that it is not uncommon for inexperienced examiners to fail to observe errors in performances. The examiner must make a special effort to listen closely. In our training procedures we have found that new examiners frequently accept spelling such as T-R-I-A-N-G-A-L-E as being correct until they have learned to listen closely to the subject's response.

The instructions begin quite simply:

I HAVE A NUMBER OF THINGS THAT I WANT TO ASK YOU TO DO. SOME OF THEM ARE VERY SIMPLE, BUT EVEN IF THEY ARE EASY FOR YOU I WANT YOU TO DO THEM CAREFULLY AND BE SURE TO DO YOUR BEST. If the subject has obvious difficulty in drawing any of the figures in the test, encourage him to proceed until it is clear that he can make no further progress. If he has not accomplished the task reasonably well on the first trial, ask him to try again, and instruct him to be particularly careful to do it as well as he can.

1. (Square) FIRST, DRAW THIS (point to square) ON YOUR PAPER. I WANT YOU TO DO IT WITHOUT LIFTING YOUR PENCIL FROM THE PAPER. MAKE IT ABOUT THIS SAME SIZE (pointing to square). The purpose in asking the subject to avoid lifting the pencil is to keep her/him from skipping around in the drawing. The task is to make steady progress in drawing the figure until it is finally completed at the original starting point. Although we permit subjects to begin the drawing at whatever point they wish, the requirement of a continuous line brings about some standardization of the problem of "closing" the drawing. If the subject shows concern about making a heavy or double line, point out that only a reproduction of the shape is required.

2. (Square) WHAT IS THAT SHAPE CALLED? or, WHAT IS THE NAME FOR THAT FIGURE?

3. (Square) WOULD YOU SPELL THAT WORD FOR ME? If the subject has not been able to name the figure, tell her/him the name so that an attempt can be made to spell the correct name.

4. (Cross) DRAW THIS (point to cross) ON YOUR PAPER. GO AROUND THE OUTSIDE LIKE THIS (examiner quickly draws a finger-line around the edge of the stimulus figure) UNTIL YOU GET BACK TO WHERE YOU STARTED. MAKE IT ABOUT THIS SAME SIZE (point to cross). Additional instructions, if necessary, should be similar to those used with the square.

5. (Cross) WHAT IS THAT SHAPE CALLED?

6. (Cross) WOULD YOU SPELL THE NAME OF IT? Again, if the subject cannot name the figure or gives a wrong name, tell the subject, SOME PEOPLE CALL THIS A CROSS. WOULD YOU SPELL CROSS FOR ME?

7. (Triangle) NOW I WANT YOU TO DRAW THIS FIGURE (point to triangle).

8. (Triangle) WHAT WOULD YOU CALL THAT FIGURE?

9. (Triangle) WOULD YOU SPELL THE NAME OF IT FOR ME?

10. (Baby) WHAT IS THIS? The stimulus figure is deliberately presented in a sideways position in order to make the problem of visual form perception a little more difficult.

11. (Clock) NOW I AM GOING TO SHOW YOU ANOTHER PICTURE BUT DO *NOT* TELL ME THE NAME OF IT. I DON'T WANT YOU TO SAY ANYTHING OUT LOUD. JUST *WRITE* THE NAME OF THE PICTURE ON YOUR PAPER. If the subject prints, let him/her finish and then ask her/him to do it again in cursive writing.

12. (Fork) WHAT IS THIS?

13. (7 SIX 2) I WANT YOU TO READ THIS. If the subject has difficulty, attempt to determine whether he can read any part of the stimulus figure.

14. (M G W) READ THIS.

15. (See the black dog.) NOW I WANT YOU TO READ THIS.

16. (He is a friendly animal, a famous winner of dog shows.) CAN YOU READ THIS? The examiner should listen carefully for omissions, additions, transposition, or mispronunciations.

17. NOW I AM GOING TO SAY SOME WORDS. I WANT YOU TO LISTEN CAREFULLY AND SAY THEM AFTER ME AS CAREFULLY AS YOU CAN. SAY THIS WORD: "TRIANGLE".

18. THE NEXT ONE IS A LITTLE HARDER BUT DO YOUR BEST. SAY THIS WORD: "MASSACHUSETTS".

19. NOW REPEAT THIS ONE: "METHODIST EPISCOPAL".

20. (Square) DON'T SAY THIS WORD OUT LOUD. (Pointing to stimulus word "SQUARE".) JUST WRITE IT ON YOUR PAPER. If the patient prints the word, ask him to write it.

21.a. (Seven) WOULD YOU READ THIS WORD?

21. Remove the stimulus card and say, NOW, I WANT YOU TO SAY THIS AFTER ME: "SEVEN".

22. I AM GOING TO SAY SOMETHING THAT I WANT YOU TO SAY AFTER ME, SO LISTEN CAREFULLY: "HE SHOUTED THE WARNING". NOW YOU SAY IT.

TELL ME IN YOUR OWN WORDS WHAT THAT MEANS. Sometimes it is necessary to amplify by asking the kind of situation to which the sentence might refer. The patient's understanding is adequately demonstrated when he brings the concept of impending danger into the explanation or illustration given.

23. NOW I WANT YOU TO WRITE THAT SENTENCE ON THE PAPER. Sometimes it is necessary to repeat the sentence so the patient understands clearly what he is to write.

24. (85 − 27) HERE IS AN ARITHMETIC PROBLEM. COPY IT DOWN ON YOUR PAPER ANY WAY YOU LIKE AND TRY TO WORK IT OUT. If the patient does not perform subtraction, ask him/her to do the problem again, and to be very careful to do it right. If the subject still does not recognize the meaning of the minus sign, question him to determine the degree of his/her confusion.

25. (17 × 3) NOW DO THIS ONE IN YOUR HEAD; WRITE DOWN ONLY THE ANSWER. If the patient has difficulty with these problems, use some simple problems in addition, subtraction, and possibly multiplication. The purpose is not to see if the patient has developed skill in dealing with complex arithmetic problems but to determine whether or not he has specific losses in his understanding of arithmetical processes. The drawback in using extremely simple problems is that the patient may respond correctly through rote memory rather than through immediate use of arithmetical processes, but some patients have such limited formal training in arithmetic that it is necessary to use very simple problems.

26. (Key) WHAT IS THIS?

27. (Still presenting the picture of the key) IF YOU HAD ONE OF THESE IN YOUR HAND, SHOW ME HOW YOU WOULD USE IT.

28. (Key) NOW I WANT YOU TO DRAW A PICTURE THAT LOOKS JUST LIKE THIS. TRY TO MAKE YOUR KEY LOOK ENOUGH LIKE THIS ONE (pointing to the picture) SO THAT I WOULD KNOW IT WAS THE SAME KEY FROM YOUR DRAWING. MAKE IT ABOUT THE SAME SIZE. Instruct patient that he may lift his pencil, but he may not erase. If he makes a serious mistake, he may start a new drawing over again; but do not erase the original error. It may be important for interpretation of the results. It is not necessary for the subject to bother with the shading. In fact, attempts to reproduce the shading sometimes conceal errors that would be important to observe.

29. (Place left hand to right ear) WOULD YOU READ THIS?

30. (Place left hand to right ear) NOW, WOULD YOU DO WHAT IT SAID? The examiner should be

sure to note any false starts or even mild expressions of confusion.

31. NOW I WANT YOU TO PUT YOUR LEFT HAND TO YOUR LEFT ELBOW. Confusion on this item often reveals minimal or subtle difficulties in right-left orientation even though the patient does not make mistakes in responding to direct requests that are within the realm of possibility. Sometimes this item elicits evidence of a very serious problem – confusion of body parts (body agnosia). This would be manifested by confusion, for example, between the shoulder and the elbow and might be evident even though right-left confusion was not demonstrated.

THE SENSORY-PERCEPTUAL EXAMINATION

The procedure for administering the Sensory-perceptual Examination is relatively simple in nature but it does require practice on the part of the examiner and close attention to detail. With sufficient practice many examiners are able to proceed quite quickly with the examination, keeping in mind errors that have been made by the subject and recording them when a natural break occurs in the testing procedure. However, if the examiner has not had sufficient experience with administration of the test, it is necessary to record errors as one goes along. As with any standardized and formal testing procedure, it is important that instructions to the subject be given in an exact and precise manner. In other words, the examiner should have memorized the instructions. The instructions may be re-stated, expanded, and so on to be sure that the subject understands exactly what is expected, but they should be given in standard form initially.

It would be advisable for a person who had not given these tests before to memorize the specific instructions, to obtain "dry run" experience with practice subjects, and finally to give the tests to an experienced and knowledgeable person in order to be sure that all aspects of the procedure are followed correctly. Secondly, if the test is routinely given by a person who does not have background and experience in the area of human brain-behavior relationships, supervision should be provided by a person who is knowledgeable with regard to the purpose of the test and the neuroanatomical and neuropathological background for interpretation of the results. In general, however, the tests can be given by any intelligent person who has been trained in the administration.

In administering the tests for perception of bilateral simultaneous stimulation, it is important that a minimal stimulus be given. The stimulus is given with the examiner's own finger, not a pencil or other object. The examiner should determine how minimal a stimulus can be given and still elicit a correct response when the stimulus is given only to one side or the other, and then give the test using the same light stimulus. An attempt should be made to continue to use this same amount of pressure when stimuli are given to both sides simultaneously, even though one side may initially have been determined to require more pressure than the other. With auditory stimulation, the same general rule is followed. Use as minimal a sound as possible that will still elicit correct responses to unilateral stimulation. A loud finger-snap is not necessary. In fact, the examiner is usually not even able to hear the stimulus although the subject is able to respond correctly. With visual stimulation a very minimal movement of only one finger is frequently sufficient to elicit correct unilateral responses. It is not necessary to wave at the subject.

The Sensory-perceptual Examination is concerned principally with evaluating the intactness of input (receptive) avenues to the brain rather than with evaluation of response (expressive) capabilities. Sometimes an individual has intact input avenues but has difficulty giving appropriate responses. This occurs particularly in persons with right-left confusion or serious impairment of the ability to pay attention. Thus, the examiner must be alert to errors in responding that are due to general confusion of the subject or specific errors in identifying the right and left sides. If a person is confused in terms of responding "right" or "left", a different response procedure should be used. In some instances, it is necessary for the subject to point to the side stimulated. With tactile stimulation it is not satisfactory to have the subject merely move the hand that was stimulated. More reliable responses are obtained when the subject is instructed to point to the location of the stimulus, even though it is necessary sometimes to point to both sides.

Finally, while homonymous visual field defects and lateralized instances of visual imperception have generally similar significance, the two findings may definitely be complementary and should not be considered as identical manifestations. Of course, if a person has a complete homonymous hemianopia, the test for visual imperception is precluded. Obviously, under such circumstances, the subject would not be able to respond to the stimuli presented on the affected (blind) side. In many instances, however, visual imperception on one side or the other occurs without a corresponding visual field deficit. In other instances, careful examining technique (as demonstrated in one of the illustrative cases in this manual) may show that visual imperception occurs in one quadrant of the affected side whereas a visual field loss involves the other quadrant on the same side. Obviously, such information would have definite significance with respect to the location of the lesion.

Instances of unilateral impairment of tactile or auditory perception are important to note, but they do not constitute a test for sensory imperception any more than does mapping of the visual fields. The principal purpose for giving unilateral stimulation initially is to determine that the individual has the capability to respond on either side when the stimulation is given to that side alone. The term "imperception" refers to a failure to report the stimulus to one side when in competition with a stimulus given to the other side. Thus, bilateral simultaneous stimulation is necessary in order to elicit a manifestation of imperception as defined by this test. Of course, unilateral impairment of tactile perception (hypesthesia) may be of definite significance with respect to lateralization of a cerebral lesion and this may possibly be true of unilateral auditory impairment as well (although unilateral auditory deficiencies are much more common, in association with peripheral rather than central hearing losses, than is true for deficits in tactile perception).

In testing for finger agnosia (impairment of tactile finger localization), the least possible stimulus should be used. Stimuli should be given to the fingers in random order, but adjacent fingers should not be tested consecutively. The examiner should always be sure that both the examiner and the subject understand the reporting system that the subject is going to use. Any reporting system is satisfactory, provided that it is unambiguous. Remember that this is a test of tactile perception rather than a test of the subject's adequacy in reporting. The stimulus is applied to the fingers by giving a distinct, light touch rather than a brushing motion.

On the finger-tip number writing perception test, the numbers are administered in the prescribed order indicated on the recording form. The numbers should be written on the palmar aspect of the hand (palm up) at the distal part of the finger. Use an instrument such as a stylus or ballpoint pen that has run out of ink. Write the numbers clearly, slowly, and distinctly, in a form that might resemble "first grade" instruction. In the case of finger-tip number writing, the examiner does not use the "least stimulus possible" but, instead, uses a steady pressure that is sufficient to leave a "trail of white" where the pen has been.

The specific instructions for administering the Sensory-perceptual Examination are as follows:

EXAMINATION FOR SENSORY-PERCEPTUAL DISTURBANCES

SENSORY IMPERCEPTION

a) *Tactile:* PUT YOUR HANDS ON THE TABLE LIKE THIS (palms down). I AM GOING TO TOUCH YOUR RIGHT HAND (touch) OR YOUR LEFT HAND (touch). The place that should be touched by the examiner is the back of the hand, just proximal to the middle knuckle. I WANT YOU TO CLOSE YOUR EYES SINCE I WANT YOU TO DEPEND ONLY ON YOUR FEELING TO TELL ME WHICH HAND I TOUCH. IF I TOUCH YOUR RIGHT HAND (touch right hand), YOU SAY, "RIGHT". THAT WAY I WILL KNOW YOU FELT IT. IF I TOUCH YOUR LEFT HAND (touch left hand) YOU SAY, "LEFT". BE SURE YOU DO NOT MAKE A MISTAKE IN TELLING ME WHICH HAND I TOUCHED. DO YOU HAVE ANY QUESTIONS?

Repeat or amplify the instructions as necessary to be sure that the patient understands the procedure.

First, touch the right hand or left hand in random sequence approximately four times each in order to determine the lightest pressure needed to obtain consistent and correct responses to unilateral stimulation. Then, touch right hand, left hand, or both hands simultaneously in random sequence until each has been tried at least four times. If the patient has more difficulty feeling the stimulus on one side or the other, this should be recorded. The important point of this test, however, is to determine whether or not the patient fails to respond to one side consistently with bilateral simultaneous stimulation even though he responds correctly on the same side with unilateral stimulation. Never warn the patient that on some trials both hands will be simultaneously touched, and do not give bilateral stimuli on consecutive trials. Some patients have so much difficulty keeping their eyes closed that it may be necessary to use a blindfold, although this rarely happens. Be sure that the responses are based upon tactile perception alone. Record errors on the form.

Using the above procedure as a model, proceed with:

NOW I'M GOING TO TOUCH EITHER YOUR HAND OR YOUR FACE, AND I WANT YOU TO TELL ME WHICH ONE I'M TOUCHING. YOU DON'T HAVE TO TELL ME "RIGHT" OR "LEFT". JUST SAY "HAND" OR "FACE". ALL RIGHT, CLOSE YOUR EYES.

Touch the right hand, left face, and both face and hand simultaneously in random sequence until each has been done at least four times. Then repeat with left hand, right face, and both.

b) *Auditory:* NOW I'M GOING TO STAND BEHIND YOU AND MAKE A NOISE LIKE THIS (a barely audible finger snap – just rubbing two fingers (thumb and another finger) *once* together should be sufficient). (Be careful not to touch the subject or the subject's hair.) I WANT YOU TO TELL ME IF THE SOUND IS BY *THIS* EAR (touch right ear) or *THIS* EAR (touch left ear). YOU CAN TELL ME WHICH EAR JUST BY SAYING "RIGHT" OR "LEFT". BE SURE TO KEEP YOUR EYES CLOSED. Use the instructions for tactile stimulation as a model for completing this test, interspersing unilateral with bilateral stimulation.

c) *Visual:* I'M GOING TO SIT IN FRONT OF YOU AND HOLD MY HANDS OUT LIKE THIS. (Place yourself about three feet in front of the patient so that you and the patient are at equal eye level; extend hands about two feet away from your body. Both the examiner and the subject should use binocular vision (both eyes open)). I WANT YOU TO LOOK DIRECTLY AT MY NOSE AND TELL ME IF I AM MOVING THIS HAND (move fingers of right hand obviously) OR THIS HAND (move fingers of left hand obviously). TELL ME WHICH HAND I MOVE BY SAYING "RIGHT" IF IT IS OVER TO *YOUR* RIGHT SIDE OR BY SAYING "LEFT" IF IT IS OVER TO *YOUR* LEFT SIDE. BE SURE TO LOOK DIRECTLY AT MY NOSE ALL THE TIME – DON'T LOOK AT MY HANDS. Administer four unilateral stimuli interspersed with four bilateral simultaneous stimuli above, at, and below patient's eye level.

It is very difficult for some patients to fixate vision on one point. However, the test is invalidated if the patient's vision is not fixated in the center of his visual field. The examiner must be alert to give the stimulus only when the subject's vision is properly fixated. First proceed with unilateral stimuli because correct responses to unilateral movement must be determined before possible failure to respond to one side or the other with bilateral simultaneous stimulation has any special significance. If the examiner suspects a possible limitation of visual fields, gross confrontation procedures or more exact methods (perimetry or use of a tangent screen) may be used to map the visual fields. In the event of homonymous hemianopsia, bilateral simultaneous visual stimulation is meaningless, but the homonymous visual field loss may have given the lateralizing information sought. Homonymous quadrantanopsia may not invalidate the test provided that the intact quadrants are used for presenting the stimulus. The test may be given at eye level, but many examiners give the test in the upper parts of the visual field, at eye level, and in the lower parts of the visual field in order to deal with partial homonymous visual field losses.

TACTILE FINGER RECOGNITION (FINGER AGNOSIA)

Ask the subject to place his right hand, *palm down,* on the table in front of him with the fingers extended and spread slightly apart. Ask the subject to close his eyes, or the examiner can shield the subject's hand with a piece of paper.

Say "I'M GOING TO NAME (NUMBER) YOUR FINGERS. WE'LL CALL THIS FINGER #1 (thumb), THIS ONE #2 (index finger), THIS ONE #3 (middle finger), THIS ONE #4 (ring finger) AND THIS ONE #5 (little finger). The examiner touches each finger with a distinct but light touch (using the examiner's own finger to control the intensity of the stimulus), just proximal to the nail bed of the subject's finger. NOW, KEEP YOUR EYES CLOSED AND TELL ME, BY *NUMBER,* WHICH FINGER I TOUCHED.

It is usually helpful initially to give a single trial to each of the fingers in a consecutive order. In this way the examiner ensures that the subject understands the reporting system and that the intensity of the stimulus (light touch) is appropriate. Then, the examiner should touch each finger in a random sequence, touching each finger a total of four times. Avoid delivering a stimulus to two adjacent fingers consecutively. It is often necessary to remind the subject that he/she should pay close attention and tell the examiner exactly what finger was touched.

Most persons can adapt to this numbering/reporting system, but it is sometimes necessary for the examiner to adapt to the limitations of individual subjects. For example, some persons prefer to name the thumb as "thumb" and then consecutively number the fingers 1 through 4 beginning with the index finger.

FINGER-TIP NUMBER WRITING

I AM GOING TO WRITE SOME NUMBERS ON YOUR FINGER-TIPS. I WANT YOU TO PAY CLOSE ATTENTION SO THAT YOU WILL BE ABLE TO TELL ME THE NUMBERS THAT I WRITE.

Illustrate on the subject's palm how the numbers will be written as follows: THIS IS THE WAY I WILL MAKE A 3; THIS IS THE WAY I WILL MAKE A 4; THIS IS THE WAY I WILL MAKE A 5; AND I WILL MAKE A 6 LIKE THIS. If the subject gives any indication that he makes the numbers differently from the examiner, the examiner's method should be adapted to the subject's method for writing the numbers. In some instances it is worthwhile to have the subject write the numbers 3, 4, 5, and 6 on paper before the illustrations are given on the subject's palm, so that the numbers can be made in the way most familiar to the subject. This illustration should not be used as a guide for the patient during administration of this procedure.

BE SURE TO KEEP YOUR EYES CLOSED BUT PAY CLOSE ATTENTION SO THAT YOU WILL BE ABLE TO TELL WHAT NUMBERS I WRITE. SINCE I AM FACING YOU, REMEMBER THAT I WILL BE WRITING THE NUMBERS UPSIDE DOWN.

Shield the patient's finger as you write each number so that he will not be able to see what is written even if he should open his eyes. Use a different finger for each trial (proceeding in order from finger #1 through #5) until four trials have been given (using the numbers indicated on the test form) for each finger of the right hand. Duplicate the procedure for the left hand. Record errors only.

TACTILE FORM RECOGNITION TEST

This test may be considered as a supplement to the Sensory-perceptual Examination because it tests for astereognosis. However, it was developed several years after the other tests and is sometimes considered to be a separate procedure.

CHAPTER 5

Identification of Deficits Elicited by the Aphasia Screening Test and Sensory-perceptual Examination

In this chapter an attempt will be made to describe a conceptual framework for classification of aphasic deficits and verbal identification of specific deficits elicited by the Aphasia Screening Test and Sensory-perceptual Examination. The reader should be forewarned that the conceptualization presented, and the terminology that stems from the conceptual framework, is somewhat different from conventional ideas and terms used by most aphasiologists.

The system for verbal identification and classification of aphasic and related deficits, used by most writers in this area, fall into three categories – aphasia, agnosia, and apraxia. The term *aphasia* is used to refer to language deficits whereas the terms *agnosia* and *apraxia* may refer to either language or non-language deficits. *Agnosia* refers to a failure to understand or comprehend either language or non-language material (input deficits) and *apraxia* refers to impairment in doing specific things such as spelling, writing, dressing, using instruments, etc. (output deficits). Input and output (receptive and expressive) deficits are recognized, of course, in the language or non-language areas. The distinction, therefore, between the terms, agnosia and apraxia essentially refers to input (receptive) deficits as contrasted with output (expressive) deficits.

A major underlying thesis of this volume is that assessment of language deficits (aphasia) may be complemented very effectively by broadening the examination to include non-language performances such as drawing of common figures and especially by inclusion of various non-language tests of input abilities (the Sensory-perceptual Examination). Such an idea is hardly new. In fact, most neuropsychologists recognize the need for evaluation of a broad range of functions in performing a clinical neuropsychological evaluation. However, the development and use of tests for aphasia, as separate instruments, has promoted a tendency to emphasize language deficits as the focus of interest rather than the broader range of functions necessary to understand brain-behavior relationships in the individual subject.

The framework we have used for developing a terminology useful in describing the deficits elicited by the Aphasia Screening Test and the Sensory-perceptual Examination is certain to be criticized, or at least be considered unconventional, because it deviates from the systems usually employed. We wish to emphasize that *any* interaction with the environment, regardless of how simple, may involve input, central processing, and output. Regardless of content (verbal or non-verbal), sensory avenues must carry information into the brain, some degree of processing of this information must occur, and if the circuit is completed, motor effectors may be involved in some form of response (output). The response necessarily is dependent on prior input and central processing, but it must be included in any testing situation in order to provide a basis for evaluation. This basic circuit is necessary regardless of the content of the stimulus or response and, in this sense, is fundamental to all behavior (even to such a primitive circuit as the patellar tendon reflex). Thus, our system of terminology broadens the use of the terms *agnosia* and *apraxia* to emphasize their input (receptive) and output (expressive) nature, regardless of the content involved. The central processing function, in turn, is identified by the nature of the deficit (reading, writing, spelling, etc.). Admittedly, this approach stems from the basic characteristics of any behavioral response circuit and is not delimited by response content. Further, this conceptualization is adaptable to emphasis on the input or output side, depending upon the characteristics of the test involved. The Sensory-perceptual Examination, for example, was deliberately designed to simplify response requirements and to emphasize sensory input and central processing.

In our earlier review of both brief and more comprehensive aphasia tests, it became clear that different tests stem from different theoretical positions, use different procedural strategies, vary with respect to content, and as a result, undoubtedly produce somewhat different results even in examination of the same subject. Thus, it is important for the individual clinician to select the procedures that will be most useful in her or his own setting. There are certain areas of examination that are regularly represented in various aphasia tests. Probably the principal areas of coverage include evaluation of free conversation; productive speech; repetition of multisyllabic words, complex sentences, or verbal sequences; word retrieval and naming of common objects; auditory comprehension; reading; and writing. In addition, many of the tests include evaluation of arithmetical abilities and evaluation of various types of apraxic deficits.

The reader should recognize that our Aphasia Screening Test is comparatively brief but covers a broad range of performances. In effect, it is a series of short, quick tests that were devised to provide a standardized basis for observing possible limitations in input, central processing, and output. It is important to recognize that these tests were not devised to permit use of a scaled scoring system, because the approach was oriented toward eliciting *abnormalities or deficits* rather than scaling level of performance. It should be equally clear that in using this approach the examiner must develop competence in observing abnormalities or deficits and in interpreting them. In fact, a basic purpose of this volume is to provide illustrative material so that the reader can become familiar with the types of deficits that are of significance with regard to impaired brain functions as contrasted with performances that do not have this kind of significance. It is also important for the reader to recognize that the Aphasia Screening Test is not fully comprehensive in covering the areas of language function that have been emphasized by many investigators. For example, free conversation and productive speech are not systematically sampled and the test is relatively limited in providing specific procedures for evaluating auditory comprehension. We had felt that the examiner might be able to gain an overall understanding of the patient's free conversation and auditory comprehension skills through interaction with the patient in administering the instructions and giving the test. However, when the test is given by a technician, failure to have included more specific methods for evaluating free conversation and tests of auditory comprehension might constitute a weakness with relation to interpretation of the results. Nevertheless, the results elicited by the Aphasia Screening Test and the Sensory-perceptual Examination, when rated by myself, produced data which differentiated between persons with and without cerebral damage as well as between groups with left, right, or generalized cerebral lesions approximately as well as did a 23-variable neuropsychological test battery (Wheeler and Reitan, 1962; Wheeler, Burke, and Reitan, 1963; Wheeler and Reitan, 1963). Thus, it would appear that the series of short, quick tests included in these procedures are fairly comprehensive in terms of their manifestations of brain functions. We must, however, emphasize the need for developing competence in recognizing the significance of deficits that are shown by individual patients.

Within the framework of input, central processing, and output, required for every response circuit, it is apparent that identification and differentiation of receptive as compared with expressive deficits is rather difficult. As recognized by most aphasiologists, nearly every patient shows elements of both types of deficits. In some cases, however, the limitation may be much more related to the receptive than the expressive avenues, or vice versa. For example, a person may not be able to name a common object when shown a picture of it because of expressive naming difficulties. Conversely, we have seen instances in which visual form discrimination was so seriously impaired that the individual was not able to name the object because he could not recognize what it was from the picture. In any instance of defective response, the limitation might be receptive, expressive, or a combination of both. Using our testing procedures it is necessary for the examiner to reach an overall judgment, based upon assessment of the types of difficulties shown on individual items, to specify the more exact nature of the difficulty.

The test booklet provides brief information with regard to the most common deficit associated with defective responses to individual items, but it may be useful to review each of the items in this regard. The first item in the test requires copying the shape of a square. Except for observing the subject's ability to understand the instructions (possibly representing a deficit in auditory comprehension), this item is not in the language or verbal area. Instead, it refers to the possibility of a deficit called constructional dyspraxia. The next item, in which the subject is required to name the figure, most commonly elicits evidence of dysnomia (naming dyspraxia). The patient next is asked to spell the name of the figure (being told the name if he was not able to give it himself), eliciting possible evidence of spelling dyspraxia. The same three procedures are used for the next stimulus figure, with the subject being asked to copy the shape of the cross (constructional dyspraxia), name the figure (dysnomia), and spell the name of the figure (spelling dyspraxia). These same procedures are also involved with the triangle. The next item, which requires identification of a picture of a baby placed in a sideways position, is aimed toward elicitation of dysnomia. The figure is deliberately turned sideways in order to make the task of visual form perception a little more difficult. The next item, which requires writing the name of a clock without speaking the name aloud, attempts to determine the presence of dysgraphia associated only with visual form perception. It is important to recognize, however, that the patient might not be able to write the name of the figure because his visual form perception is so defective that he cannot recognize the figure. However, it usually is possible to discern, in the individual case, that the person knows what he is attempting to write even when the writing effort is typically characteristic of dysgraphia. The next item (naming a fork) is relatively simple and a defective response nearly always indicates dysnomia. Reading 7 SIX 2 is a useful item in that some persons, with impairment of ability to respond to the symbolic significance of letters in the form of words, fail to recognize that the stimulus figure actually presents three numbers. Thus, this item sometimes elicits evidence of visual number dysgnosia, visual letter dysgnosia, and possible dyslexia. The next item, which requires identification of M G W, is intended to elicit evidence of visual letter dysgnosia.

It is clear that the Aphasia Screening Test does not provide an intensive or extended examination in any particular area. In fact, specific reading items are really quite limited. Nevertheless, these items frequently do elicit evidence of difficulties in reading that are useful in assessment. The next two items require reading skills at the second to third grade level and the fifth to sixth grade level. Obviously, these items are intended to elicit evidence of dyslexia (visual word dysgnosia). The next three items require the subject to enunciate, after the examiner, the words TRIANGLE, MASSACHUSETTS, and METHODIST EPISCOPAL. The purpose in these tests is to elicit evidence of central dysarthria. The patient is next presented with the printed letters SQUARE and asked to write the word, without reading it aloud. This is another test for dysgraphia. A simple additional reading test is given by presenting the word SEVEN (dyslexia). A very simple test for word repetition, under conditions when it should never be failed by anyone, is given next by having the patient repeat SEVEN after the examiner. A more complex test of repetition is given when the patient is asked to repeat HE SHOUTED THE WARNING. In addition, the subject is asked to explain the meaning of this sentence. These procedures are intended to gain information with respect to the subject's ability to understand oral verbal communication and to test for auditory comprehension. The symptom elicited, when the patient is not able to understand the meaning of the sentence, is identified as auditory verbal dysgnosia. In addition, the enunciation of the subject, when he repeats the sentence, in some cases shows further evidence of central dysarthria. Next, the patient is asked to write the sentence HE SHOUTED THE WARNING, a procedure designed to show evidence of dysgraphia. Simple arithmetical computational procedures are next tested in order to provide possible evidence of dyscalculia (computational dyspraxia). The next item, which requires naming, demonstrating the use of, and drawing a key tests for dysnomia, ideo-kinetic dyspraxia, and constructional dyspraxia. An additional reading item (PLACE LEFT HAND TO RIGHT EAR) provides additional evidence with respect to dyslexia. The final two items are intended principally to elicit evidence of right-left confusion. However, when the subject is asked to place his left hand to his left elbow (final item), failure to understand the verbal communication sometimes demonstrates evidence of auditory verbal dysgnosia and, in some instances, confusion of body parts provides evidence of body dysgnosia.

The reader will note that the system for terminology described above permits identification of any particular deficit in terms of the basic nature of the deficits (agnosia and apraxia), the sensory avenue involved in receptive deficits, and the nature or content of the deficit (naming, spelling, writing, etc.). Thus, if one observes that the patient is impaired in his ability to understand the symbolic significance of individual letters of the alphabet, the deficit can be described as a visual letter dysgnosia. In the same sense, dyslexia or specific impairment in reading ability may be described as a visual word dysgnosia. The first term, based on this system, is used to identify the sensory avenue involved, the second term identifies the content of the deficit, and the third term characterizes the general nature of the deficit. Expressive deficits (apraxia) require only two terms. The first refers to the content and the second term identifies the general nature of the deficit. For example, dysgraphia can be described as writing dyspraxia.

Deficits elicited by the Sensory-perceptual Examination are not conventionally identified in this same terminological framework. Instead, we have elected to use more directly descriptive terms. The sensory-perceptual tests basically involve perception of bilateral simultaneous tactile, auditory, and visual stimuli (referred to as tactile, auditory, or visual imperception), tactile finger recognition (sometimes referred to as finger dysgnosia), and impairment of finger-tip number writing recognition.

CHAPTER 6

Brain Correlates of Aphasic and Sensory-perceptual Deficits

Chapter 2 summarized some of our research contributions to a basic question regarding the nature of aphasia centering on the relationship of aphasic deficits to intellectual losses. The results of various studies indicated that certain general losses occur in persons with cerebral damage and that a more specific kind of loss, in the area of language and communicational processes, is present in persons with aphasic deficits. Investigation directed toward the nature of aphasia obviously can represent only a partial explanation of brain-behavior relationships because aphasia represents only one of the kinds of losses that may occur with cerebral damage. The more general question of how the brain subserves neuropsychological functions must also be considered in an attempt to understand the special case of aphasic deficits.

Exploration of the interrelationship between language losses and the more general characteristics of impaired brain functions opens a considerably broader perspective. It is hardly possible to understand the interrelationships of aphasic symptoms and brain functions without asking about losses in other areas. Since this manual is directed toward language deficits and language performances as related to brain functions, the full range of behavioral aspects of brain functions is beyond our present scope of presentation and other sources are available for such information. As was noted earlier, however, it should be mentioned that a much more extensive set of examinations is required in order to reveal brain-behavior relationships than measures restricted to the area of language functions. A study of the relationships between deterioration of language function and the biological condition of the brain contributes additional understanding of how the brain represents language functions in addition to providing a more general insight into the entire area of brain-behavior relationships. A study of language losses as related to cerebral lesions provides something of a basis for understanding the organization of language and verbal communicational skills in terms of their dissolution. Obviously, it is not necessary to be an aphasic person in order to understand the nature of aphasia, but it may be helpful to know something about the brain-related basis for impairment of language and verbal communicational skills. Thus, this chapter will be concerned with an evaluation of the types of language difficulties that occur most frequently with cerebral lesions as contrasted with those types of deficits that occur less frequently and only in the presence of other disorders; the intercorrelations of various manifestations of organic language deficits; the types of deficits and their degree of dependence upon lateralized cerebral functions; and development of information that provides a basis for evaluating the integrity of brain functions as shown by performances on our Aphasia Screening Test.

An evaluation of the frequency of occurrence of various kinds of aphasic deficits, provided there is a difference in frequency, would suggest that the brain is differentially related to various aspects of language and communicational functions. The types of deficits that occur most frequently would be those that are most susceptible to some kind of impairment with *any* damage of the language area of the cerebral cortex whereas those kinds of deficits that occur less frequently may require more severely disruptive cerebral lesions for their manifestation. Beyond this, however, the differential frequency of occurrence of aphasic symptoms might even imply the presence of a hierarchical organization of language functions. It would appear, in one sense, that those kinds of aphasic difficulties that occur most frequently are less closely dependent on the biological integrity of the cerebral cortex and that those deficits that occur less frequently are more closely and deeply rooted in brain functions. It might even be possible, in this sense, to suggest that the more readily disrupted aspects of language function might be those abilities that were gained most recently whereas the most resistive aspects of language functions were those that had been gained earlier in life and were more securely established. This kind of postulate prompts the often made observation that persons who are competent in two languages and become aphasic may show more serious losses in the language that was last acquired whereas the initial language may not show much aphasic disruption at all. The broader question, however, may relate to the structural organization of language skills as manifested by inter-correlations between various types of aphasic deficits.

FREQUENCY OF OCCURRENCE OF APHASIC DEFICITS

It is somewhat difficult to estimate the frequency of occurrence of aphasic symptoms because most normal individuals do not demonstrate brain-related abnormalities of language functions. It would be rather meaningless to postulate the frequency of particular aphasic symptoms in the population as a whole because the great majority of normal persons would far outnumber those with brain lesions that have caused organic language deficits. This problem stems basically from the fact that aphasic difficulties represent distinct abnormalities in language capabilities whereas many other types of abilities may be scaled and evaluated within the distribution of the normal population. When the incidence of definite abnormalities is considered in the context of total occurrence within the overall population, a tendency occurs to obscure the significance of the problem because of the great number of persons who fall in the normal range and do not show evidence of the abnormality. An example of this problem was shown in an extensive study (Broman and Kennedy, 1974) concerned with correlation between specific variables and IQ. These investigators demonstrated a correlation between the occurrence of Down's syndrome and mental retardation of 0.06. Obviously, this is a very misleading statistic inasmuch as nearly all persons with Down's sysndrome show evidence of mental retardation. When the influence of Down's syndrome was considered in the context of the great number of persons who do not have Down's syndrome and fall within the normal range of intelligence, little effect of the variance due to Down's syndrome remained to influence the total distribution. Thus, a question exists with respect to just how one should proceed when dealing with behavioral manifestations that represent specific abnormalities in comparison with normal functions. If one considers the abnormality in the context of the great number of persons with normal functions, one may lose the significance of the abnormality almost entirely.

In an attempt to deal with this problem, we decided that we would identify the types of aphasic and sensory-perceptual disorders that might be elicited from the Reitan-Indiana Aphasia Screening Test and the Reitan-Kløve Sensory-perceptual Test; base our results only on persons with independently established neurological evidence of cerebral disease or damage; and include only those persons who showed at least one positive manifestation of deficit. Following these criteria, we screened possible candidates until we had composed a group of 174 persons. Feeling that this might be an adequate number on which to base an initial generalization, we reviewed the test results for these 174 persons and determined the frequency of various kinds of abnormalities. These frequencies are given in Table 1.

In reviewing the percentages given in Table 1 it is apparent that certain types of deficits, at least as represented by our examining procedures, occur much more frequently than do others. Table 1 may give some clue with regard to whether or not earlier acquired abilities show less frequent evidence of deficit, but we must caution in this regard that our examining procedures may possibly over-represent one type of deficit as compared with another. In other words, the *Reitan-Indiana Aphasia Screening Test* and the *Sensory-perceptual Examination* may or may not provide an

Table 1.

Frequency of occurrence of positive findings on the Reitan-Indiana Aphasia Screening Test and the Reitan-Kløve Sensory-perceptual Examination among 174 brain-damaged subjects each of whom demonstrated at least one positive deficit.

Deficit	%
Constructional dyspraxia	47
Dyscalculia	45
Central dysarthria	39
Dysgraphia	39
Right-left confusion	35
Spelling dyspraxia	33
Dysnomia	32
Dyslexia	28
Finger dysgnosia – right	22
Visual letter dysgnosia	20
Finger dysgnosia – left	18
Dysstereognosis – right	17
Tactile imperception – left	14
Dysstereognosis – left	13
Auditory imperception – left	11
Visual imperception – left	10
Visual number dysgnosia	8
Body dysgnosia	7
Auditory verbal dysgnosia	5
Tactile imperception – right	5
Visual imperception – right	<5
Auditory imperception – right	<5

equivalent examination for the various types of symptoms listed in Table 1. In fact, it obviously is difficult to compare rates of frequency of occurrence of these types of difficulties because one can scarcely have any confident assurance that each of these difficulties has been evaluated in a perfectly comparable manner. Nevertheless, it would appear that there are substantial differences in frequency inasmuch as certain types of the deficiencies occurred in nearly one-half of the sample and others occurred in less than 5%. Table 1 thus may provide some kind of guidance with respect to the overall comparative frequency of deficits in persons with cerebral damage and be useful in this sense as a general guide. The clinical significance of the individual deficit, however, when it actually occurs, must be evaluated in a rather different context as will be described in a later section of this volume.

INTERCORRELATIONS OF APHASIC SYMPTOMS

The interrelationships or intercorrelations of aphasic symptoms contribute to an understanding of the nature of aphasia and even provide some insight into the organization of higher-level abilities as related to the brain. One would expect certain types of deficits to be closely associated. For example, if the subject had demonstrated impaired ability in recognizing the symbolic significance of individual letters (visual letter dysgnosia) one would certainly expect that person to have significant difficulties in reading (dyslexia). Thus,

Table 2

Intercorrelational Matrix between Aphasic and Sensory-perceptual Deficits.

SYMPTOM	1	2	3	4	5	6	7	8	9	10	11	12	13	14	15	16	17	18	19	20
1. Visual number dysgnosia	....																			
2. Visual letter dysgnosia	.84																			
3. Visual word dysgnosia	.76	.78																		
4. Auditory verbal dysgnosia	.30	.30	.62																	
5. Body dysgnosia	.67	.68	.72	.33																
6. Right-left confusion	.39	.60	.59	.30	.64															
7. Naming dyspraxia	.86	.64	.80	.58	.69	.63														
8. Spelling dyspraxia	.40	.44	.67	.10	.50	.38	.64													
9. Writing dyspraxia (dysgraphia)	.49	.76	.84	....	....	.70	.78	.66												
10. Calculation dyspraxia (dyscalculia)	.59	.69	.52	.18	....	.53	.57	.48	.63											
11. Enunciatory dyspraxia	.32	.54	.58	.02	.60	.48	.63	.66	.61	.53										
12. Constructional dyspraxia	−.13	−.29	−.38	−.08	−.06	−.03	−.36	−.32	−.28	−.08	−.28									
13. Dysstereognosis (right)	.66	.43	.35	.35	.42	.40	.45	.30	.51	.61	.42	.10								
14. Finger dysgnosia (right)	.25	.48	.36	.48	.64	.59	.43	.29	.73	.43	.38	−.11	.64							
15. Tactile imperception (right)	....	....	−.12	....	....	.30	.10	.08	.02	.18	.02	−.08	.58	−.03						
16. Dysstereognosis (left)	.00	....	−.45	....	....	−.36	−.50	−.33	−.40	−.35	−.28	.10	−.03	....	....					
17. Finger dysgnosia (left)	....	.43	−.25	....	−.08	.08	−.44	−.46	−.10	−.30	−.10	.15	−.17	.00	.32	.70				
18. Tactile imperception (left)	−.03	−.35	.46	....	.00	−.24	−.51	−.36	−.60	−.51	−.30	.28	−.30	−.18	....	.62	.58			
19. Visual imperception (left)	....	.00	−.14	....	.40	−.08	−.20	−.20	−.30	−.08	.18	.33	.07	−.04	....	.37	.40	.73		
20. Auditory imperception (left)	....	....	....	....	....	−.48	....	....	....	−.42	−.34	.10	....	....	....	.48	.48	.78	.80	

one would postulate a relatively high correlation between the presence of visual letter dysgnosia and dyslexia. Certain other kinds of difficulties, however, might show lesser relationships. For example, if a subject showed evidence of impairment in being able to recognize and identify various parts of the body (body dysgnosia), would such a deficit be positively related, unrelated, or negatively related to the types of language difficulties associated with left cerebral damage? Answers to questions such as these may be derived in part from a study of the interrelationships among various aphasic manifestations. In Table 2, an overall tetrachoric correlation matrix for various specific deficits involving losses of language abilities dependent upon brain function (aphasia), losses in ability to copy simple spatial configurations (constructional apraxia), and various sensory-perceptual skills is presented.

It is difficult to comprehend this entire table, however one can facilitate comprehension of the intercorrelations by subdividing the table. The first six variables represent deficits which are frequently receptive in nature inasmuch as they depend upon appreciation of the symbolic significance of incoming information to the brain. Table 3 presents intercorrelations among these variables.

Table 3

Tetrachoric Intercorrelations between Receptive Aphasic Symptoms, Body Dysgnosia and Right-Left Confusion.

SYMPTOM	1	2	3	4	5
1. Visual number dysgnosia	....	....	....	....	....
2. Visual letter dysgnosia	.84	....	....	....	....
3. Visual word dysgnosia	.76	.78	....	....	....
4. Auditory verbal dysgnosia	.30	.30	.62	....	....
5. Body dysgnosia	.67	.68	.72	.33	....
6. Right-left confusion	.39	.60	.59	.30	.64

It is apparent that there is quite a striking intercorrelation among these variables. In fact, the median coefficient among these indicators, all of which are principally dependent on the biological status of the left cerebral hemisphere, was 0.62. Auditory verbal dysgnosia (impairment in the ability to understand the communicational significance of language through the auditory avenue) tended to show the lowest correlation among the six variables, although this symptom was closely associated with reading difficulties (dyslexia or visual word dysgnosia). It would appear, however, that receptive difficulties in the language area are rather intimately associated with each other. It is particularly noteworthy that deficits dependent upon visual mediation of symbolic stimulus material (variables 1, 2, and 3) had intercorrelations that tended to be quite high.

Table 4

Tetrachoric Correlations between Receptive and Expressive Aphasic Symptoms.

SYMPTOM	Naming Apraxia (Dysnomia) 7	Spelling Dyspraxia 8	Writing Dyspraxia (Dysgraphia) 9	Calculation Dyspraxia (Dyscalculia) 10	Enunciatory Dyspraxia (Central Dysarthria) 11	Constructional Dyspraxia 12
1. Visual number dysgnosia	.86	.40	.49	.59	.32	−.13
2. Visual letter dysgnosia	.64	.44	.76	.69	.54	−.29
3. Visual word dysgnosia (alexia)	.80	.67	.84	.52	.58	−.38
4. Auditory verbal dysgnosia	.58	.10	....	.18	.02	−.08
5. Body dysgnosia	.69	.50	....	....	.60	−.06
6. Right-left confusion	.63	.38	.70	.53	.48	−.03

One should also note that body agnosia had high correlations with these variables.

Table 4 presents correlations of the variables included in Table 3 (mainly receptive aphasic symptoms) with a number of apraxic deficits (losses in ability to perform certain purposeful movements of a symbolic nature).

The reader will note that the apraxic manifestations involve verbal and numerical symbolic material for variables 7 through 11 but that variable 12 represents the subject's ability to comprehend and draw spatial configurations. (Correlations between certain variables had to be omitted because of failure to meet technical requirements of the method for computing tetrachoric coefficients of correlation). The verbal and language variables relate to the integrity of the left cerebral hemisphere whereas constructional dyspraxia is more dependent upon the status of the right cerebral hemisphere, as will be indicated by results presented in a later section. The median coefficient, 0.58, among the verbal and numerical variables (left hemisphere indicators) was nearly as large as the median coefficient for the results in Table 3. Again, auditory verbal receptive difficulties tended in some instances to have rather low correlations with other verbal variables. It should be noted, however, that in general the correlations based on calculating difficulties (dyscalculia) were quite substantial with the verbal variables.

One outstanding result occurred. Correlations of constructional dyspraxia with the other variables were consistently negative. Undoubtedly this finding reflects the dependence of constructional skills on the status of the right cerebral hemisphere whereas verbal and numerical symbolic abilities are dependent upon the left cerebral hemisphere. This finding needs to be considered carefully with relation to the fact that the group of 174 subjects was composed of brain-damaged persons, all of whom had at least one symptom among those being considered. Among normal subjects it is very likely that a *positive* (rather than negative) correlation between abilities dependent upon either the left or right cerebral hemisphere would be obtained. In this instance, however, the correlations did not reflect the *level of skill* on various abilities, but instead on the *occurrence of abnormalities* in performance that were produced by brain lesions. Such a procedural condition may have a very pronounced and decided effect on the direction of the relationships. Instead of finding that a person who is good at one thing is good at another (a positive correlation among abilities even though they are differentially dependent upon the cerebral hemispheres), the results suggest that in a brain damaged group if the deficit is due to damage of the left cerebral hemisphere there is a lessened prospect of eliciting symptomatology due to right cerebral damage, and vice versa.

Table 5 presents intercorrelations between expressive deficits. Variables 7 through 11 are left cerebral indicators whereas Variable 12 (constructional dyspraxia) is a right cerebral indicator. Again, consistently positive coefficients were obtained between the left cerebral indicators, with a median coefficient of 0.63. Constructional dyspraxia, on the other hand, had negative relationships with each of the other variables in every instance, showing a median coefficient of −0.28.

Table 5

Tetrachoric Intercorrelations between Expressive Aphasic Symptoms.

SYMPTOM	7	8	9	10	11
7. Naming dyspraxia (dysnomia)	....	....	....	....	....
8. Spelling dyspraxia	.64	....	....	....	....
9. Writing dyspraxia (dysgraphia)	.78	.66	....	....	....
10. Calculation dyspraxia (dyscalculia)	.57	.48	.63	....	....
11. Enunciatory dyspraxia (central dysarthria)	.63	.66	.61	.53	....
12. Constructional dyspraxia	−.36	−.32	−.28	−.08	−.28

Table 6

Tetrachoric Correlations between Aphasic Symptoms and Sensory-perceptual Deficits of the Right and Left Sides of the Body.

	Visual Number Dysgnosia	Visual Letter Dysgnosia	Visual Word Dysgnosia (Dyslexia)	Auditory Verbal Dysgnosia	Body Dysgnosia	Right-Left Confusion	Naming Dyspraxia (Dysnomia)	Spelling Dyspraxia	Writing Dyspraxia (Dysgraphia)	Calculation Dyspraxia (Dyscalculia)	Enunciatory Dyspraxia (Central Dysarthria)	Constructional Dyspraxia
SYMPTOM	**1**	**2**	**3**	**4**	**5**	**6**	**7**	**8**	**9**	**10**	**11**	**12**
13. Dysstereognosis (right)	.66	.43	.35	.35	.42	.40	.45	.30	.51	.61	.42	−.10
14. Finger dysgnosia (right)	.25	.48	.36	.48	.64	.59	.43	.29	.73	.43	.38	−.11
15. Tactile imperception (right)	....	....	−.12	....	....	.30	.10	.08	.02	.18	.02	−.08
16. Dysstereognosis (left)	.00	....	−.45	....	....	−.36	−.50	−.33	−.40	−.35	−.28	.10
17. Finger dysgnosia (left)	....	.43	−.25	....	−.08	.08	−.44	−.46	−.10	−.30	−.10	.15
18. Tactile imperception (left)	−.03	−.35	.46	....	.00	−.24	−.51	−.36	−.60	−.51	−.30	.28
19. Visual imperception (left)	....	.00	−.14	....	.40	−.08	−.20	−.20	−.30	−.08	.18	.33
20. Auditory imperception (left)	....	....	....	....	....	−.48	....	....	....	−.42	−.34	.10

The data, thus far considered, indicates a striking degree of consistency among the left cerebral indicators in spite of the fact that some are much more closely associated than others. Receptive deficits dependent upon the left cerebral hemisphere had a median coefficient of 0.62, expressive deficits had a median coefficient of 0.63, and expressive as compared with receptive deficits had a median coefficient of 0.58. Thus, it would appear that these various types of deficits are about equally related to each other. The impressive finding is that the coefficients are consistently so high.

Table 6 presents intercorrelations between the variables previously considered (variables 1 through 12) and measures dependent upon sensory-perceptual functions, listing these latter variables according to whether the deficits occurred on the right side of the body (pointing toward left cerebral damage) or on the left side of the body (pointing toward right cerebral damage). The variables previously considered were left hemisphere indicators (variables 1 though 11) and a right hemisphere indicator (variable 12). Among the 29 coefficients given in Table 6 that involve language functions and losses on the right side of the body, 28 were positive and only one negative. Conversely, constructional dyspraxia (variable 12), a right hemisphere indicator, had small negative coefficients in each instance with variables 13, 14, and 15. Variables reflecting sensory-perceptual skills on the left side of the body, on the other hand, were predominantly negative in their relationships to variables that reflected language or numerical symbolic losses. Omitting those variables that had zero coefficients, 31 of 36 of these intercorrelations were negative. Coefficients which reflected the relationship between constructional dyspraxia (variable 12) and variables that measured left-sided sensory-perceptual losses were consistently positive.

Finally, Table 7 reveals intercorrelations between sensory-perceptual losses on the right side of the body versus those on the left. In summarizing this table, losses on the right side were substantially correlated among themselves in two of three instances. Similar substantial coefficients were present for variables 16 through 20, representing losses on the left side of the body. However, when losses on the right side were correlated with losses on the left side, five of eight

Table 7

Tetrachoric Intercorrelations between Sensory-perceptual Deficits of the Right and Left Sides of the Body.

SYMPTOM	13	14	15	16	17	18	19
13. Dysstereognosis (right)	....	....	....	....	....	....	....
14. Finger dysgnosia (right)	.64	....	....	....	....	....	....
15. Tactile imperception (right)	.58	−.03	....	....	....	....	....
16. Dysstereognosis (left)	−.03	....	....	....	....	....	....
17. Finger dysgnosia (left)	−.17	.00	.32	.70	....	....	....
18. Tactile imperception (left)	−.30	−.18	....	.62	.58	....	....
19. Visual imperception (left)	.07	−.04	....	.37	.40	.73	....
20. Auditory imperception (left)	....	....	....	.48	.48	.78	.80

coefficients were negative, two were positive, and the remaining coefficient was zero.

In addition to demonstrating a substantial degree of relationship between various kinds of deficits dependent upon brain functions, the results are generally consistent in pointing toward differential deficits associated with damage of the two cerebral hemispheres. This situation may very well tend to create a significant problem in statistical analysis of data, considering the fact that the coefficient of correlation is the basic statistic. In other words, if the relationships among variables are negative or positive depending upon lateralization of cerebral damage, it is entirely possible that inclusion of persons with differentially lateralized lesions in the same group would tend to have a cancelling or at least confounding effect on the resulting coefficient. Correlations that would ordinarily be positively correlated may have zero or even negative correlations depending upon the status of the cerebral hemispheres that produced the data. This bewildering fact must be viewed with concern. It would appear that our methods of data analysis, which depend upon a presumption of positive correlations among similar types of measures, do not necessarily fall in a framework that is consistent with the organization of brain functions. The problem is indeed serious. The possibility exists that we either can cancel and confound our understanding of the organization of brain functions through application of basic statistical methods of analysis or we can recognize the problems of the differential functions of the two cerebral hemispheres and attempt to gain an understanding of them possibly in spite of the misleading consequences that may be implicit in statistical analyses.

The correlational analysis presented above permits several conclusions as listed below. We would also suggest that the reader may wish to inspect and organize the coefficients in more detail than was done in this report. We wished to avoid attribution of special significance to what may have been chance variations in individual coefficients and, instead, to have taken only a broader look. Nevertheless, there may be some heuristic value in a more specific inspection and analysis of the overall correlation matrix.

1. Aphasic symptoms must be viewed generally as representing a complex and diversified range of deficits, even though the intercorrelation of these symptoms is sufficiently high to presume that they tend in general to be consistent with one another rather than to occur in isolation or to be incompatible. Incompatibility (inverse relationship) comes about only in terms of deficits differentially dependent upon the biological status of the two cerebral hemispheres.

2. The correlation of receptive symptoms within a single sensory avenue tends to be high. However, correlations between sensory modalities are certainly no higher, and perhaps not as high, as those between receptive and expressive deficits.

3. The correlations between receptive and expressive deficits are quite high in spite of the fact that there has been a strong historical and current tendency in the

literature on aphasia (Schuell, et al., 1964; Albert, et al., 1981) to differentiate between these types of losses. The high correlation, however, suggests that such deficits are frequently present at the same time and rule out the possibility of any simple categorization of persons, for clinical purposes, along these dimensions. The coincidence of receptive and expressive deficits in individual patients is the rule rather than the exception. This finding would call into question the tendency to postulate refined and separate classifications of aphasic disorders.

4. Sensory-perceptual disturbances on the right side of the body are generally rather closely correlated with aphasic symptoms that involve language and numerical symbolic losses whereas sensory-perceptual disturbances on the left side of the body tend to be negatively related to such deficits. Constructional dyspraxia, on the other hand, is negatively associated with aphasic symptoms but positively related to sensory-perceptual disorders on the left side of the body.

Comparisons of groups with left, right or generalized cerebral lesions:

It is possible, of course, to inquire more specifically with relation to the differential effects of right and left cerebral lesions by composing groups with lateralized damage and investigating the differential frequency of occurrence of various types of deficits in such groups. In fact, an investigation of this kind, in which the independent variables represented lateralized cerebral damage and the dependent variables represented deficits previously shown to be differentially dependent on the cerebral hemispheres, permitted us to gain a more exact understanding not only of the nature of deficits as they are related to the status of the brain but also of the interrelationships of deficits and frequency of their occurrence. It must be recognized, however, that results obtained in such a study with subjects carefully selected according to brain lesions, will yield somewhat different frequencies of occurrence of specific deficits than would be the case following the procedure in the previous section where any person with a brain lesion and at least one of the deficits in question qualified for inclusion. It is important to recognize that the percentage of subjects with deficits will vary depending upon how the groups were composed.

Heimburger and Reitan (1961) investigated the frequency of occurrence of difficulties in copying simple geometric figures as contrasted with difficulty in writing as demonstrated on the Aphasia Screening Test. Groups of subjects were composed with left cerebral lesions, right cerebral lesions, and generalized or bilateral involvement of both cerebral hemispheres. These groups were composed solely on the basis of neurological evidence that was sufficient for individual classification, using results from the history, physical neurological examination, electroencephalography, X-ray contrast studies, surgery, or autopsy. Obviously, not all of these sources of evidence was available for every subject, but a subject was not used unless the evidence was convincing with regard to classification of the patient into one of the three groups. Types of lesions were variable in nature and probably tended to exclude certain categories in which the evidence of cerebral damage was not strongly positive. The number of subjects totaled 239 and were distributed as follows: Left cerebral hemisphere damage, 78; Right cerebral damage, 92; and Generalized damage, 69. The performance of each subject was judged independently of neurological evidence with respect to the presence of deficits in copying the shape of a square, cross, and triangle from the Aphasia Screening Test and a judgment was also made as to whether the subject had significant brain-related difficulties in the simple writing tasks that are included in the test. The results of this study are presented in Table 8.

It is apparent that there is a great difference in the percentage of subjects with one type of difficulty or another among the groups with lateralized cerebral damage. Ten percent of the subjects with left cerebral damage had some difficulty in copying geometric figures but did not show any significant difficulty in writing tasks. These subjects tended to have lesions in the posterior part of the left cerebral hemisphere. In contrast, 48% of the subjects with right cerebral lesions had difficulties copying the geometric figures. An intermediate percentage of subjects with involvement of both cerebral hemispheres (30%) had difficulty with copying the figures but no difficulty with writing. In

Table 8

Distribution according to difficulties in copying geometric figures or writing in 239 patients with lesions of the brain.

LESION	LEFT CEREBRAL HEMISPHERE			RIGHT CEREBRAL HEMISPHERE			BOTH CEREBRAL HEMISPHERES			TOTALS		
Type of Difficulty	No.	Per Cent	Per Cent Aphasic	No.	Per Cent	Per Cent Aphasic	No.	Per Cent	Per Cent Aphasic	No.	Per Cent	Per Cent Aphasic
Difficulty with geometric figures only	8	10	50	44	48	5	21	30	48	73	31	22
Difficulty with writing only	35	45	100	0	0	0	12	17	100	47	20	100
Both difficulties	13	17	100	9	10	100	12	17	100	34	14	100
Neither difficulty	22	28	50	39	42	15	24	35	12	85	36	24
TOTALS	78	33	81	92	38	18	69	29	54	239	100	49

contrasting the types of difficulties (difficulty with writing but no difficulty in copying the geometric figures), 45% of the subjects with left cerebral damage showed positive evidence and no subject with right cerebral damage had difficulty with writing alone. Again, an intermediate number of subjects with generalized cerebral damage (17%) had difficulty only with writing. The occurrence of both types of difficulties in a single subject with lateralized cerebral damage tended to occur relatively infrequently (17% with left cerebral lesions and 10% with right cerebral lesions). Among subjects with generalized damage 17% had difficulty with both types of tasks. The greater frequency of writing difficulties with left cerebral lesions and difficulty in drawing geometric figures with right cerebral lesions, as contrasted with the intermediate percentages for persons with generalized involvement, reflects the fact that lateralized lesions tend to be more focal and more specifically destructive and, as a result, are more commonly associated with specific deficits. Finally, it should be noted that a substantial proportion of persons in each group showed no difficulties on these simple tasks. Twenty-eight percent of the subjects with left cerebral lesions had no discernable difficulties on these tasks whereas 42% of those with right cerebral lesions had no difficulties. Nevertheless, when difficulties do occur they are fairly specific with respect to indicating cerebral damage and are useful even in lateralizing lesions. These results suggest that the use of even a few items from the aphasia examination, perhaps done at bedside, may be of some diagnostic significance. Of course, the entire examination can frequently be done at bedside and when the test is used by neurologists and neurological surgeons such a practice may be the rule rather than the exception.

The most definitive study regarding the presence and laterality of brain damage based on results from the Aphasia Screening Test was performed by Wheeler and Reitan (1962). This study was based on an analysis of results obtained in examination of 47 subjects with damage to the left cerebral hemisphere, 57 subjects with right cerebral damage, 54 subjects with diffuse or bilateral damage, and 104 subjects who showed no past or present evidence of cerebral damage. The types of brain lesions involved were heterogenous in nature and probably are fairly representative of the types of brain lesions and diseases that are customarily encountered. Forty of the control subjects were functioning normally and 64 had various kinds of diagnoses including neurosis, 25; paraplegia, 24; surgical conditions that did not involve the nervous system, 12; and medical conditions not involving the nervous system, 3. These subjects were assigned to their appropriate groups only when the evidence, based on thorough neurological evaluation, was considered to be definitive. Those subjects who did not meet independent criteria for classification to one of these groups were omitted from the study. Thus, the results of the study should be referable specifically to differences in the independent variables. Each subject was assigned to his appropriate group on the basis of neurological criterion material without reference to results obtained on the Aphasia Screening Test. The Aphasia Screening Test was given by carefully trained technicians who did not have access to the neurological criterion material. Test results, including the responses of each subject, were recorded by the examiners. The test protocols were then later evaluated by myself in complete absence of any knowledge of the neurological criterion data or the group to which the subject was assigned.

The groups were generally comparable with respect to age and education, even though some minor differences, which probably were without significance regarding the test results, were present. The tasks involved in the Aphasia Screening Test are relatively simple in nature and can usually be done satisfactorily by normals with even limited education. The percentages of each group with less than a sixth-grade education were: left, 0%; right, 5%; diffuse, 4%; and controls, 2%.

It should be noted, at this point, that evaluation of the subjects' responses represented a critical aspect of this study and the evaluations were done by a person (myself) on the basis of a very considerable amount of past experience with the test data. There is no assurance or guarantee that similar evaluations of the subjects' responses would be made by persons who did not have comparable experience. In fact, one of the limiting conditions in the effective use of the Aphasia Screening Test undoubtedly relates to the experience of the person who evaluates the results. Many people do not have this background of experience. One of the principal purposes of presentation of cases in this manual is to provide experience along this line.

The study by Wheeler and Reitan (1962) postulated: (1) that the number or frequency of positive signs generated by each subject on the Aphasia Screening Test would provide a valid basis for predicting the presence or absence of cerebral damage; (2) that a subset of test variables could be identified that would characterize left or right cerebral damage and that a preponderance of positive signs in one set or the other would provide a valid basis for prediction of laterality of cerebral damage in individual patients; and (3) that the occurrence of nearly equal numbers of positive signs in a set of left indicators and a set of right indicators would provide a valid basis for prediction of diffuse or bilateral cerebral damage.

Table 9 presents the frequency of occurrence of positive signs on the Aphasia Screening Test for each of the groups and total groups with or without cerebral damage. Inspection of this table makes it quite clear that the group with left cerebral damage showed the greatest number of positive signs (as would be expected in consideration of the predominance of verbal and numerical symbolic material included in the test), that the group with diffuse damage showed a striking incidence of positive findings although to a lesser extent than the group with left cerebral damage, that a significant number of deficits were present in subjects with right cerebral damage, and that the majority of

Table 9

Subject Frequency, Percentages of Each Criterion Group and of Total Group for 0, 1, 2, 3 and 4 or More Positive Signs Over 18 Aphasia Test Variables.

CRITERION GROUPS	N	MEASURE	NUMBER OF POSITIVE SIGNS				
			0	1	2	3	4+
Control	104	f	71	29	2	2	0
		% Crit.	68.3	27.9	01.9	01.9	00.0
		% Total	27.1	11.1	00.8	00.8	00.0
Right Damage	57	f	14	13	6	10	14
		% Crit.	24.6	22.8	10.5	17.5	24.6
		% Total	05.3	05.0	02.3	03.8	05.3
Left Damage	47	f	3	6	6	3	29
		% Crit.	06.4	12.8	12.8	06.4	61.7
		% Total	01.1	02.3	02.3	01.1	11.1
Diffuse Damage	54	f	7	12	4	12	19
		% Crit.	13.0	22.2	07.4	22.2	35.2
		% Total	02.7	04.6	01.5	04.6	07.3
All-damage	158	f	24	31	16	25	62
		% Crit.	15.2	19.6	10.2	15.8	39.2
		% Total	09.2	11.8	06.1	09.5	23.7
Total	262	f	95	60	18	27	62
		% Total	36.3	22.9	06.9	10.3	23.7

control subjects had no difficulty with the task at all. In fact, every one of the control cases showed fewer than four signs, 96.2% of them showed one sign or less, and 68.3% of them gave no positive responses at all. Of the subjects with cerebral damage, 84.8% showed one or more signs, 65.2% showed two or more, and 39.2% gave four or more positive responses.

Table 10 provides conditional probabilities which permit an estimate of the percentage of correct classifications to be expected on a positive-sign frequency basis for brain-damaged versus non-brain-damaged subjects. On a combined basis (see note) these probabilities give the very striking value of 78.3% correct classifications.

Table 11 gives more detailed information regarding the frequencies of positive signs that occur above and below each cut-off point between positive sign frequencies for each group used in the study. These results show that use of a frequency cut-off for predicting brain-damage versus non-brain-damage in no instance gave a higher percentage of correct classification than 78.3%,

Table 10

Percentage of Each Sign Frequency Group Occurring in Each Criterion Group; Conditional Probability Estimate of Percentage of Correct Damage or Non-Damage Predictions.

CRITERION GROUPS	NUMBER OF POSITIVE SIGNS (Sign Frequency Groups)				
	0	1	2	3	4+
Controls	74.7	48.3	11.1	07.4	00.0
All-damage	25.3	51.7	88.9	92.6	100.0
Column Total	100.0	100.0	100.0	100.0	100.0
N of Ss in Col. as % of N (N=262)	36.3	22.9	06.9	10.3	23.7

Note – Calculation of conditional probability: (74.7 × 36.3) + (51.7 × 22.9) + (88.9 × 06.9) + (92.6 × 10.3) + (100.0 × 23.7) = 78.3%; an estimate of correct predictions of damaged and non-damaged cases. $X^2 = 109.39$, df = 4, $p < .001$.

the value that occurred between 0 and 1 positive signs. This result means that the best cut-off point occurs between 0 and 1 positive signs and this point appears to be the best criterion to use for a general classification of this type. It is also perfectly clear that while use of this criterion may affect general classification, it is hardly adequate to provide any degree of clinical understanding of the behavioral correlates of impaired brain functions in the individual subject. Thus, a considerably more detailed analysis should be followed.

Hypotheses two and three concerning laterality of cerebral damage and generality of cerebral damage, as shown by the Aphasia Screening Test, are evaluated by results presented in Table 12. The percentage of subjects in each group showing positive signs are listed in Table 12 and a set of Left cerebral indicators and Right cerebral indicators are shown. It may be noted that there are just more than twice as many left as right indicators, but the average number of responses per variable in the left indicator set was 32.6 and in the right indicator set was 30.3 over all of the subjects. While the Aphasia Screening Test may be weighted more heavily toward left than right cerebral damage in terms of the test content itself, the results suggest that when right cerebral damage is present positive test findings are about as frequent as with left cerebral damage. In summary terms, the group with left cerebral damage showed evidence of one or more left indicators in 91.5% of the subjects while only 17% of the subjects with left cerebral lesions showed positive results on the right cerebral indicators. In the group with right cerebral damage, 71.9% gave one or more positive responses to the right indicators but only 31.6% of them responded to left indicators. In the group with diffuse or generalized damage, 75.9% made one or more responses to left indicators and 55.6% of them responded to right indicators. The positive responses for control subjects were 23.1% for left indicators and 10.6% for right indicators.

The principal finding shown in Table 12, however, relates to the striking differences between the groups with left and right cerebral damage. Taking Dysnomia, for example, we find that 53% of the subjects with left cerebral damage showed evidence of this type of deficit on the Aphasia Screening Test whereas none (0%) of the group with right cerebral damage had this kind of difficulty. In fact, if the deficit related to verbal or language communicational skills there was practically no incidence of significant impairment in persons with right cerebral damage except for evidence of central dysarthria (ennunciatory skills). It should also be noted, however, that calculating difficulties occurred about four times as frequently with left cerebral lesions as with right.

In the group with right cerebral lesions, constructional dyspraxia stood out as being a very common type of difficulty. However, about 15% of subjects with left cerebral lesions also showed evidence of definite difficulty in copying simple spatial configurations. An analysis of these cases has indicated that most of them had lesions that fell in the posterior part of the left cerebral hemisphere, especially involving the posterior temporal area. Thus, instead of being confused by the occurrence of constructional dyspraxia in patients with left cerebral lesions, one may use the presence of constructional dyspraxia, in a patient with left cerebral damage, as an indication of posterior left cerebral involvement. Before being able to use this point of information in individual evaluation it is necessary still to have some criteria for deciding on the side of damage. In this respect, we observed that all patients with left cerebral lesions who showed evidence of constructional dyspraxia also demonstrated distinct evidence of pronounced language deficits of an aphasic type. Thus, if one finds clear evidence of aphasic difficulties, such indications take precedence in pointing toward left cerebral damage. Simultaneous evidence of constructional dyspraxia would suggest that the left cerebral damage is posterior in its area of involvement within the left cerebral hemisphere. We realize that details of this kind go beyond the interpretations that are possible based only on the results as shown in Table 12. It is perfectly clear, however, that a great deal of consistency exists in the correlation of lateralization of cerebral damage and the types of deficits that are shown.

Results in Table 12 represent some of the earlier definitive indications of differential functions of the two cerebral hemispheres. While there has been a great deal of more recent literature in this area, these results, published first in 1962, were the first to cover in a systematic manner a broad range of functions. Later

Table 11

Subject Frequency, Percentage of Each Criterion Group, and Percentage of Total Group Falling Above or Below Division Points Between Positive Sign Frequencies; Conditional Probabilities of Correct Damage and Non-Damage Predictions.

CRITERION GROUPS	MEASURE	POSITIVE SIGN FREQUENCY CUT-OFF POINTS							
		0/1+		0,1/2+		0,1,2/3+		0,1,2,3/4+	
Control	f	71	33	100	4	192	2	104	0
(N=104)	% Crit.	68.3	31.7	96.1	03.9	98.1	01.9	100.0	00.0
	% Total	27.1	12.6	38.2	01.5	38.9	00.8	39.7	00.0
Left Damage	f	3	35	9	38	15	32	18	29
(N=47)	% Crit.	06.4	74.5	19.1	80.9	31.9	68.1	38.3	61.7
	% Total	01.1	13.3	03.4	14.5	05.7	12.2	06.9	11.1
Right Damage	f	14	43	27	30	33	24	43	14
(N=57)	% Crit.	24.6	75.4	47.4	52.6	57.9	45.1	75.4	24.6
	% Total	05.3	16.4	10.3	11.4	12.6	09.2	16.4	05.3
Diff. Damage	f	7	47	19	35	23	31	35	19
(N=54)	% Crit.	13.0	87.0	35.6	64.8	42.6	57.4	64.8	35.2
	% Total	02.7	17.9	07.2	13.4	08.8	11.8	13.4	07.2
All-Damage	f	24	134	55	103	71	87	96	62
(N=158)	% Crit.	15.2	84.8	34.8	65.2	44.9	55.1	60.8	39.2
	% Total	09.2	51.1	21.0	39.3	27.1	33.2	36.6	23.7
Total	f	95	167	155	107	173	89	200	62
(N=262)	% Total	36.3	63.7	59.2	40.8	66.0	34.0	76.3	23.7
		CELL PROPORTION OF COLUMN TOTAL							
Controls		.747	.198	.645	.037	.590	.022	.520	.000
All-damage		.253	.802	.355	.963	.410	.978	.480	1.00
Conditional p*		.783		.775		.722		.634	
X^{2}**		76.42		97.72		78.92		56.67	

*Conditional probability was calculated as follows: 0/1 + Positive Sign: (.747 × .363) + (.802 × .637) = .783; 0,1/2 + Positive Sign: (.645 × .592) + (.963 × .408) = .775; 0,1,2/3 + Positive Sign: (.590 × .660) + (.978 × .340) = .722; 0,1,2,3/4 + Positive Sign: (.520 × .763) + (1.00 × .237) = .634.
**$p < .001$, df=1.

Table 12

Percentage of Each Criterion Group Showing a Positive Sign for Each Aphasia Test Variable; Left and Right Indicators Separated and Listed by Rank – Order of Percentage Response in Appropriate Group; Over-All Frequencies of Positive Signs for Each Variable, Last Column.

TEST VARIABLE; LEFT INDICATOR	CRITERION GROUPS					TOT.	OVER-ALL
	Left	Right	Diffuse	Control	All-damage		f
Dyscalculia	55.32	14.04	20.37	00.00	28.48	17.18	45
Central Dysarthria	55.32	10.53	37.04	08.65	32.91	23.28	63
Dysnomia	53.19	00.00	16.67	00.96	21.52	13.36	35
Dysgraphia	51.06	01.75	25.93	00.00	24.68	14.89	40
Spelling Dyspraxia	48.94	05.26	16.67	06.73	22.15	16.03	42
Dyslexia	46.81	00.00	20.37	00.00	20.89	12.60	34
Right-Left Disorientation	42.55	05.26	29.63	09.62	24.68	18.70	49
Right Finger Dysgnosia	36.17	01.75	25.93	00.96	20.25	12.60	34
Right Dysstereognosis	29.79	01.75	09.26	00.00	12.66	07.63	19
Visual Letter Dysgnosia	25.53	00.00	07.41	00.00	10.13	06.11	17
Right Tactile Imperception	14.89	00.00	18.52	00.00	10.76	06.49	17
Auditory Verbal Dysgnosia	12.77	00.00	07.41	00.00	06.33	03.82	10
Visual Number Dysgnosia	10.64	00.00	01.85	00.00	03.80	02.29	6*
TEST VARIABLE; RIGHT INDICATOR	**Left**	**Right**	**Diffuse**	**Control**	**All-damage**	**TOT.**	**OVER-ALL f**
Construction Dyspraxia	14.89	61.40	44.44	07.69	41.77	28.24	75
Left Dysstereognosis	02.13	29.82	11.11	00.00	15.19	09.16	25
Left Finger Dysgnosia	00.00	28.07	16.67	02.88	15.82	10.67	28
Left Tactile Imperception	02.13	21.05	14.81	00.00	13.29	08.02	21
Left Visual Imperception	02.13	15.79	07.41	00.00	08.86	05.34	14
Left Auditory Imperception	02.13	14.04	18.52	00.00	12.03	07.25	19
AVERAGE % RESPONSE OF GROUPS TO SETS OF VARIABLES							
Left Indicators	37.11	03.10	18.23	02.07	18.40	11.92	
Right Indicators	03.90	28.36	18.83	01.76	17.83	11.45	
Total Set	26.60	11.08	18.42	01.97	18.22	11.77	

*Variables showing f < 10: Visual Number Dysgnosia, Body Dysgnosia, Right Auditory Imperception, Right Visual Imperception, Paragrammatism, Color Dysgnosia, Number Dyspraxia and Ideo-kinetic Dyspraxia. Number Dysgnosia (f=6) is included in some calculations of this study.

studies, based on persons with surgical section of commissural fibers, also pointed toward differential functions of the two cerebral hemispheres, but the results probably in general were not quite as consistent as those shown in Table 12. The reason for the very striking differences in groups with left and right cerebral lesions, as shown in Table 12, probably relates to the fact that our subjects had the advantage of normal growth and development of brain functions and sustained cerebral damage only after having reached physical maturity. Such a conclusion cannot be consistently claimed in the split-brain human studies nor in studies of persons with, for example, temporal lobe epilepsy or focal epileptogenic lesions of the frontal lobes. In all of these groups it is entirely likely that at least some of the subjects included in reported studies have had lesions that date back to early childhood if not infancy. In other words, many studies have reported results of the organization of brain function that were influenced by inclusion of subjects with damage sustained early in life. There is probably general agreement that early damage may result in a somewhat different organization of brain-behavior relationships, even with the possibility of the right cerebral hemisphere being involved in subserving language functions. The subjects represented in Table 12, however, were persons who had developed normally and had sustained cerebral damage only after completion of physical growth and development. Thus, our findings suggest that when normal growth and development of brain functions is possible, the left cerebral hemisphere is very heavily involved in language and related verbal symbolic functions, whereas the right cerebral hemisphere has little if any role to play in this regard. In fact, the data represented in Table 12 appear to permit generalization to *normal* adult brain functions. Young children who sustain brain damage have never had the advantage of normal brains, in a biological sense, with which to develop their abilities whereas persons who have not sustained brain damage presumably have basically a normal biological potential. Thus, results on the kinds of patients that were studied by Wheeler and Reitan (1962) would appear to be more representative of how the brain is organized among normal individuals than might be true for persons who had sustained damage early in life.

Additional analyses have been carried out with respect to results obtained on the Aphasia Screening Test. Wheeler (1963) used the data recorded above for the same 262 subjects and subjected them to an analysis by discriminant functions. He compared the power of this analysis with the discriminant ability reported in the previous study (Wheeler and Reitan, 1962) and a discriminant function analysis based on 23 variables from the Halstead-Reitan Battery (Wheeler and Reitan, 1963). Linear discriminant function analysis of the three groups with cerebral damage (left, right, and generalized) together with the control group, arranged in seven two-way comparisons, gave an overall percentage of correct prediction that ranged between 77.5% and 93.4%. Of course, cross-validation of such a study is necessary and one might expect the values to diminish by ten to twenty percentage points. Wheeler (1963) also devised a method for classifying each subject to a single one of these four neurological categories using four mutually exclusive and exhaustive, non-linear rules. The results of application of this four-rule system were essentially similar to the results achieved with linear discriminant function analysis. Of special interest was the fact that the correctness of classification achieved from the aphasia test alone was essentially similar to that achieved when using 23 variables from the Halstead-Reitan Battery. Of course, this result does not indicate that the neuropsychological analysis possible from the aphasia examination is comparable to that derived from the Halstead-Reitan Battery, but the results do suggest that the Aphasia Screening Test covers a sufficiently broad range of brain-related variables and that the results obtained permit a high level of accuracy with regard to classifying subjects into left, right, generalized, or control groups. Again, the reader must be reminded that interpretation of a subject's performances on the Aphasia Screening Test requires experience and, if the person who reviews the test results is unfamiliar with the types of deficits associated with cerebral damage, the results will be essentially meaningless. In this sense it is especially important that the reader who may not have familiarity with the manifestations of cerebral damage on the Aphasia Screening Test study the cases presented in this report repeatedly and in careful detail.

CHAPTER 7

Results for Individual Patients

The following section of this manual presents results for 25 adult patients that illustrate the kinds of deficits that occur on the Aphasia Screening Test and the Sensory-perceptual Examination. All of these patients, as will be noted, have diagnosed diseases or injuries involving the brain. Cases were selected deliberately to demonstrate positive findings and thus they present deficits more commonly than is customarily seen in persons with cerebral disease more generally considered. We have deliberately selected cases that have previously been used in various study manuals and have included the complete test results from the Halstead-Reitan Neuropsychological Test Battery, so the reader who has studied these cases elsewhere, and has these manuals available, will be able to compare the types of conclusions that can be drawn from the Aphasia Screening Test and the Sensory-perceptual Examination alone, as contrasted with the complete neuropsychological examination. As was noted in the section on research results, it seems that the relatively simple items included in the Aphasia Screening Test, in spite of their simple nature, provide nearly as accurate a basis for assigning subjects to a control group or groups with right, left, or generalized cerebral damage as does the entire test battery (Wheeler and Reitan, 1962; Wheeler, 1963). However, there is much more involved in neuropsychological testing than mere identification and localization of structural brain lesions. Probably the majority of persons with cerebral disease or damage do not, in fact, have focal lesions. More pointedly, neuropsychological examination is rarely needed for purposes of neurological diagnosis. Neurologists, neurosurgeons, neuroradiologists, and others are really quite expert in establishing neurological diagnoses without the aid of neuropsychological testing. The principal contribution of neuropsychological testing concerns the information that may be gained regarding a domain of brain-related evidence that is not contained in electroencephalographic tracings, x-rays, etc., namely, data concerned with the adaptive skills and abilities that represent higher brain functions. Information of this type must be obtained to understand the most important aspects of brain functions and to take appropriate steps toward remediation, retraining of brain functions, and rehabilitation. Most persons with brain disease or damage do not have strictly focal lesions but, instead, have generalized or multi-focal lesions that frequently are relatively stabilized (or, at most, slowly progressive) in a biological sense. Thus, it must be pointed out that the rather simple procedures involved in the Aphasia Screening Test and the Sensory-perceptual Examination are quite useful, when positive results are obtained, for drawing conclusions about the biological condition of the brain but do not constitute, in and of themselves, an adequate neuropsychological examination as far as higher-level aspects of brain functions are concerned. One will note in studying the complete set of test results for these patients (if one has the available manuals) that the rest of the test battery provides information regarding highly significant aspects of behavioral correlates of brain functions including, in comparison with the Aphasia Screening Test and Sensory-perceptual Examination, a more detailed assessment of input (sensory-perceptual or receptive) and output (motor or expressive) adaptive abilities, a more extensive evaluation of verbal abilities, a more complete assessment of visuo-spatial problem-solving skills, measures of alertness and ability to maintain concentrated attention to tasks, various memory measures, and probably most importantly, measures of abstraction, concept formation, logical analysis, and reasoning. Thus, in spite of the usefulness of the findings to be shown in the following 25 cases, it is important to recognize that a comprehensive neuropsychological examination is necessary to understand more fully the behavioral correlates of brain functions for the individual patient.

We should again mention that in evaluating the performances of these 25 patients, we have concentrated on identification and description of deficits related to impaired brain functions as shown in results of performances using a standard testing procedure rather than adopting a heavy dependence upon the use of specific terminology. We have felt first of all that selection of an appellation (naming something) does little implicitly to clarify the nature of the deficit. Secondly, we take seriously the problem in intra-individual variability of responses noted by Head and many other serious students of aphasia (see Chapter 1). While some degree of classification of defective responses is necessary, a review of Chapter 5 should be sufficient to acquaint the reader with the necessary terminology. Our principal purpose will be to identify brain-related response abnormalities and to comment on their significance with regard to brain pathology.

A word of information is necessary with respect to how the data were recorded for the individual patients. Familiarity with the test will make clear the relevance of the content of the recording form. However, we should note that even with impaired patients many responses can be given quite satisfactorily. Thus, when no entry occurs in a particular space, the reader can assume that the subject's response was within normal limits. We have made entries when the subject's response was open to question or was abnormal. No entry necessarily has been made for items that can be evaluated by reference to the subject's written or non-verbal responses. As the reader is aware, for example, the subject is required to copy the shapes of several figures. Customarily no entry has been made for these items because the drawings have been reproduced and the reader may inspect and evaluate the actual performances. We have not included any examples of entirely normal results because such instances would be represented by blank entries. As noted in the presentation of research findings, nearly all normal subjects show normal results on these relatively simple tasks. Recent research has also shown that aging effects, for neurologically normal older persons, are minimal on these tasks. Lorin Meyerink has completed a doctoral dissertation entitled, "Intellectual Functioning: The Nature and Pattern of Change with Aging," in which he evaluated groups of normal subjects numbering 25 in each instance, that fell in each decade from the 20's through the 60's. Results on the Aphasia Screening Test and the Sensory-perceptual Examination contributed little to the variance because the older as well as younger subjects were able to perform these simple tasks essentially without difficulty. Of course, all of the subjects in this part of Meyerink's study had been examined neurologically and were well within normal limits even though more than half of the subjects had significant emotional problems of adjustment or diagnosed medical illnesses that did not involve the nervous system. We should note, however, that aging is not entirely without some kind of influence on even these simple kinds of performances. Deficits, in association with pathological involvement of the brain, do appear clinically to be somewhat accentuated in older age groups.

The 25 cases to be presented range from those with serious to relatively mild deficits. It is important to be able to recognize *definite abnormalities* in performances even though they are relatively mild. In other words, an abnormal or pathological performance is not necessarily a seriously defective performance. Examples of this kind will be shown. Finally, one cannot hope to cover all variations of responses in a sample of 25 subjects. It will be necessary for the reader to gain additional experience, even though careful and detailed study of the 25 cases should provide a good start in developing clinical competence.

In each case there are two important steps. First, one must be able to identify those aspects of the patient's performances that represent brain damage or dysfunction as contrasted with poor or deficient performances that may stem from many other influences. If brain-dependent deficits are not correctly identified, interpretation of the findings in a neuropsychological context will be misleading. Secondly, the significance of brain-related deficits must be understood with relation to the question of brain dysfunction or damage for the individual subject. In this respect the neuropsychologist must raise questions concerning the meaning of the deficits with respect to brain impairment. These questions may concern biological impairment of brain functions (Is brain damage present?); regional localization of damage (Where is the lesion?); and status of the lesion (Has significant cerebral damage occurred recently?). The neuropsychologist should also be concerned as to whether the deficits imply the presence of a progressive condition of immediate medical significance or point toward a relatively stabilized condition of the brain.

In each of the following cases we will focus first upon the data (identification of brain-related deficits) and then upon their interpretation (the significance of the deficits). The cases begin with persons who have intrinsic brain tumors.

INTRINSIC BRAIN TUMORS

REITAN-INDIANA APHASIA SCREENING TEST

Form for Adults and Older Children

Name: J.A. Age: 54 Date: ______ Examiner: ______

Copy SQUARE	Repeat TRIANGLE "Triango."
Name SQUARE	Repeat MASSACHUSETTS "Massaschusses"
Spell SQUARE "S-square"(pause)"S-W-I-W-L-E" (pause)"Or A-R-E. Square, S-R-I-I-E-R."	Repeat METHODIST EPISCOPAL "Methodis mesical pesical"
Copy CROSS	Write SQUARE Verbalized, "S-Q-U-A." (Pause) "S-Q-U-A-S-E."
Name CROSS "Square (pause) 4-way side (pause) I can't say it."	Read SEVEN "S-S-U-E (pause) wait, S-E-V-E-N (pause) seven, seven."
Spell CROSS "Cross-cross-k-cross-s-let's see. Cross (pause) this is a cross."(Points)	Repeat SEVEN
Copy TRIANGLE	Repeat/Explain HE SHOUTED THE WARNING.Repeated "He shouteth the waining." Explained:"Show something that you're doing when you're not doing it."
Name TRIANGLE "I know what it is but I can't say it; same as number 1 (pause) hector."	Write HE SHOUTED THE WARNING.
Spell TRIANGLE "Triangle, no, go to the left and this way once and back that way. T-R-I, T-R-I, T-R-A-N-E, triangle, angle, B-A-L-G-E-R."	Compute 85 - 27 = Verbalized "27" as he wrote down the problem. Made errors in arithmetic (see).
Name BABY "Boy, isn't it? Little boy."	Compute 17 X 3 = Copied and worked problem. Then, examiner gave 12x5. Patient wrote and worked problem but verbalized, "5x13 (pause) 5 threes is 9 and, that is 3x15?"
Write CLOCK Verbalized "Watch?" Kept verbalizing, "W-A-G-E-S, that don't sound right."Examiner finally emphasized he write his response.	Name KEY
Name FORK "A war-a-a-watch, no (pause) waste, not a waste."	Demonstrate use of KEY
Read 7 SIX 2	Draw KEY Patient said, "Very poorly done."
Read MGW	Read PLACE LEFT HAND TO RIGHT EAR. "Place left land to right edge."
Reading I "See the black dock-dock-D-O-G-dark."	Place LEFT HAND TO RIGHT EAR Patient slow to understand. Instructions repeated often.
Reading II "Let's see; he is a friend, hm, I can't get that one, but it's a family (points to famous), this is show (points to show)." "I can't see anymore."	Place LEFT HAND TO LEFT ELBOW "I can't, other people might."

REITAN-KLØVE SENSORY-PERCEPTUAL EXAMINATION

(Instance indicated where stimulus was not perceived or was incorrectly perceived.)

TACTILE:

RH					LH					Both: RH					LH					
RH					LF					Both: RH					LF					
LH					RF					LH					RF					

AUDITORY:

RE			X		LE					Both: RE					LE				

VISUAL:

	X	X	X	X						Both:										– (Above eye level)
RV	X	X	X	X	LV					RV					LV					– (Eye level)
	X	X	X	X																– (Below eye level)

TACTILE FINGER RECOGNITION:

Right:	1					2	3	3			3	2				4	2		3		5	3	4	4	3	9 / 20
Left:	1					2				4	3			2		4	2	2	2	3	5	1	1			8 / 20

COMMENTS: Often responded with wrong word such as "face, right, left, and hand."

FINGER-TIP NUMBER WRITING PERCEPTION:

	4	6	3	5	3	5	4	6	6	5	4	3	5	4	6	3	6	3	5	4	
Right:		5																			1 / 20
Left:	5																				1 / 20

COMMENTS:

VISUAL FIELDS:

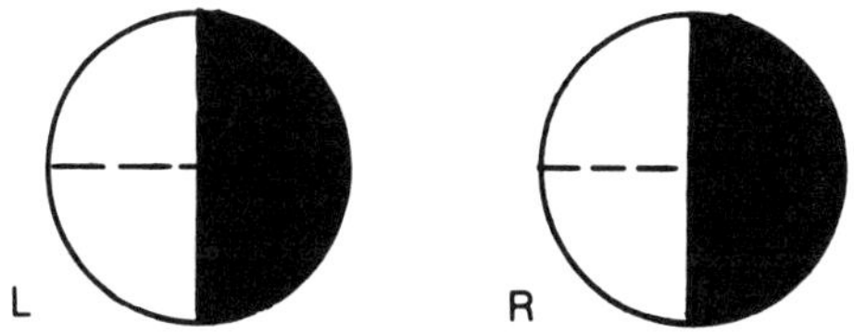

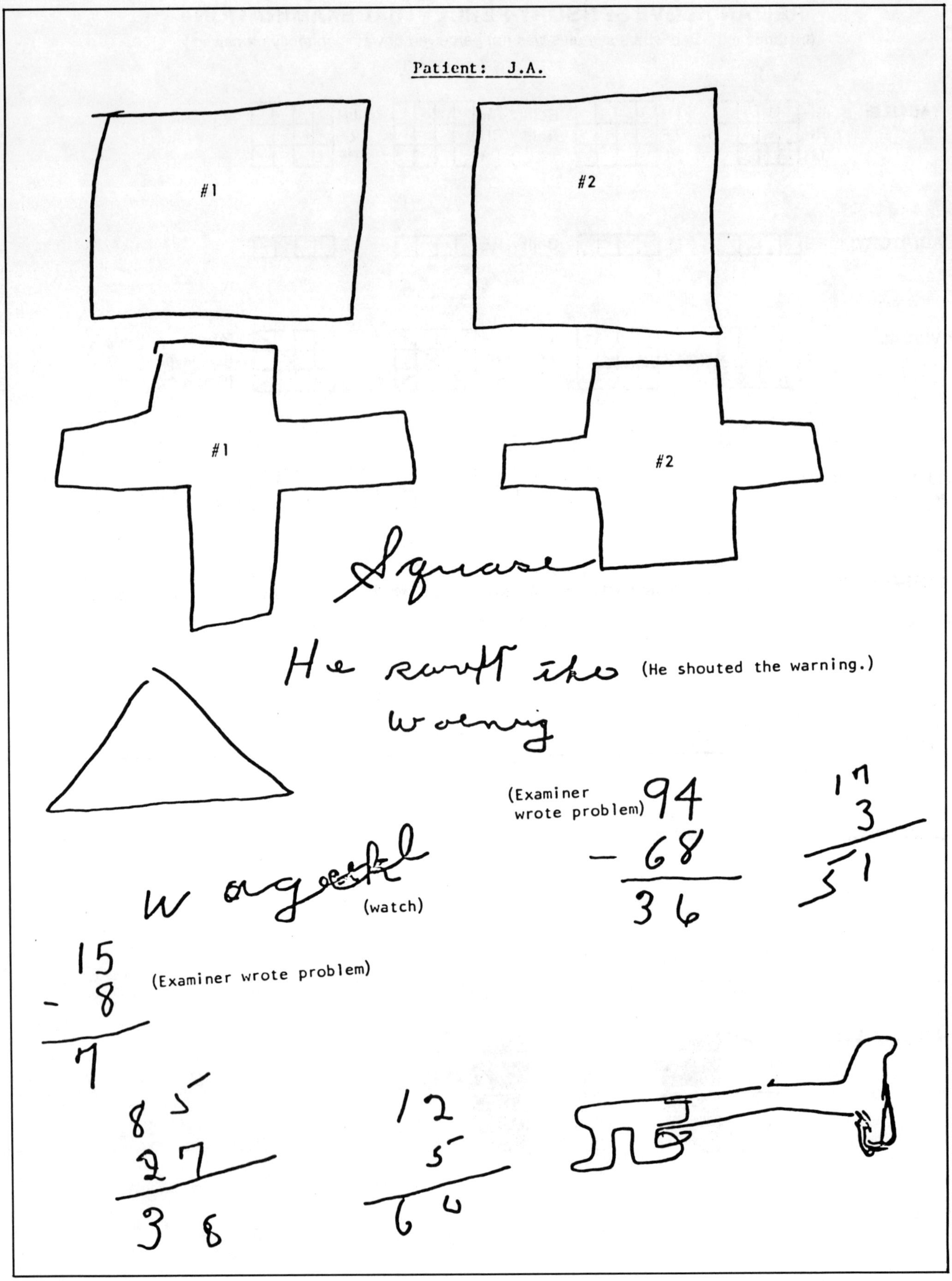
Patient: J.A.
#1
#2
#1
#2
(He shouted the warning.)
(Examiner wrote problem)
(watch)
(Examiner wrote problem)

J.A. – A 54-year-old right-handed male bartender with a twelfth grade education.

Identification of brain-related deficits:

For purposes of convenience we will review the entries on the form for the Aphasia Screening Test initially, then refer to the page that shows the patient's drawings, writings, and calculations, and finally review the results of the Sensory-perceptual Examination.

Reference to the form for the Aphasia Screening Test immediately indicates that the patient had a number of problems. If the performances had been done correctly and without difficulty, the spaces on the form would have been blank. The first space to be considered, involved in naming the square, was blank, and we can assume from this that the patient had no difficulty in naming this object. However, when asked to spell the name, he had clear difficulty. He began with "s," then said the word "square," and went on to try to identify individual letters that were appropriate. It was apparent that he was able to begin with "s," but beyond that the letters made little sense and did not relate to the phonic structure of the word. As is not uncommon in persons who have previously known how to spell the word in question, this man was able at one point to name the last three letters. Then he said the word again and began to try to spell it a final time, but again his effort represented confusion and complete deviation from phonic correspondence. This is a very typical example of serious spelling dyspraxia.

The patient demonstrated an obvious dysnomia in his attempt to name the cross. First he called it a square, then said, "four-way side," and finally said that he was unable to give the name. It is not uncommon for a person with serious aphasia to show perseveration in the language area. Thus, the patient first gave the word "square," which was the correct identification of the previous item. Since he was not able to name the cross, the examiner told him the name in accordance with standard instructions. He was then requested to spell that word. He began by repeating the word two times, then inserting the letter "k," saying the word again, saying the letter "s," and not being able to make further progress in spelling. Again, we have a typical example of spelling dyspraxia.

When asked to name the triangle the patient gave a response very typical of aphasic patients. He indicated that he knew what the object was, and in all probability this was quite true. Nevertheless, he said that he was not able to say the word. Aphasic patients frequently say that they know what the object is but can't get the word out. Sometimes a word or sound is mentioned that may possibly have some relation to the actual name of the object. In this case the subject said, "Hector." While it is not possible to relate this word very easily to "triangle," there might in fact actually be some such relationship.

When asked to spell the word "triangle," the patient said the word, made some verbal comments that may relate to the procedure in drawing the figure, began to try to spell and actually named the first three letters, but finally became completely confused with respect to the spelling.

In attempting to name the picture of the baby, the patient was fairly close but instead of calling the picture a baby called it a boy. It is not uncommon among aphasic patients for them to come fairly close to the word required but actually not be quite accurate.

On the next item the patient was asked not to say anything aloud but instead merely to write the name of the figure that he observed. However, he did not follow these instructions. While the picture obviously is one of a clock, the patient said "Watch?" He kept verbalizing the word, tried to spell it but did so incorrectly, and realized that his spelling was not accurate. As will be noted when we refer to the patient's writings and drawings, he was quite confused in his attempt to write a name for the object, although in all probability he was attempting to write "watch." It is sometimes difficult to differentiate between spelling dyspraxia and dysgraphia, because if a person does not know the correct letters he ends up with quite a confused attempt at writing. We tend to differentiate between the two by referring to incorrect letter sequences as spelling dyspraxia and to failure in forming letters correctly as evidence of dysgraphia. Such examples will be identified later in this person's responses on the Aphasia Screening Test.

When shown a picture of a fork and asked to name it, the patient perseverated with regard to the previous item. He showed evidence of a clear naming deficit, in this instance not being able to say "watch" correctly in his initial attempt. However, the object (fork) did not call for this word, and this probably was a basis for the patient's difficulty in actually giving the name. Thus, while he was able to say "watch" correctly when looking at a clock, he perseverated in an attempt to say the same word when looking at a fork but, with a fork as a visual stimulus, was not able to state the word correctly. Finally, he was able to identify the object only as a "waste."

On the next item, reading 7 SIX 2, the patient had no difficulty. Many aphasic persons do have special difficulties in reading this item. In fact, this has turned out to be a very fortunate item for inclusion in the test. It is not uncommon for patients with language difficulties to fail to recognize that SIX represents a number just as do the 7 and 2. In this case, however, the patient had no difficulty. He also was quite able to read the letters MGW.

On the next item, however, when he was required to read a simple sentence, the patient demonstrated a distinct deficit in dealing with symbolic material. It often is difficult to differentiate between naming problems (dysnomia) and reading deficits (dyslexia). In this case the patient became confused in reading the word "dog." At first he called it a "dock," spelled the letters individually, and finally said "dark." In this instance it seems likely that the patient actually realized that the word was "dog," and he may well have been demonstrating a naming deficit rather than a problem in reading. On the next reading item, however, the patient demonstrated distinct difficulties. On this item, he was asked to read the sentence, "He is a friendly animal, a famous winner of dog shows." The patient's response in this instance, particularly including his admission that he was not able to understand the sentence, probably constitutes evidence of definite dyslexia. Finally, his statement, "I can't see anymore" again represents a dysphasic admission of confusion with respect to reading the item.

The next three items are ones in which the patient was requested to repeat the words triangle, Massachusetts, and Methodist Episcopal. The first response of this man was probably within normal limits. It is not uncommon for many normal subjects to finish the word "triangle" with an "o" sound at the end. The patient's response to Massachusetts also was nearly within normal limits. However, when a patient adds a sound, transposes sounds, or omits sounds, we interpret the results as evidence of central dysarthria. Cases of central dysarthria are frequently associated with damage to the left cerebral hemisphere. Peripheral dysarthria, which is represented only by slurring of the sounds involved, occurs among many persons, especially including those with relatively limited educational background and verbal experience. Thus, slurring of the sounds does not constitute a brain-related type of deficit. In this instance, however, the patient added an "s" sound in the middle of the word just before the "ch" sound. This is abnormal and unusual and probably a manifestation of mild central dysarthria. On the next item the patient had more obvious difficulty. Omitting the "t" sound from "Methodist" is not particularly unusual. However, the difficulties encountered by the patient from this point on clearly represented more than slurring of the sounds involved. In fact, he demonstrated a tendency toward mixing the sounds of the two words ("mesical"). This example is quite typical of central dysarthria and occurs in persons with left cerebral damage.

On the next item, when the patient was asked to write printed letters representing the word "square," he proceeded to attempt to verbalize the letters. Even though the stimulus material was directly in front of him on the stimulus card, he still had difficulty and made a mistake by substituting an "s" for an "r." We will inspect his writing of the word "square" when we examine his written performances.

When the patient was asked to read the word "seven" he had apparent difficulty and began by attempting to identify the individual letters. Finally, he responded correctly. The neuropsychologist might question whether the patient was demonstrating a reading difficulty (dyslexia) or a naming difficulty (dysnomia). Since he began with an attempt to identify individual letters rather than a name word, it is likely that his basic problem was one of dyslexia. However, prior results have already indicated that both of these difficulties were present. As indicated by the blank space for the next item, the patient was able to repeat "seven" correctly after the examiner.

The next item is particularly important. The patient was asked to repeat the sentence, "He shouted the warning." The patient responded, "He shouteth the waining." If this difficulty could be judged to be based on failure to understand the symbolic meaning of the sentence, the results would show evidence of auditory verbal dysgnosia and would tend to implicate the posterior part of the left cerebral hemisphere, especially involving the posterior left temporal area. In this case, however, it is difficult to know whether a naming deficit (dysnomia) was responsible for the problem experienced by the patient or whether it may have been an auditory receptive deficit (auditory verbal dysgnosia). A naming deficit (dysnomia) is more commonly associated with anterior temporal and posterior-inferior frontal involvement, and a difficulty in understanding the symbolic significance through the auditory avenue (auditory verbal dysgnosia) is more commonly associated with posterior involvement. Next, the patient was asked to explain the meaning of the sentence. He was not able to respond to this request in any meaningful way. Failure of response, as contrasted with a defective response, is difficult to interpret. If the patient had given a response that demonstrated failure of understanding and confusion in terms of understanding the meaning of the sentence, we would have had positive evidence of auditory verbal dysgnosia. However, an absence of any kind of response fails to yield positive evidence for interpretation. Since the aphasia examination is based on elicitation of deficits in performance, as contrasted with absence of performance, it is most important that the examiner try to elicit some type of response even though the patient has obvious difficulties.

The patient's next effort, in attempting to write the sentence mentioned above, will be considered when we look at the patient's written responses as will his attempts to do simple computations.

The patient was able to name the key, demonstrate its use, and made an attempt at drawing the figure. Drawing the figure is related to the status of the right cerebral hemisphere and will be considered when we evaluate the patient's written responses.

The patient's reading difficulties were again clearly demonstrated on the next item. Instead of reading, "Place left hand to right ear," he read, "Place left land to right edge." It is possible that confusion between the word "hand" and the verbalization of "land" may have represented something of a naming deficit. However, it is quite likely that confusion of "ear" and "edge" represented a clear deficiency in understanding the meaning of written language. Thus, it seems likely that the response in this instance does demonstrate evidence of dyslexia.

The next item is particularly important inasmuch as it probably demonstrates the presence of auditory verbal dysgnosia. The subject was asked to place his left hand to his right ear. He was slow to do so, instructions had to be repeated often, and it was clear that the patient had difficulty understanding this verbal communication. Such difficulty constitutes a basis for concluding that the patient had evidence of impairment in understanding incoming (auditory) verbal symbols and, as stated above, this type of deficit is frequently associated with posterior left temporal lobe damage. On the final item the patient was able to respond adequately.

The patient's drawing and writing, together with arithmetical computations, are demonstrated on the next two pages. The first attempt in drawing the square resulted in something of a rectangle. This is not uncommon among many persons. The second attempt came closer to achieving sides of equal length and probably was a satisfactory reproduction of the square. However, the patient had some clear difficulty in attempting to draw the cross. The first attempt at drawing the cross represents a rather typical example of mild constructional dyspraxia. The patient failed to achieve symmetry with respect to the extensions of the figure. The right side of the figure is not grossly deficient except for the length of the upper extremity. However, the left side of the figure lost a great deal of symmetry and is typical of persons with cerebral damage. The second attempt in drawing the figure comes much closer to the types of performances shown by persons with normal brains, even though the lateral extremities are not nearly as wide as the upper and lower extensions of the figure. It is not particularly uncommon among normals to find this kind of deviation, with symmetry being maintained only for the opposing extremities. Thus, it is interesting to note that the first attempt at drawing the cross was a "brain-damaged" attempt whereas the second attempt probably could not be interpreted in this way with confidence. The patient failed to close his drawing of the triangle, but this is not uncommon among many persons with normal brain functions. Thus, the drawing of the triangle must be considered within normal limits. Moving on to the next page and considering the drawing of the key, the patient showed clear deficits. He became confused with respect to the lines needed to effect the spatial configuration. Thus, on the basis of the first cross and the drawing of the key, we would have to conclude that this man showed evidence of mild constructional dyspraxia. A question still exists, however, as to whether these deficits may be associated with (1) aphasic difficulties or with (2) damage of the right cerebral hemisphere.

Returning to the first page, the patient had some difficulty in forming the "r" in his writing of the word "square." This kind of deviation from normality probably is a manifestation of left cerebral dysfunction. However, the patient showed this type of difficulty much more clearly when required to write from dictation. His attempts to write, "He shouted the warning" and the word "watch" showed serious difficulties. He was not able to form the letters properly for the words "shouted," "warning," or "watch." This is a typical example of dysgraphia. It was not just a matter of spelling deficiency but, instead, the patient had actual difficulty in forming the appropriate letters. Further, one can tell from the writing of "square," "He," and "the" that the patient has had some prior experience in writing and in the past had learned to write. In comparing what the patient was able to do correctly with his defective performances, the neuropsychologist can draw the judgment quite confidently that there has been some distinct impairment in the patient's ability to form letters to represent words (dysgraphia).

The patient showed evidence of calculating deficiencies (dyscalculia) in his attempts to solve simple arithmetic problems. His efforts show that he has had some prior arithmetical ability, but he became seriously confused on the problem 85 − 27 = ____. The examiner wrote additional problems for the patient. On 94 − 68, the patient made a mistake only in failing to borrow. This kind of mistake sometimes occurs among persons with poor educational backgrounds, but we would estimate in this instance that it probably represents a deficit rather than a failure of prior acquisition. On the next page the patient attempted multiplication and performed satisfactorily. This finding, in its own right, reinforces the impression that the patient has had some adequate training in simple arithmetical procedures and should have been able to perform better on the simple subtraction problems. While dyscalculia is not strictly a left hemisphere manifestation, it occurs approximately four times as frequently with left as compared with right cerebral lesions.

This completes a review of the actual performances of this subject on the Aphasia test. The interpretation and significance of these findings will be considered in the evaulation of the results for J.A.

The results on the Sensory-perceptual Examination are often particularly helpful in supplementing the findings of the Aphasia test. J.A. did not show any deficits in his responses to either unilateral or double simultaneous tactile stimulation. In other words, he responded correctly in each instance. While findings of this kind may occur even in some persons who have parietal lobe involvement, the negative results tend to be a favorable sign in this regard. With respect to auditory stimulation, the patient made one mistake in identifying a unilateral stimulus. On the third trial using the right ear alone, the patient responded that the stimulus had been given on the left side. This is an unusual type of mistake, but an isolated error, particularly when it occurs with unilateral stimulation, cannot be given much significance. Thus, we are essentially in a position of having to conclude that results with unilateral and bilateral simultaneous auditory stimulation also were essentially within the normal range. However, with visual stimulation the patient was not able to respond toward his right side. In fact, in confrontation testing of the visual fields, the patient showed evidence of a right homonymous hemianopsia, failing to be able to respond with either eye toward the right side. Thus, administration of the test for double simultaneous visual stimulation was definitely precluded.

In evaluating tactile finger recognition, the patient made errors on both sides. Nine errors occurred on the right hand and eight erors occurred on the left hand. However, two of the eight errors on the left hand were on the fifth finger and the patient identified these trials as the first finger. It is likely that this was a confusion in offering a response rather than a tactile-perceptual deficit (a *response* problem representing some degree of confusion rather than a *perceptual* deficit). Thus, a careful analysis of the errors would suggest that the patient did have somewhat more perceptual difficulty on the right hand than the left hand. Nevertheless, bilateral deficits clearly were present. It is necessary, in an instance of this kind, to give further attention to whether the errors occurred as a result of tactile-perceptual difficulties or whether a reporting difficulty was present. This patient showed a tendency to have difficulty in making appropriate responses, confusing his intended response with words such as "face, right, left, and hand." This finding exemplifies the difficulty that sometimes occurs in reaching a conclusion as to whether the deficit represents a loss in input, output, or central processing. It is possible that the output (response) requirement was sufficiently difficult for this man that the errors, at least in some instances, may have been attributable to this factor. A comparison of results obtained on various types of testing procedures sometimes helps to answer this question. In finger-tip number writing perception the patient made only one mistake on each hand. Customarily, a greater requirement in concentration and central processing characterizes performances on finger-tip number writing perception than on tactile finger recognition. Since the patient was able to respond correctly in 19 of 20 items on each hand in finger-tip number writing perception, we must presume that he had the basic capabilities to report which fingers were touched. Thus, there does seem to be an element of confusion in tactile finger recognition involving the left hand as well as the right hand. Since more errors usually occur in the test of finger-tip number writing perception than tactile finger recognition, the errors in tactile finger recognition with the left hand, in fact, take on some added significance as an indicator of impaired brain functions. This will be a factor that must be considered with respect to the interpretation of the possibility that the right cerebral hemisphere is damaged in addition to the left.

Interpretation of the results for the Aphasia Screening Test and the Sensory-perceptual Examination for J.A.

A review of the deficits shown by this man clearly implicate the left cerebral hemisphere. However, a question exists as to whether the lesion may involve the right cerebral hemisphere as well. The possible right cerebral indicators include the drawing of the first cross, the drawing of the key, and the evidence of tactile finger recognition deficits on the left hand. The preponderance of evidence, however, involves aphasic disorders and difficulties on the right side of the body.

The patient shows many instances of organic language deficits including dysnomia, spelling dyspraxia, dysgraphia, dyslexia, central dysarthria, auditory verbal dysgnosia, and mild dyscalculia. Perhaps the most reliable indicator of left cerebral damage on the sensory-perceptual examination was the right homonymous visual field loss. A right homonymous hemianopsia definitely implicates the geniculostriate pathway in the left cerebral hemisphere. A second factor was present in that tactile finger recognition difficulties (finger dysgnosia) appeared to be a little more prominent on the right than the left hand. In the main, however, the results from the sensory-perceptual examination tended to downgrade an inference regarding parietal lobe involvement. It would be possible, considering the pronounced evidence of dysphasia and definitely lesser tactile-perceptual losses, that the lesion was principally located in the left temporal lobe and included some aspects of the adjacent (inferior) left parietal lobe. Thus, the results of the Sensory-perceptual Examination, in this instance, were particularly useful in limiting the location of the lesion principally to the left temporal lobe.

Both expressive and receptive aphasic deficits were present. The patient had clear naming problems as well as spelling problems but also had difficulties in reading and in auditory perception of verbal communication. In my experience the one type of receptive difficulty that is particularly significant in pointing to involvement of the posterior part of the language area is the occurrence of auditory verbal dysgnosia. Dyslexia may occur with lesions in many areas, even though it is dependent upon visual input of language material. Failure to be able to understand the significance of verbal communication through the auditory avenue, however, when it is rather prominently displayed by the subject and goes beyond an interpretation related to possible general confusion, almost certainly implicates the posterior part of the left cerebral hemisphere and probably particularly the posterior temporal area. Thus, the clear evidence of auditory verbal dysgnosia as shown by this patient suggests that the lesion does extend fairly far posteriorly. The extensive nature of the aphasic difficulties, including clear manifestations of expressive losses, suggests the strong probability that the anterior temporal area is involved as well. Probably many persons would postulate that the presence of naming deficits (nominal aphasia or Broca's aphasia) necessarily implicates the posterior-inferior frontal area (Broca's area). In my experience this is not necessarily true. Clear expressive aphasic manifestations may be shown by people with anterior temporal lobe lesions that do not necessarily, in a structural sense, even involve the frontal lobe. Thus, from the interpretation of the aphasic symptoms and the sensory-perceptual losses, one would conclude that this man has a serious structural lesion principally involving the left temporal lobe.

As noted above, a question exists as to whether this lesion may also involve the right cerebral hemisphere. This could be possible either by postulating the presence of metastatic carcinoma (with the principal lesion in the left cerebral hemisphere but a secondary lesion in the right cerebral hemisphere) or a rapidly developing intrinsic tumor that had crossed to the right cerebral hemisphere through the corpus callosum. It is difficult to answer this question. Evidence pointing toward involvement of the posterior part of the language area presents a complicating factor inasmuch as some persons with damage in this area also have difficulty copying simple spatial configurations. Reference to Table 12 indicates that about 15% of persons with left cerebral lesions show evidence of constructional dyspraxia. However, in most such instances the difficulties manifest themselves as a rather general kind of confusion in the drawing rather than specific and selected distortions of the spatial configuration. However, most persons with left cerebral lesions who show difficulties in drawing the figures used in the Aphasia test have lesions that involve the posterior part of the language area and, of course, also show very definite signs of dysphasia. The problem in this instance is that the deficits in the drawings are not quite typical of what is usually seen in persons with left cerebral damage, although some of the confusion demonstrated in the drawing of the key is suggestive of this possibility. I believe that it would be difficult to draw a definite conclusion as to whether the right hemisphere was involved or whether the drawing difficulties were part of the total picture of involvement of the left hemisphere, including the posterior part of the language area. It is possible that results on the complete neuropsychological examination would provide assistance in resolving this question. In any case, the test results show positive evidence for involvement of the left cerebral hemisphere with a structural lesion that is located principally in the left temporal lobe.

It is difficult from the aphasia examination and the sensory-perceptual results, considered alone, to draw a confident conclusion regarding the type of lesion. However, in this instance, there are several factors that point toward a neoplastic type of lesion rather than a vascular lesion. First, while the deficits are pronounced and severe in the language area, they are not as pronounced and severe in the area of sensory-perceptual deficits. This kind of disparity is much more often seen with neoplastic lesions than with vascular lesions. If a stroke had caused the language deficits shown by this man, it is entirely likely that more extensive losses, including some deficits in double simultaneous tactile and auditory testing, would have been present. It is also entirely unlikely that this man would have done as well in finger-tip number writing perception if he had experienced a stroke of the left hemisphere. However, the severity of the deficits certainly point toward structural tissue damage and a serious type of lesion that would call for neurological and possibly neurosurgical evaluation had this not already been done. In the context of the question regarding right as well as left hemisphere involvement, it is interesting to note that autopsy findings (see below) about nine months later showed that the tumor had invaded the right cerebral hemisphere at the time of death. Right cerebral involvement at the time of our examination, however, remains unanswered because the crossing could have occurred in the ensuing nine months.

J.A.

NEUROLOGICAL SUMMARY

Symptoms:

J.A., a 54-year-old male bartender and country club manager who complained about headaches and difficulties with memory and vision. These had progressed over an eight to ten month period and had become so severe that he was forced to give up his job. At the time of hospital admission he had great difficulty remembering names and appeared somewhat confused.

Signs:

Very slight right facial weakness.
Weakness and clumsiness of right hand.
Positive Hoffman's sign on the right.
Questionable positive Babinski sign on the right.
Possible diminution of abdominal reflexes on the right.
Right homonymous hemianopsia.

Diagnostic Tests:

EEG: Delta waves, left frontal and temporal areas.
Radioisotopic brain scan: Large area of increased activity in the left temporo-parietal region.
Cerebral angiogram: Extensive tumor stain from the left anterior temporal area to the left occipital area, but not involving much of the left parietal area.
Neuropsychological examination done two days before surgery.

Treatment:

Craniotomy and ablation of entire left temporal lobe. Tumor could be seen extending superiorly and posteriorly following the temporal lobe removal.

Postoperative Course:

The patient did extremely well in the immediate post-operative period. X-ray therapy was instituted and continued for nine weeks. Patient readmitted for chemotherapy seven months after surgery, but began to show rapidly progressive deterioration and died seven weeks later.

Diagnosis:

Glioblastoma multiforme principally of the left temporal lobe but also extending posteriorly and superiorly. Autopsy revealed that the tumor had crossed into the right cerebral hemisphere via the splenium of the corpus callosum.

REITAN-INDIANA APHASIA SCREENING TEST

Form for Adults and Older Children

Name: V.S. Age: 56 Date: Examiner:

Copy SQUARE	Repeat TRIANGLE
Name SQUARE	Repeat MASSACHUSETTS "Mass-a-mass-a (pause) no"
Spell SQUARE "S-Q-U-U-A-R-E-E"	Repeat METHODIST EPISCOPAL "Methus auntispisctness."
Copy CROSS	Write SQUARE
Name CROSS "Scross", then responded correctly.	Read SEVEN
Spell CROSS "S-Q-U-I-S (pause) now then."	Repeat SEVEN
Copy TRIANGLE	Repeat/Explain HE SHOUTED THE WARNING. Patient confused and could not understand. Unable to repeat or explain.
Name TRIANGLE	Write HE SHOUTED THE WARNING.
Spell TRIANGLE Patient wrote instead of spelling orally, but made a mistake.	Compute 85 – 27 =
Name BABY	Compute 17 X 3 =
Write CLOCK	Name KEY "Krey"
Name FORK "Knife"	Demonstrate use of KEY
Read 7 SIX 2	Draw KEY
Read MGW	Read PLACE LEFT HAND TO RIGHT EAR.
Reading I	Place LEFT HAND TO RIGHT EAR Doubt about location of ear.
Reading II "He is a family animal, a famous winner of dog shows."	Place LEFT HAND TO LEFT ELBOW Mild confusion regarding location of elbow.

REITAN-KLØVE SENSORY-PERCEPTUAL EXAMINATION

(Instance indicated where stimulus was not perceived or was incorrectly perceived.)

TACTILE:

RH					LH					Both: RH	X	X	X	X	LH				
RH					LF					Both: RH	X	X	X	X	LF				
LH					RF					LH					RF	X	X	X	X

AUDITORY:

RE					LE					Both: RE	X	X	X	X	LE				

VISUAL:

																				– (Above eye level)
RV					LV					Both: RV					LV					– (Eye level)
																				– (Below eye level)

TACTILE FINGER RECOGNITION:

Right:	1					2		X	X	X	3	X	X	X	X	4	X	X	X		5	X	X	X	X	14/20
Left:	1					2					3					4				X	5		X		X	3/20

COMMENTS:

FINGER-TIP NUMBER WRITING PERCEPTION:

	4	6	3	5	3	5	4	6	6	5	4	3	5	4	6	3	6	3	5	4	
Right:	X	X	X	X	X	X	X	X	X	X	X	X	X	X	X	X	X	X	X	X	20/20
Left:		X	X	X	X	X	X	X	X	X	X	X	X	X	X	X	X	X		X	18/20

COMMENTS:

VISUAL FIELDS:

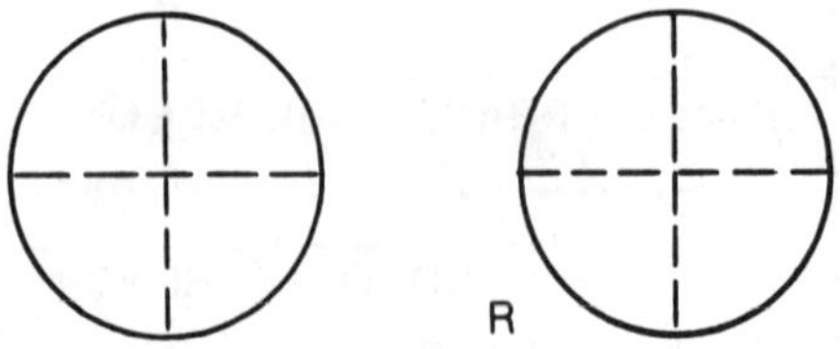

L R

FULL

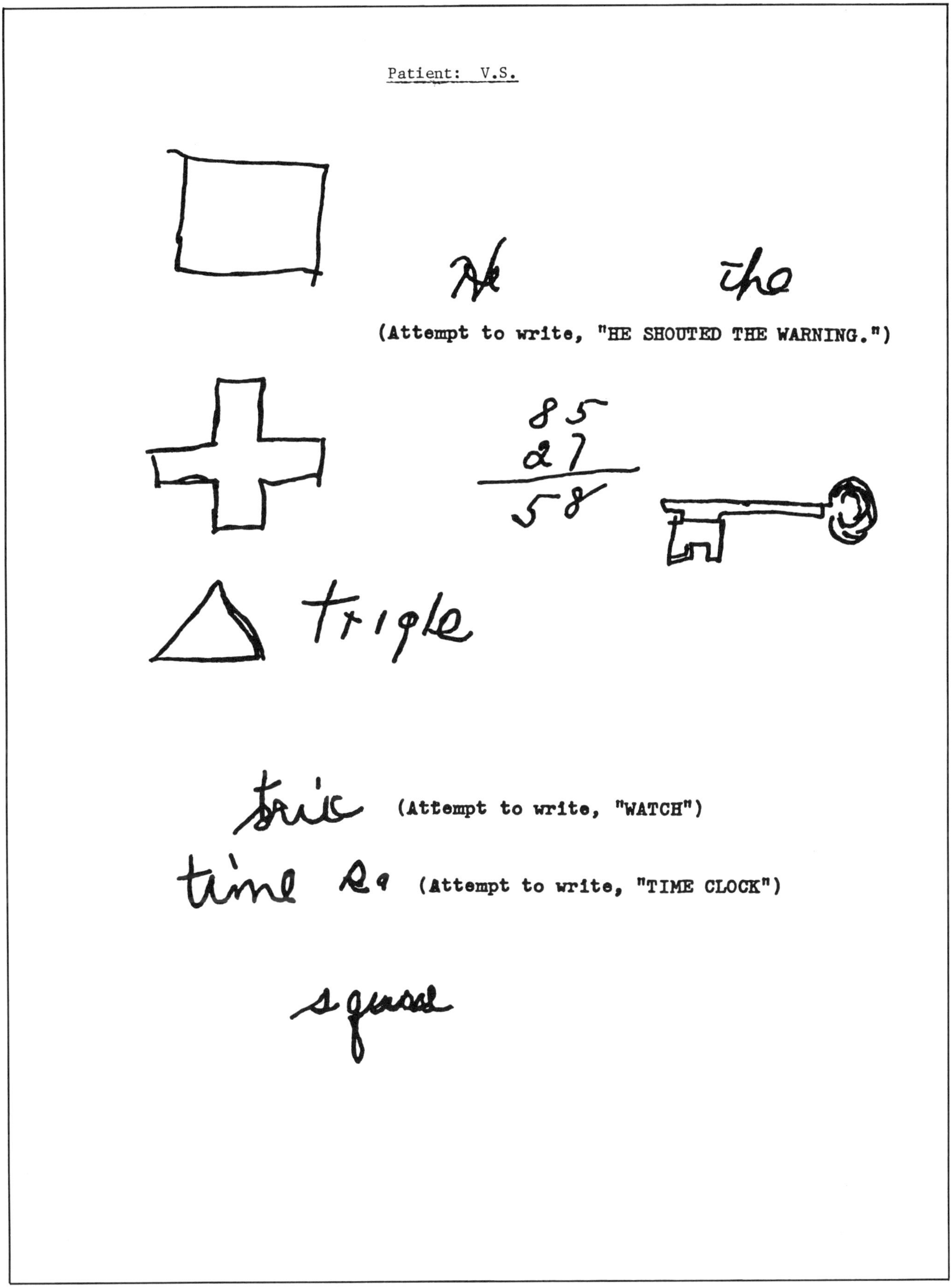
Patient: V.S.
(Attempt to write, "HE SHOUTED THE WARNING.")
(Attempt to write, "WATCH")
(Attempt to write, "TIME CLOCK")

V.S. – A 56-year-old right-handed female bookkeeper with an eighth grade education.

Identification of brain-related deficits:

This woman had some definite aphasic symptoms although she was not as profoundly handicapped as was the previous patient. She was able to name the square correctly but, when asked to spell "square", had difficulty that included repetition of the "u" and the "e." When she was then asked to name the picture of the cross she showed a mild perseverative tendency, probably from the word SQUARE, responding "scross." She recognized her mistake and was able to correct it. However, correction of a mistake of this kind does not delete the significance of the original mistake. In fact, the ability of this subject to make a correction suggests that the mistake should not have occurred in the first place. Thus, corrections often tend to document the validity of the abnormality in response, considering that the test requirements are basically simple and most persons can respond correctly the first time. When the patient was asked to spell CROSS she definitely deviated from a normal response. In fact, she was not even close to the correct word and again demonstrated perseveration with regard to the previous response. This is a rather typical oranic language deficit and, in its own right, would point toward some left cerebral dysfunction.

Continuing with items on the scoring form, it can be seen that she made a mistake on the next item. It is not at all uncommon for the word "family" to be substituted for the word "famous," but this kind of mistake nevertheless is clearly a manifestation of left cerebral dysfunction. The patient was able to repeat "triangle" but had great difficulty with the word "Massachusetts." She was able to make no progress in attempting to repeat "Methodist Episcopal." Thus, the patient showed definite evidence of central dysarthria. She also was completely unable to repeat the sentence, "He shouted the warning." When the subject is not able even to make an attempt at repeating spoken material, a question must be raised regarding the possible presence of auditory verbal dysgnosia. When the limitation is expressive in nature, the patient may make mistakes in attempting to repeat the sentence, but when no response at all is possible for the subject, a definite possibility exists that the incoming symbolic content just did not register. One must also recognize, however, that absence of information (no response) is more difficult to interpret than a defective response. She demonstrated difficulty in naming when she was asked to give the name of the key. Finally, she became confused when asked to place her left hand to her right ear. Sometimes it is difficult to judge whether confusion on this item stems from input problems or output problems. In other words, there may be a question as to whether this woman was able to understand the instructions. Her deficit, therefore, may have represented an auditory verbal dysgnoisa. On the other hand, perhaps the performance of the act was the limiting factor, in which case we could conlcude that he patient had at least a degree of body dysgnosia. In this case the examiner felt that the patient seemed to understand the instructions but was confused with relation to her body parts. She was not quite able to figure out where her ear was as contrasted with other parts of the body. Thus, we concluded that the patient did demonstrate a mild body dysgnosia. This is quite a serious symptom inasmuch as it does not occur very often, occurs only with a rather serious lesion, and is frequently accompanied by rather prominent aphasic deficits of other types. One can speculate in this regard as to whether abilities that are learned early in life, such as identifying body parts, are among the last to go as a result of cerebral damage. In any case, body dysgnosia is not frequently seen and, when it is present, is quite a serious sign of left cerebral damage.

In referring to the patient's drawings and writing, she was able to draw the general shape of the square, cross, and triangle relatively well. The fact that she did not draw exactly straight lines is not of particular significance. However, in her drawing of the key she did show some deficits that must be noted. She was not able to close the handle properly and this rarely happens in persons with normal brain functions. In addition, she showed a little confusion with respect to symmetry involving the teeth of the key. Thus, one would have to judge the drawing as showing definite abnormalities and, again, one might raise a question as to whether right cerebral damage was present.

In comparison with her drawings, the patient had much more serious difficulties in her attempts to deal with language material. She was not even able to begin to write the words "shouted" and "warning" in her attempt to write the sentence. Because the patient was not able to spell "triangle" verbally, she was asked by the examiner to write the word (even though it is not a formal part of our standard testing procedure) and the patient demonstrated definite confusion.

When looking at the picture of the clock, the patient made it clear that she was trying to write the word "watch." However, she was completely confused at this point and was not able to write anything that was legible. This is a clear instance of dysgraphia. Next, she decided that she would try to write "time clock." She was able to write the word "time" correctly but then became quite confused, and was not able to get "clock" started correctly.

Finally, the patient became confused in writing even when she had the word "square" directly before her. She attempted to write the word, became confused with respect to making the letters, went back and tried to correct her writing, but only made the whole situation look worse.

Results on the Sensory-perceptual Examination were clearly in the abnormal range. This woman showed very profound losses in perception on the right side during double simultaneous tactile stimulation. She had no difficulty in any instance when the stimulus was delivered unilaterally, but when stimuli were delivered to both sides simultaneously her left cerebral hemisphere was not able to process the information to the point that perception of the stimulus occurred. The patient showed the same kind of deficit in auditory stimulation. These findings would point toward left temporal and parietal involvement. However, the patient had no difficulty with either unilateral or bilateral simultaneous visual stimulation.

This woman had difficulty on both hands in tactile finger recognition (finger agnosia), but had more difficulty on the right hand than the left hand. We do not have an accurate recording of the precise results in this case, but fingers 2, 3, 4, and 5 of the right hand were clearly deficient. However, the patient also had some difficulty and confusion of fingers 4 and 5 of the left hand. The fact that finger 5 of the left hand was included among the two fingers on which errors were made is of definite significance. Most errors occur on fingers 2, 3, and 4 and errors occur much less frequently on fingers 1 or 5. Thus, a question must be raised in this instance of the possibility of some degree of bilateral involvement. This woman was not able to make any progress in fingertip number writing perception on her right hand but she also consistently made mistakes on her left hand. It seems likely that either the reporting problem was beyond her or that she did not have the ability to focus her concentration sufficiently well to be able to perform this task. If this task was essentially too difficult for the patient, regardless of the hand being tested, the results cannot be used for comparison of the two cerebral hemispheres.

Interpretation of results:

The results definitely implicate the left cerebral hemisphere. The question regarding possible involvement of the right cerebral hemisphere, on the basis of the drawing of the key and some errors on fingers 4 and 5 of the left hand in tactile finger recognition, probably cannot be resolved from these data alone. Results of the complete neuropsychological examination might be of specific help. The problem in this regard pertains to the need for comparisons of motor proficiency on the two sides of the body together with evaluation of the integrity of higher-level functions related to right hemisphere functioning. As noted previously, the results of the aphasia examination and the sensory-perceptual examination, taken by themselves, do not constitute a complete neuropsychological examination.

This woman showed evidence of both expressive and receptive aphasic deficits. She had evidence of spelling dyspraxia, dysnomia, dyslexia, dysgraphia, central dysarthria, auditory verbal dysgnosia, and mild body dysgnosia. We should note particularly that the patient showed clear evidence of difficulty in appreciating and understanding auditory verbal communications. This indication of auditory verbal dysgnosia probably points toward involvement of the posterior part of the language area. In this case, however, there were quite clear signs from the sensory-perceptual examination of very strong tactile deficits as well as auditory impairment in perceiving double simultaneous stimulation. Thus, one might well postulate that the parietal lobe had more direct, structural damage than in the previous case although temporal lobe involvement, especially in the posterior part, was also quite clear.

It would appear possible to draw a rather confident inference regarding the type of lesion, considering the overall results. The lesion, in this case, almost certainly would be an intrinsic tumor and probably a fairly rapidly growing one. The reason for this inference relates both to the positive and the negative evidence. The patient had distinct evidence of dysphasia of the type that is seen in persons with actual serious structural damage but she did not have any deficits with respect to either primary aspects of her visual fields (both visual fields were full on confrontation testing) nor on the test of double simultaneous visual stimulation. It is entirely unlikely that a person with a stroke, and such definite deficits in other respects, would have escaped a homonymous right visual field loss. This question, however, frequently can be answered more confidently when results of the entire neuropsychological examination are available. In any case, the severity of the deficits as well as their nature point toward a seriously destructive lesion of the left cerebral hemisphere, at least involving the parietal and posterior temporal areas.

V.S.

NEUROLOGICAL SUMMARY

Symptoms:

Two months prior to admission patient began to make mistakes in her bookkeeping.
One month prior to admission developed some difficulty with writing and some dysphasia.
Progressive confusion, 2 weeks.

Signs:

Aphasia.
Right hemihypesthesia.
Stereognosis and finger writing poor bilaterally.
Motor functions adequate bilaterally.

Handedness:

Right.

Diagnostic Tests:

X-rays: Skull films negative.
Angiogram: Left Parietal mass.
Neuropsychological examination done 7 days before surgery.

Treatment:

Craniotomy. Partial removal of glioblastoma, left parietal area.

Postoperative Course:

Patient developed right-sided seizures and increasing hemiparesis and aphasia. Wound reopened one month later. Brain was edematous. Dura left open and bone flap left free. Improved slowly but complete paralysis of right upper extremity remained. Some function was present in the right lower extremity. Marked aphasia and perseveration. Treated with X-ray therapy. Discharged on anticonvulsants. Patient died at another hospital, five months after craniotomy.

Diagnosis:

Glioblastoma multiforme, left parietal area.

REITAN-INDIANA APHASIA SCREENING TEST

PATIENT: J.B.

Copy SQUARE	Repeat TRIANGLE
Name SQUARE	Repeat MASSACHUSETTS
Spell SQUARE	Repeat METHODIST EPISCOPAL Patient stuttered, but said the words.
Copy CROSS	Write SQUARE
Name CROSS	Read SEVEN
Spell CROSS	Repeat SEVEN
Copy TRIANGLE	Repeat/Explain HE SHOUTED THE WARNING.
Name TRIANGLE	Write HE SHOUTED THE WARNING.
Spell TRIANGLE	Compute 85 – 27 =
Name BABY	Compute 17 X 3 = Patient attempted the problem verbally but could not do it.
Write CLOCK	Name KEY
Name FORK	Demonstrate use of KEY
Read 7 SIX 2	Draw KEY
Read MGW	Read PLACE LEFT HAND TO RIGHT EAR.
Reading I	Place LEFT HAND TO RIGHT EAR
Reading II "He is a very friendly" then self-corrected.	Place LEFT HAND TO LEFT ELBOW

REITAN-KLØVE SENSORY-PERCEPTUAL EXAMINATION

(Instance indicated where stimulus was not perceived or was incorrectly perceived.)

TACTILE:

RH		LH		Both: RH	X X X X	LH	
RH		LF		Both: RH	X X X	LF	
LH		RF	X X X	LH		RF	X X X

AUDITORY: RE [ ] LE [ ] Both: RE [X X X] LE [ ]

VISUAL:

RV	X X X X / X X X X / X X X X	LV		Both: RV	(crossed out)	LV	(crossed out)

– (Above eye level)
– (Eye level)
– (Below eye level)

TACTILE FINGER RECOGNITION:

Right:	1	2	2	3 1	3	2 2 4 2	4	X 3	5	X 2	11/ 20
Left:	1		2		3		4	3	5	4 4	3/ 20

COMMENTS:

FINGER-TIP NUMBER WRITING PERCEPTION:

	4	6	3	5	3	5	4	6	6	5	4	3	5	4	6	3	6	3	5	4	
Right:		3		X	5	4		X	3		5	4				5	4				10/ 20
Left:				X																	1/ 20

COMMENTS:

VISUAL FIELDS:

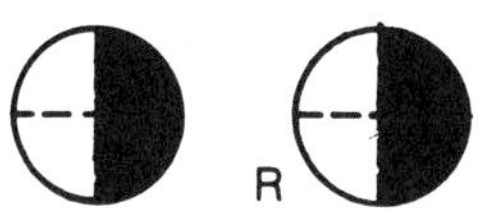

L R

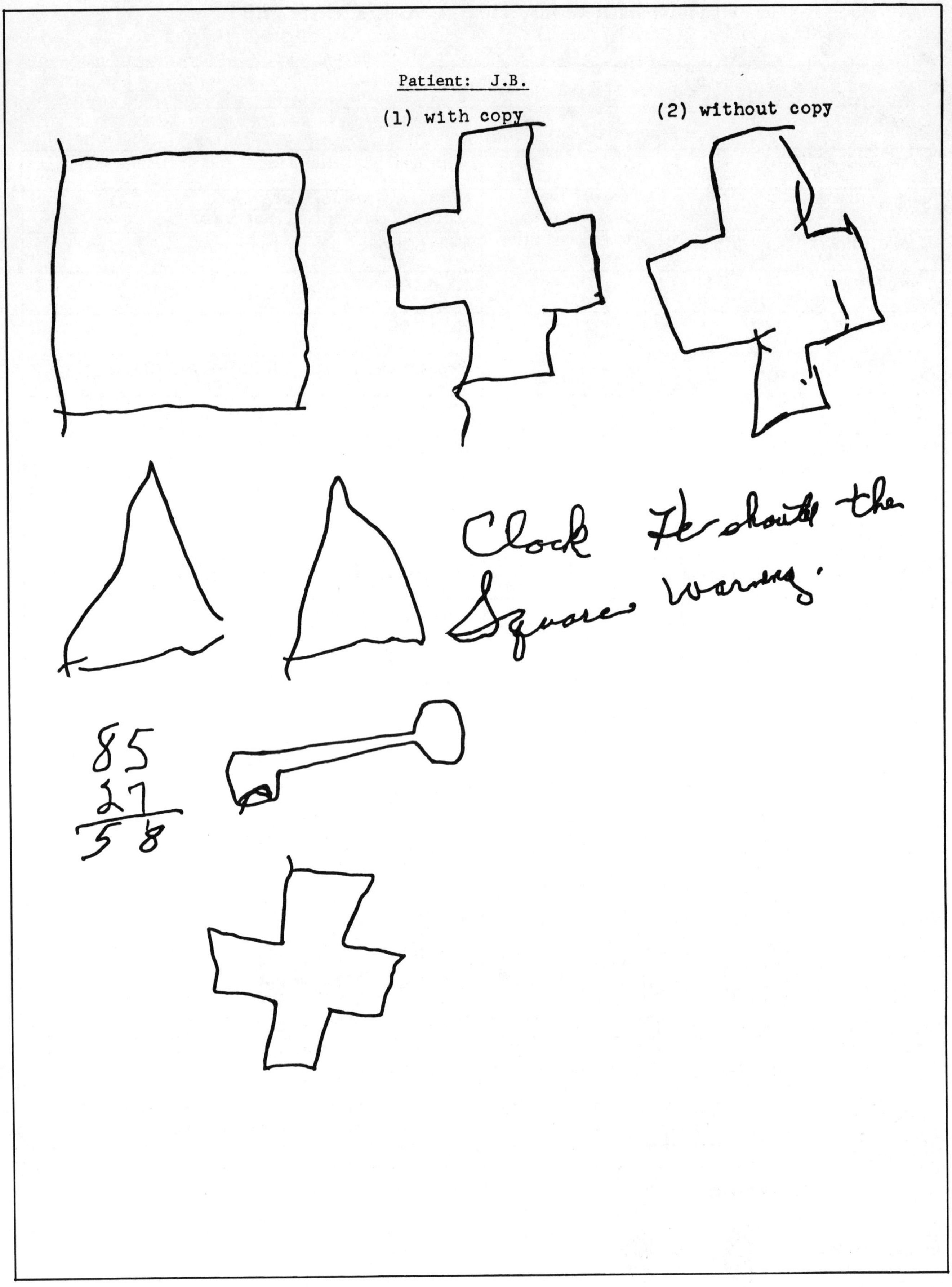
Patient: J.B.
(1) with copy
(2) without copy
Clock
85
27
58

J.B. – A twenty-year-old right-handed female homemaker with an eleventh grade education.

Identification of brain-related deficits:

The recording form for the Aphasia Screening Test does not reveal many instances of failure. On the second reading item the patient inserted the word "very" and corrected herself. This error is a little suspicious and suggests that the patient may have mild difficulty with language material, but it is not enough by itself to conclude that she has any significant left cerebral dysfunction. The patient also stuttered when attempting to repeat METHODIST EPISCOPAL, but was able to say the words correctly. Stuttering does not constitute a significant indication of brain dysfunction and the correct enunciation must be considered as an adequate performance. The patient had some difficulty in doing the problem "17 x 3" in her head. She repeated the problem and attempted to work it out in her verbalizations, but she was not able to reach any answer. It is possible that this item was too difficult for her. It would have been advisable to try simpler items although this was not done. In terms of the results obtained, one could not conclude that a failure to solve this problem necessarily represented any type of brain dysfunction.

Turning to the patient's writing and drawings, it is immediately apparent that she had some difficulties with motor control. She had a problem in drawing straight lines and in controlling her pencil. The first cross, done while looking at the sample figure, shows all four extremities in approximately equivalent relationships, although the lateral extremity on the right suggests that the patient had somewhat of a problem. The curved line at the bottom probably represents nothing more than a motor control problem. Out of general interest, the examiner had the patient attempt to draw the figure a second time with the stimulus figure removed from sight. The patient had more difficulty under these circumstances and one would be inclined to interpret some aspects of the drawing as representing difficulty with the spatial configuration over and beyond the obvious problems with motor control. This is particularly true considering the vertical line involving the lower part of the right lateral extremity. It would appear that the subject started to draw this extremity without sufficient length, changed her mind, and made it somewhat longer. However, the four extremities are still fairly distinct and obvious and in approximately appropriate relationships. The final cross drawn by the subject is probably better than either of the two previous attempts, and although not very good should be considered within normal limits. The triangles are basically adequate even though the problem of motor control is apparent. The subject's drawing of the key is lacking in detail. It is not uncommon for many persons, even though we attempt to overcome the problem with the instructions, to draw a simplified version of the key. When this happens it is difficult to draw conclusions regarding impairment of ability in dealing with spatial relationships. In this instance we can only conclude that the drawing was quite simplified and cannot reach specific conclusions about possible impairment of brain functions. An example of this kind serves to reinforce the recommendation that every effort be made to get the subject to perform as carefully and adequately as possible. If a careful effort is not made it becomes next to impossible to identify brain-related deficits.

The patient's writing appears to be fairly close to normal limits although one could raise a question about the "ed" on "shouted" and possibly the "ni" in "warning". It would be difficult to be sure that these deviations from the expected performance have particular significance for left cerebral dysfunction. Thus, the total impression from the aphasia examination is that this woman might have very mild language difficulties, but it is difficult to be sure that they represent actual abnormalities as contrasted with merely falling in the lower part of the normal range.

Results on the sensory-perceptual examination quite clearly demonstrated distinct abnormalities in performance. The patient showed definite indications of failure to perceive a stimulus to the right side of the body when given simultaneously with a stimulus on the left side. Over and beyond this, the patient had some primarily tactile insensitivity (hypesthesia) of the right side of the face. The patient had similar difficulties on the right side with auditory stimulation. While she did not make any mistakes with unilateral stimulation on either side, she failed to perceive the stimulus on the right side in three of four instances when the stimulation was given bilaterally. In addition to this, the patient was not able to respond toward her right side to visual stimulation at all. Confrontation examination indicated that she had a striking visual field loss involving the right visual field for each eye (right homonymous hemianopsia).

The patient also had definite difficulty in tactile finger recognition, failing in 11 of 20 trials with her right hand and 3 of 20 trials with her left hand. In an instance of this kind one might raise the question as to the significance of the three errors on the left hand. In terms of clinical interpretation, they probably are not sufficient to postulate a lesion of the right cerebral hemisphere, although the 11 errors on the right side clearly indicate that the parietal lobe of the left hemisphere is deficient. The patient also had a good deal of difficulty on her right hand in finger-tip number writing perception, being unable to perceive the number in 10 of the 20 trials. With her left hand she had difficulty only in one instance. Thus, results on this procedure were very striking in their lateralizing significance.

Interpretation of the results:

There can be no doubt that J.B. has a significant lesion of the left cerebral hemisphere, even though she does not have any striking impairment of language abilities as shown, at least, on the Aphasia Screening Test. The right homonymous hemianopsia, tactile and auditory imperception on the right side, and evidence of much greater difficulty in tactile finger recognition and finger-tip number writing perception on the right than the left side all point toward left cerebral damage. These results are enough so that one would postulate that some structural damage had occurred in the left cerebral hemisphere. The problem in interpretation involves the striking sensory-perceptual losses, which often are associated with rather serious destruction of brain tissue, and the absence of any striking aphasic deficits. In instances of this kind one must consider both sources of evidence. The sensory-perceptual deficits clearly indicate left cerebral damage and the relative absence of aphasic difficulties may suggest that the language area is relatively spared but also very probably, and perhaps even more significantly, suggests that the lesion is not acutely destructive but, instead, perhaps gradually progressive.

It would be of great advantage to have additional test results for this woman. One would wonder about possible differences between Verbal and Performance intelligence values, the severity of generalized impairment of higher-level brain-related abilities, and about evidence of motor impairment particularly on the right side of the body. One might, on the basis of the results of the Aphasia Screening Test and the Sensory-perceptual Examination, be inclined to postulate that the lesion is probably not vascular in nature. If the lesion were vascular, considering the patient's age, one would suspect that it was a congenital anomaly. As noted above, the striking sensory-perceptual deficits would suggest that actual tissue damage in the left cerebral hemisphere had occurred. Tissue damage from a vascular lesion would, very probably, have brought about corresponding deficits in the language area. However, residual damage from a penetrating head injury or a slowly growing tumor could have caused results of this kind. In fact, the patient did have a slowly growing intrinsic tumor that was quite extensive in the left cerebral hemisphere. The present results focus particularly on the left parietal area whereas, in fact, the lesion was more extensive than this as was discerned from results on the entire test battery.

It is possible that the mild difficulty in dealing with spatial configurations related to involvement of the posterior part of the left cerebral hemisphere, but it would be difficult in this instance to be sure of this. In any case, considering the overall test results, there certainly was not enough positive information in total to postulate specific structural involvement of the right cerebral hemisphere.

J.B.

NEUROLOGICAL SUMMARY

Symptoms:

J.B. was a 20-year-old woman who had experienced episodes of numbness in her right arm for about six years. During the last year the numbness had increased and some impairment of motor functions had also occurred. In addition, she had developed severe headaches.

Signs:

Physical neurological examination: Right hemiparesis, right hemihypesthesia, hyperative deep tendon reflexes on the right, impairment in form recognition and figure and number writing on the right hand, and a right homonymous hemianopsia.

Handedness:

Right

Diagnostic Tests:

EEG: Delta waves, Grade II, left frontal-parietal area. Carotid angiogram: Pronounced shift from left to right, suggesting a mass lesion possibly in the left parietal area. Neuropsychological examination was done 7 days before surgery.

Treatment:

Craniotomy with partial removal of a large tumor from the left cerebral hemisphere. The lesion appeared to extend from the posterior frontal area through the parietal lobe and nearly to the occipital pole.

Postoperative Course:

The patient did very poorly after surgery and expired.

Final Diagnosis:

Ependymoma of left occipital-temporal-parietal area.

REITAN-INDIANA APHASIA SCREENING TEST

PATIENT: P.H.

Copy SQUARE	Repeat TRIANGLE
Name SQUARE	Repeat MASSACHUSETTS
Spell SQUARE	Repeat METHODIST EPISCOPAL
Copy CROSS	Write SQUARE
Name CROSS	Read SEVEN
Spell CROSS	Repeat SEVEN
Copy TRIANGLE	Repeat/Explain HE SHOUTED THE WARNING.
Name TRIANGLE	Write HE SHOUTED THE WARNING.
Spell TRIANGLE	Compute 85 − 27 =
Name BABY	Compute 17 X 3 = "54" then corrected.
Write CLOCK	Name KEY
Name FORK	Demonstrate use of KEY
Read 7 SIX 2	Draw KEY
Read MGW	Read PLACE LEFT HAND TO RIGHT EAR. "Place right hand to right ear."
Reading I	Place LEFT HAND TO RIGHT EAR Right hand to left ear; self-corrected.
Reading II	Place LEFT HAND TO LEFT ELBOW Left hand to right elbow; self-corrected.

REITAN-KLØVE SENSORY-PERCEPTUAL EXAMINATION

(Instance indicated where stimulus was not perceived or was incorrectly perceived.)

TACTILE:

RH		LH		Both: RH		LH	X X X X
RH		LF		Both: RH		LF	X X
LH		RF		LH	X X X X	RF	

AUDITORY:

RE		LE		Both: RE		LE	X X X X

VISUAL:

RV		LV	X X X X	Both: RV	(crossed out)	LV	(crossed out)	– (Above eye level)
			X X X X					– (Eye level)
			X X X X					– (Below eye level)

TACTILE FINGER RECOGNITION:

	1	2	3	4	5	
Right:						0 / 20
Left:			X X X X			4 / 20

COMMENTS:

FINGER-TIP NUMBER WRITING PERCEPTION:

	4	6	3	5	3	5	4	6	6	5	4	3	5	4	6	3	6	3	5	4	
Right:																					___/___
Left:																					___/___

COMMENTS: Patient confused and test not done.

VISUAL FIELDS:

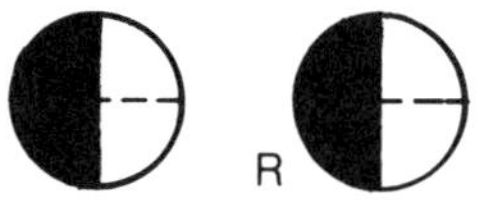

L R

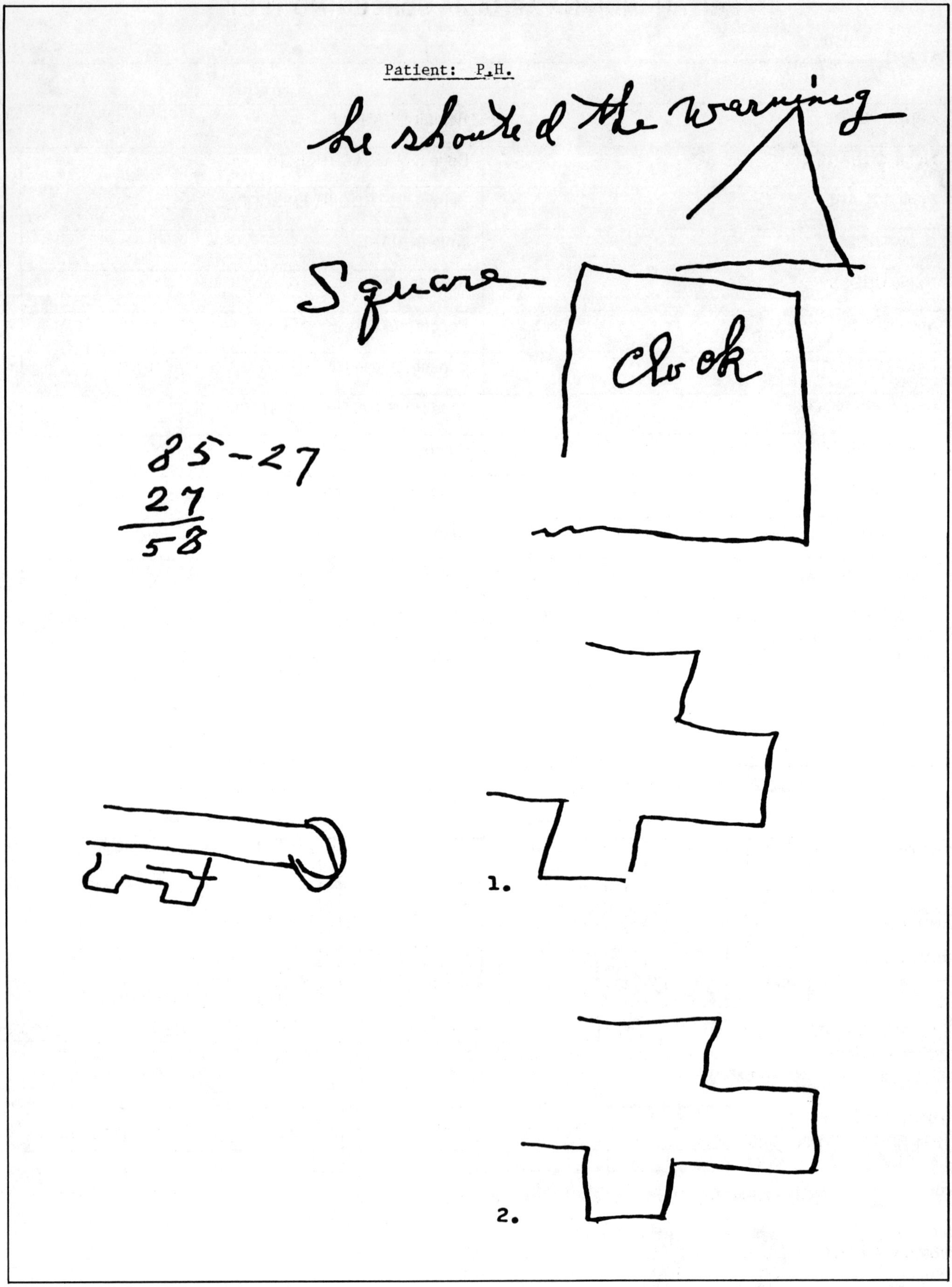
Patient: P.H.
he shouted the warning
Square
Clock
85-27
27
58
1.
2.

P.H. – a 67-year-old right-handed male with sixteen years of education.

Identification of brain-related deficits:

Review of the Aphasia Screening Test form indicates that this man had no difficulty with most of the items that involved language and communicational skills. He made a mistake in performing 17 x 3 but corrected himself. There is no evidence that his answer of "54" was anything other than the usual type of arithmetical problem that many people have. He did make a mistake in reading PLACE LEFT HAND TO RIGHT EAR and this is somewhat suspicious. However, it stands pretty much in isolation and thus is difficult to use as a confident indicator of left cerebral dysfunction. When asked to put his left hand to his right ear he made a mistake in right-left orientation, placing his right hand to his left ear. He was able to correct this himself, but we must consider the error as a genuine mistake. He also demonstrated some mild right-left confusion when asked to place his left hand to his left elbow. Again, he was able to correct himself but it does appear that the patient has mild right-left confusion.

Referring to the patient's writing and drawings, he had somewhat unusual handwriting, reminding one of the type of writing that might be done by some older persons or possibly by a person whose initial language had not been English. However, the major difficulties clearly related to the drawings. In his attempt to draw the square the patient made a mistake on the third line, coming down too far, and then having a problem with respect to effecting closure. He had this same kind of problem on the triangle. In his attempt to draw the cross, the patient did fairly well until he reached a point where he became confused. The patient seemed to be a relatively conservative man and he was unwilling to attempt to continue the drawing because he did not know which way to draw the line. Finally, he was asked to do the drawing again and he had exactly the same kind of problem as he had initially. In his attempt to draw the key it is apparent that the patient had a serious problem involving spatial relationships. Finally, it should be noted that he regularly had his difficulties on the left side of the figure. This is not uncommon in persons with right cerebral lesions. However, difficulty on the left side of the figure in association with right cerebral damage is sometimes tempered by a problem in closure. If the subject draws the figure in a counter-clockwise direction the closure problem frequently occurs on the right side of the figure. The problem of closure constitutes a difficulty in its own right and, thus, the most deficient aspect of the drawing may in some instances be on the right side. However, when the subject draws the figure in a clockwise direction, having to close the figure on the left side, and in addition has a right cerebral lesion that may constitute special problems in perceiving and understanding the spatial configuration on the left side, both factors operate against the subject. In this instance one would judge that both closure of the figure and probably especial difficulty in appreciating the spatial configuration on the left side were significant factors. The difficulty experienced by this man in drawing simple figures (constructional dyspraxia) was certainly much more prominent and striking than the mild difficulty he had in right-left orientation.

The patient showed definite and distinct difficulties on the Sensory-perceptual Examination. He had a pronounced tendency to fail to perceive stimuli to his left hand or left face when given in competition with stimuli to the other side of the body. Nevertheless, he had no difficulty with unilateral stimulation on either side. Exactly the same situation was present with respect to perception of double simultaneous auditory stimuli. These findings were quite profound and definitely imply the presence of a serious lesion of the right cerebral hemisphere. In addition, the test for double simultaneous visual stimulation was precluded by the presence of a left homonymous hemianopsia.

The patient had relatively little difficulty in tactile finger recognition except for the third finger of the left hand. In every trial on this finger the patient was confused and not able to give a correct response. Finger-tip number writing perception was difficult for this patient and he manifested confusion on both sides. Sometimes this test is just a little too complex for some persons. We would postulate that the subject probably was poorer on the left hand than the right hand, but because he was confused on both sides, there is no way to be sure about this. In effect, this test probably was somewhat inappropriate for this man, being too difficult for him to perform on either hand.

Interpretation of the results:

These test results quite clearly point toward significant damage of the right cerebral hemisphere. One would draw such a conclusion from the strikingly defective figure drawings. This man not only had difficulty with the spatial relationships but had additional difficulty on the left side of the figures. The Aphasia Screening Test alone might be interpreted to suggest the presence of some left cerebral damage as well, considering the fact that the patient did have some definite right-left confusion. As noted in Table 12, right-left confusion does not ordinarily occur any more commonly among persons with right cerebral lesions than among control subjects but is quite common in persons with left cerebral lesions. However, the figure drawing difficulties were much more pronounced than the right-left confusion.

Results on the Sensory-perceptual Examination were quite clear and distinct in their lateralizing significance. Tests of double simultaneous tactile and auditory stimulation, together with evidence of a definite left homonymous hemianopsia, all point strongly toward seriously destructive damage of the right cerebral hemisphere, particularly involving the area behind the Rolandic fissure. It is surprising that the patient did not have more difficulty on his left hand in tactile finger recognition. However, in the face of the severe constructional dyspraxia and pronounced evidence of left-sided imperception, the failure to find more evidence of left finger dysgnosia strongly inclines the interpretation toward a neoplastic rather than a vascular lesion. As shown by Hom (1982), vascular lesions customarily show the most pronounced sensory-perceptual deficits, intrinsic neoplasms also show consistent deficits but not as strikingly, and traumatic lesions are less striking than either of the other two lesion categories. Thus, one would postulate that this man has a seriously destructive lesion, possibly an intrinsic neoplasm that might be rapidly growing, and located probably in the parietal area of the right cerebral hemisphere. Without more evidence of left cerebral involvement than indicated by the mild right-left confusion, one would be hesitant to postulate any structural involvement of the left cerebral hemisphere.

P.H.

NEUROLOGICAL SUMMARY

Symptoms:

Three months prior to admission patient complained of dizziness, fatigue and blurring of vision. Had glasses changed 3 times in past 3 months.
Three weeks prior to admission he developed severe frontal headaches.
During the week prior to admission he developed left sided weakness and numbness.

Signs:

Physical examination: Normal.
Neurological examination: Sluggish and apathetic.
Discs flat.
Left homonymous hemianopsia.
Left central facial paresis.
Left spastic hemiparesis involving upper extremity more than lower.
Left hemihypalgesia.
Reflexes increased on left.
Babinski positive, left.
Sensory suppression, left; astereognosis, left; finger agnosia, left.
Acalculia.

Handedness:

Right.

Diagnostic Tests:

CSF: Protein, 120 mgm %, 100% lymphs, 190 WBC, sugar, 54.
Serology negative.
EEG: Delta Grade III, right temporal-frontal-parietal area. Dysrhythmia Grade II, generalized, maximal right. Asymmetry Grade I.
X-ray: Skull films, negative.
Angiogram: Right occipital-parietal-temporal mass.
Incidental finding: Aneurysm of internal carotid, right.
Neuropsychological tests administered 16 days after surgery.

Treatment:

Craniotomy and occipital lobectomy. Additional tumor also removed from parietal area.

Postoperative Course:

Hemiparesis cleared almost completely one week postoperatively. Astereognosis cleared. Still had marked dressing apraxia. Considerable difficulty telling time. Given X-ray therapy.

Diagnosis:

Astrocytoma Grade III, right parietal-temporal-occipital area.

REITAN-INDIANA APHASIA SCREENING TEST

Form for Adults and Older Children

Name: C.B. Age: 45 Date: ______ Examiner: ______

Copy SQUARE	Repeat TRIANGLE
Name SQUARE	Repeat MASSACHUSETTS
Spell SQUARE	Repeat METHODIST EPISCOPAL
Copy CROSS	Write SQUARE
Name CROSS	Read SEVEN
Spell CROSS	Repeat SEVEN
Copy TRIANGLE	Repeat/Explain HE SHOUTED THE WARNING.
Name TRIANGLE	Write HE SHOUTED THE WARNING.
Spell TRIANGLE Spelled and also wrote.	Compute 85 – 27 =
Name BABY	Compute 17 X 3 =
Write CLOCK	Name KEY
Name FORK	Demonstrate use of KEY
Read 7 SIX 2 "SIX 2." (Examiner questioned her.) "SIX 2." (Examiner pointed to 7, then responded correctly.)	Draw KEY
Read MGW	Read PLACE LEFT HAND TO RIGHT EAR.
Reading I	Place LEFT HAND TO RIGHT EAR
Reading II "Friendly famous dog shows." Notice that the patient read only the words on the right side.	Place LEFT HAND TO LEFT ELBOW

REITAN-KLØVE SENSORY-PERCEPTUAL EXAMINATION

(Instance indicated where stimulus was not perceived or was incorrectly perceived.)

TACTILE:

RH					LH					Both:	RH					LH						
RH					LF					Both:	RH					LF						
LH					RF						LH					RF						

AUDITORY:

RE					LE					Both:	RE					LE				

VISUAL:

																	X		X		– (Above eye level)
RV					LV			X		Both: RV						LV	X			X	– (Eye level)
						X	X	X	X								X	X	X	X	– (Below eye level)

TACTILE FINGER RECOGNITION:

Right:	1					2					3					4					5					0 / 20
Left:	1					2					3					4					5					0 / 20

COMMENTS:

FINGER-TIP NUMBER WRITING PERCEPTION:

	4	6	3	5	3	5	4	6	6	5	4	3	5	4	6	3	6	3	5	4	
Right:																					__/__
Left:																					__/__

COMMENTS: Not done.

VISUAL FIELDS:

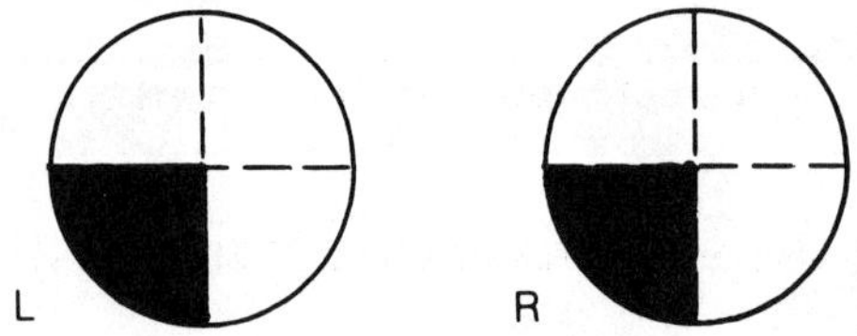

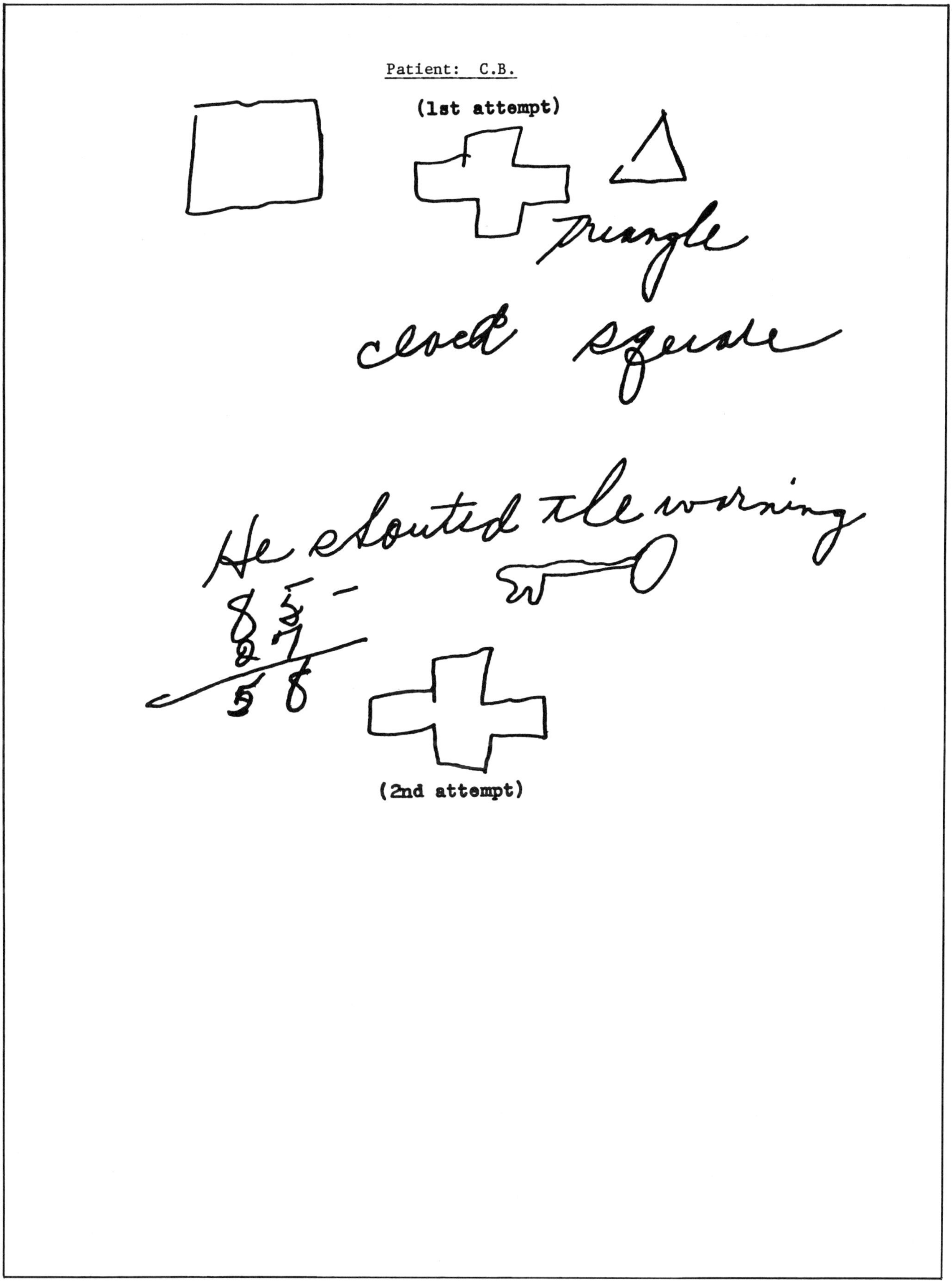
Patient: C.B.
(1st attempt)
(2nd attempt)

C.B. – A 45-year-old right-handed female homemaker with a twelfth grade education.

Identification of brain-related deficits:

This woman was feeling ill at the time of our examination and the technician felt that she might encounter difficulties in doing the testing because the patient became dizzy when she sat up. As a result, the examination was performed by Hallgrim Kløve and myself in the patient's hospital room. Because of some discomfort that was being experienced by the patient, we did not perform the finger-tip number writing perception test. However, the other parts of the Aphasia Screening Test were given as well as the Sensory-perceptual Examination. Having administered the tests personally, it will be possible to provide a description of certain responses on a first-hand basis.

As noted on the recording form, this woman had few difficulties on the verbal parts of the aphasia test. However, when responding to the item "7 SIX 2," the patient first said only SIX 2. She was questioned about her response and she looked at the stimulus figure again and repeated her first response, SIX 2. At that time I pointed to the seven, calling it specifically to the patient's attention. Then she responded correctly. It was apparent that the patient had a tendency to fail to respond to the left side of the stimulus configuration.

The only other mistake she made was in responding to the second reading item. She read only the words on the right half of the configuration – friendly famous dog shows. Again, it was apparent that she was responding only to the right side and showed a definite tendency to ignore the left side of the stimulus material.

It can be noted from the patient's drawings and writing that her writing was done quickly and spontaneously and that she had no noticeable problems. It is necessary for the examiner to observe in many instances the writing of the items included in this test because there are personal idiosyncracies in writing this material as with any other material. Thus, some judges might feel that the patient may have made a mistake on the "k" in the word "clock", perhaps have had difficulty with the "h" in the word "shouted", with the "h" in the word "the", and with the "a" in the word "warning." However, these appear to be personal idiosyncrasies in writing and merely represent the patient's normal writing style. One of the great advantages in using a formal test, as contrasted with presenting any stimulus items that might come to mind, is that one becomes familiar with the personal writing styles of individual subjects and learns quickly to differentiate between manifestations of pathology and normal variations.

The patient's drawings show definite abnormalities. The square was within normal limits but the patient's attempt to draw the cross showed a distinct deviation from normality. The upper and lower extremities were not in the same plane and this was even more apparent for the lateral extremities. In the patient's attempt to draw the triangle, her second line was too long and, when she drew the bottom line, she found it necessary to go back in the direction of the first line in order to close the figure. This kind of mistake is clearly indicative of right cerebral damage, although the overall spatial distortion of the figures is not extremely pronounced. At the end of the examination we had the patient draw another cross and she made exactly the same kind of mistakes as she had made the first time. It is difficult to judge the drawing of the key because the patient did not go into enough detail. Nevertheless, the mistakes on the two crosses and the triangle are quite typical of right cerebral hemisphere damage.

The patient had no difficulty with tactile or auditory tests of double simultaneous stimulation. However, when the visual test was administered I thought at first that the patient had a complete left homonymous hemianopsia. She tended to fail to respond to any stimulus toward her left side. However, on some trials I was able to elicit a correct response in the upper part of the visual field on the left side. I realized that I was eliciting a combination of deficits including a visual field loss in in the lower quadrant and a very strong tendency toward imperception in the upper quadrant on the left side. I proceeded to map the visual fields by confrontation testing, being extremely careful that there were no competing stimuli within the patient's visual field. With very careful administration of single stimuli I was able consistently to elicit correct responses in the upper part of the left visual field for each eye but never in the lower part. It was apparent, therefore, that the basic loss in the visual fields was represented by a left lower homonymous quadrantanopsia. In addition, however, the patient had left-sided imperception. She frequently failed to respond in the middle and the upper part of the left visual field when a competing stimulus was given on the right side. Being able to establish that a primary visual field loss was present only in the lower quadrant turned out to be quite important with respect to the overall intepretation of the findings. In fact, I learned later, in reviewing the patient's chart, that prior confrontation testing of the visual fields had been done by both a neurologist and a neurological surgeon and, in each instance, they had concluded that the patient had a complete left homonymous hemianopsia.

Interpretation of the results for C.B.:

The tendency shown by this woman to ignore, or at least fail to respond to, the left side of stimulus configurations represents quite a significant type of mistake inasmuch as it is associated with seriously destructive lesions of the right cerebral hemisphere. This manifestation is seen most frequently in persons with intrinsic tumors or strokes. A frequent presumption is that a visual field defect is a necessary or responsible condition as a basis for such deficits. This is not the case. Many patients with right cerebral lesions show such deficits even though their visual fields are full. Thus, the perceptual disorder manifested is not a result of primary sensory deficit, but instead represents a more complex perceptual phenomenon.

The errors in drawing the cross and the triangle were quite definite and characteristic of right cerebral damage. Nevertheless, the four extremities were present on each cross and the drawings were not as distinctly impaired as is the case with many persons having seriously destructive right cerebral lesions. Thus, there is a mild incompatibility between the strong tendency shown by this woman to ignore the left side of spatial configurations and the adequacy of drawing of the cross and triangle. If the lesion had been in the posterior part of the right cerebral hemisphere, one would certainly have expected the patient to have more difficulty in copying these figures. The fact that her difficulty was not extremely prounounced would be more compatible with frontal than posterior involvement in the right cerebral hemisphere. However, if the patient had a complete left homonymous hemianopsia, one would have to postulate a rather complete interruption of the geniculostriate tract. A frontal lesion would be less likely to cause a complete left homonymous visual field defect because the fibers of the geniculostriate tract are not structurally located within the frontal lobe. Thus, it would have been difficult to have resolved the relatively mild, though definite, impairment in drawing the figures with a left homonymous hemianopsia. We also would have had a problem in that we failed to find any evidence of impairment of tactile finger recognition on either hand. If the posterior part of the cerebral hemisphere had been involved, giving rise to the tendency to fail to perceive the left side of stimulus configurations and mild but definite drawing difficulties, one would certainly have expected some difficulty with finger localization on the left hand. However, with a frontal lesion, not directly or extensively involving the parietal area, one could postulate that tactile difficulties of this type might not be present.

Considering these overall factors, the critical point of information was that the patient appeared to have a primary visual field loss on the left side of each eye that involved only the lower quadrant. A frontal lesion may often extend to involve the anterior part of the white matter in the parietal lobe, thus interrupting only some of the fibers in the geniculostriate pathway and, as a result, causing only a partial homonymous visual field loss. If fibers of the geniculostriate pathway are involved in the parietal area, the visual field loss is customarily in the lower part of the visual fields whereas involvement of the temporal lobe customarily causes losses in the upper part of the visual field. The lower quadrants were lost in this instance, suggesting that a frontal lesion, invading the parietal area in its most anterior aspects, could well have been responsible. A frontal lesion would also fit the relatively mild deficit shown on the drawings of the cross and triangle better than a posterior lesion. Thus, the test results were quite indicative of a lesion involving principally the frontal lobe of the right cerebral hemisphere.

The importance of careful examination is clearly indicated in this case. In fact, clinical examination of this woman by persons who had interpreted imperception in the upper part of the left visual field, together with a primary visual field loss in the lower part, as evidence of a left homonymous hemianopsia had been inclined, on the basis of clinical evaluation, to place the lesion in the posterior part of the right cerebral hemisphere. One can note from these results that important inferences can be drawn and a good deal can be learned in the individual case from evaluating the degree of deficit and the combination of deficits in terms of their complementary meaning.

The types of deficits shown by C.B. have serious implications. This is especially true in consideration of the patient's tendency to fail to perceive and respond to the left side of certain spatial configurations. As noted above, this tends to happen with intrinsic tumors and with strokes, although it sometimes occurs in persons with traumatic damage. In this case the likely postulate would be that this woman had a right frontal intrinsic tumor. We would judge that the lesion was a tumor rather than a cerebral vascular accident because of the complete absence of any difficulty in tactile finger recognition with the left hand. If the patient had experienced a stroke it is likely that she would have had some deficiencies of this type on the left side. It should be clear from this example, as well as others, that we use both positive and negative findings as a basis for drawing conclusions in the individual case.

C.B.

NEUROLOGICAL SUMMARY

Symptoms:

Headaches and lethargy.
Two years prior to admission patient had a generalized seizure.
Six weeks prior to admission she developed severe headaches and blurring of vision.
Memory had been impaired for an indefinite period.
For two weeks prior to admission she had become progressively more lethargic and confused.

Signs:

Lethargic, memory poor, confused and disoriented.
Disk margins blurred, left lower quadrant field defect, suppression on left, left Hoffman and left Babinski.

Handedness:

Right.

Diagnostic Tests:

EEG: Delta Grade II, maximal right Sylvian.
X-rays: Skull films negative. Chest films negative.
Ventriculogram: Large tumor in right frontal-parietal area with displacement of ventricular system to left and depression of frontal horn.
Neuropsychological tests administered 6 days before surgery.

Treatment:

Craniotomy, right frontal. Large oligodendroglioma found.
Frontal lobectomy done.

Postoperative Course:

Expired second postoperative day.

REITAN-INDIANA APHASIA SCREENING TEST

PATIENT: V.N.

Copy SQUARE	Repeat TRIANGLE
Name SQUARE "Box"; (Examiner questioned, then responded correctly.)	Repeat MASSACHUSETTS "Massachusesss"
Spell SQUARE	Repeat METHODIST EPISCOPAL
Copy CROSS	Write SQUARE
Name CROSS	Read SEVEN
Spell CROSS	Repeat SEVEN
Copy TRIANGLE	Repeat/Explain HE SHOUTED THE WARNING.
Name TRIANGLE	Write HE SHOUTED THE WARNING.
Spell TRIANGLE	Compute 85 – 27 =
Name BABY	Compute 17 X 3 =
Write CLOCK	Name KEY
Name FORK	Demonstrate use of KEY
Read 7 SIX 2	Draw KEY
Read MGW	Read PLACE LEFT HAND TO RIGHT EAR.
Reading I	Place LEFT HAND TO RIGHT EAR
Reading II	Place LEFT HAND TO LEFT ELBOW

REITAN-KLØVE SENSORY-PERCEPTUAL EXAMINATION

(Instance indicated where stimulus was not perceived or was incorrectly perceived.)

TACTILE:

RH					LH					Both: RH					LH	X			
RH					LF					Both: RH					LF				
LH					RF					LH					RF				

AUDITORY:

RE					LE					Both: RE					LE	X		X	

VISUAL:

																				– (Above eye level)
RV					LV					Both: RV					LV					– (Eye level)
																				– (Below eye level)

TACTILE FINGER RECOGNITION:

Right:	1					2					3					4					5					0/20
Left:	1					2					3					4			5		5					1/20

COMMENTS:

FINGER-TIP NUMBER WRITING PERCEPTION:

	4	6	3	5	3	5	4	6	6	5	4	3	5	4	6	3	6	3	5	4	
Right:	X																				1/20
Left:	2			3																	2/20

COMMENTS:

VISUAL FIELDS: L R FULL

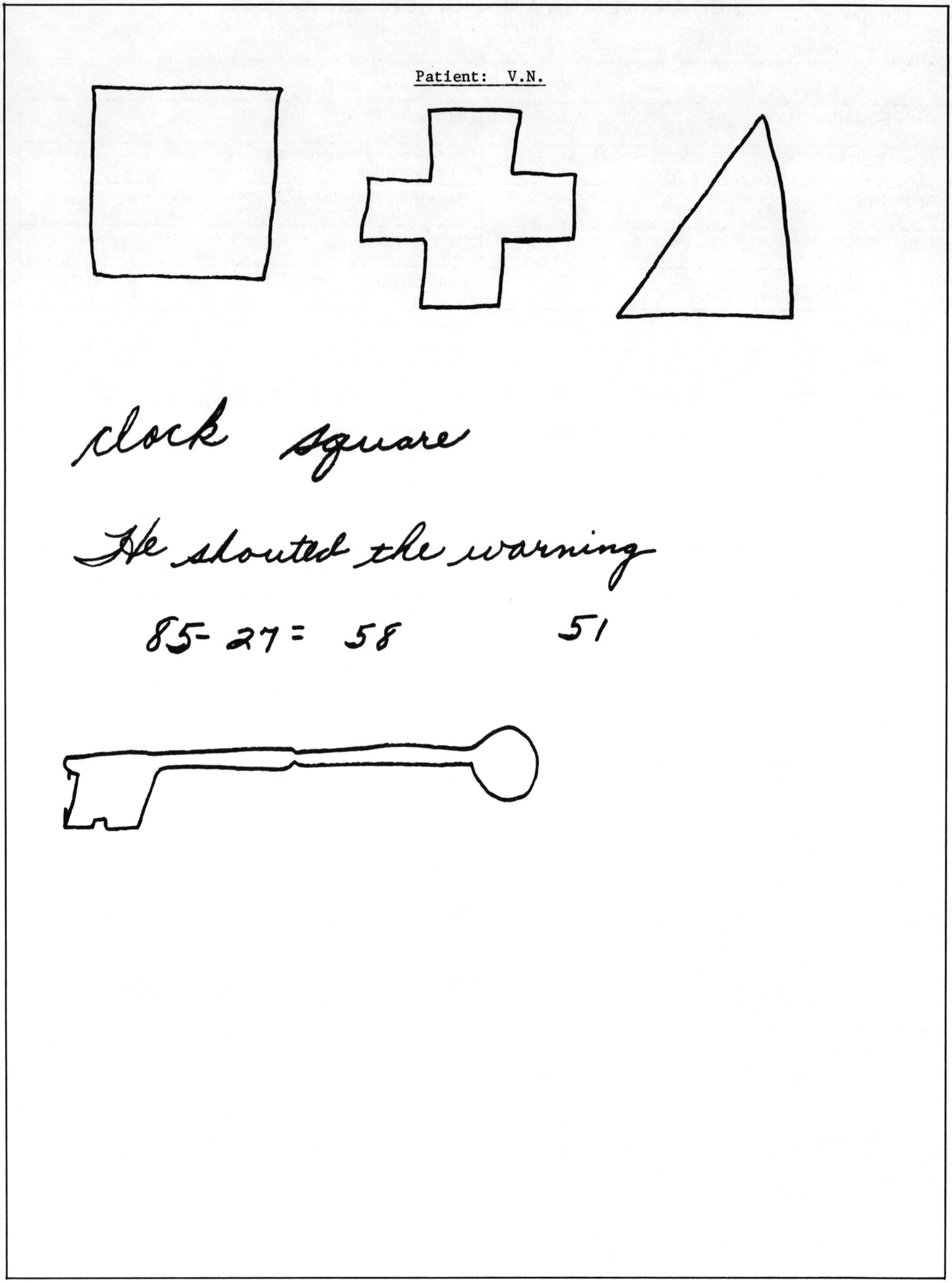
Patient: V.N.
clock square
He shouted the warning
85-27= 58
51

V.N. – A 40-year-old right-handed female cook with a twelfth grade education.

Identification of brain-related deficits:

This woman showed relatively few deficits. As noted on the form for the Aphasia test, she identified the SQUARE as a "box." When she was questioned by the examiner and asked if she could think of another name, she identified it correctly. She had just a mild degree of slurring in her repetition of MASSACHUSETTS, but her response was within normal limits.

Observation of the patient's writing and drawings shows that she did quite well. It is clear that she has excellent handwriting and has received adequate and proper training. Her drawings of the square, cross, and triangle were also within normal limits. However, her drawing of the key showed deficits that probably have some significance. Inexperienced persons refer immediately to the fact that she did not draw the inside part of the handle. However, this kind of mistake is made by many persons, including normals. For some reason people sometimes do not pay much attention to the handle. The elongation of the stem is also cited by inexperienced persons as being a sign of brain damage. However, this is not necessarily the case. Many persons make a rather short or a rather long stem. The "teeth" of the key, in this instance, do not give enough detail to permit one to draw conclusions about brain functions. However, the small lines at the extreme left side of the figure are probably pathological. This is particularly true of the upper line extending from the "nose" of the key. One scarcely ever would see a mistake of this kind in a person with normal brain functions. While the error seems minimal, and many persons would be inclined to think that I was engaging in over-interpretation, I can say on the basis of extensive experience that the odds are extremely minimal that one would find an error of this kind among normal controls. One certainly does find poorly drawn keys, but not this particular kind of error. However, this was the only abnormal manifestation up to this point.

The Sensory-perceptual Examination yielded a little additional information. The patient failed to report a tactile stimulus to her left hand in one instance when both hands were stimulated. One mistake is really not enough to use as a basis for drawing conclusions about impaired brain functions. However, with auditory stimulation she made mistakes in two of four trials on her left side. These results are probably enough to begin to be concerned about the status of the right cerebral hemisphere. The patient made only one mistake with her left hand and no mistakes with her right hand in tactile finger recognition and had only minimal difficulties in finger-tip number writing perception. These findings are probably not enough, by themselves, to feel confident about implicating the right cerebral hemisphere, although when added to the three instances of left-sided imperception, one might begin to have some question. This woman did not show evidence of any constriction of her visual fields on confrontation testing.

Interpretation of the results:

One could raise a question about some impairment of right cerebral functions on the basis of these results, but I would be disinclined to use them in any strongly confident way. This woman did have an intrinsic tumor of the right frontal lobe. It is important to recognize, as noted repeatedly above, that the Aphasia Screening Test and the Sensory-perceptual Examination are based upon elicitation of positive "signs," and it is not uncommon for persons, even with significant brain lesions, sometimes to fail to show positive evidence when only simple examining procedures are used. However, this woman did show evidence of definite impairment on the complete Halstead-Reitan Battery, even though the results were somewhat difficult to interpret with relation to localization.

V.N.

NEUROLOGICAL SUMMARY

Symptoms:

Headaches for six months which were becoming progressively more severe.

Signs:

Physical examination normal.
No papilledema.

Diagnostic Tests:

EEG: Slow wave activity in the right frontal area. This finding led to the hospitalization of the patient.
Physical examination: Normal.
Radioisotopic brain scan: Significant uptake in right frontal area suggesting the possibility of a tumor.
Repeat EEG and radioisotopic exams yielded the same results.
Bilateral carotid angiogram: A 16 mm. shift of right anterior cerebral artery from right to left suggesting a right frontal mass lesion.
Neuropsychological testing was done three days before the angiogram.

Treatment:

Right frontal craniotomy 9 days after admission. Incomplete removal of a right frontal glioma, especially involving the medial portion. Pathological examination of the tissue indicated that it was ependymomatous in nature, but it had a sufficient degree of nuclear atypism and vascular proliferation to classify it as Grade III in the Kernohan system. Some oligodendroglial foci and some rather anaplastic astrocytic foci were observed which pointed toward a glioblastoma multiforme.

Postoperative Course:

The patient did extremely well, showed no evidence of papilledema or neurological deficits on physical examination, was up and about three days after surgery and was discharged from the hospital eight days after the operation.

REITAN-INDIANA APHASIA SCREENING TEST

Form for Adults and Older Children

Name: W.P. Age: 69 Date: ______ Examiner: ______

Copy SQUARE	Repeat TRIANGLE "Tri (long pause) angle"
Name SQUARE	Repeat MASSACHUSETTS "Mashashooshess"
Spell SQUARE "C-Q-U-A-R-E." Patient knew "C" was wrong but couldn't correct it.	Repeat METHODIST EPISCOPAL "Methodist Epistical"
Copy CROSS	Write SQUARE
Name CROSS	Read SEVEN Patient counted on fingers, then responded correctly.
Spell CROSS "S-R-O-C (pause) S-R-O-S-S (pause) C-R-O-C-R-O-C-S-S"	Repeat SEVEN
Copy TRIANGLE	Repeat/Explain HE SHOUTED THE WARNING Repeated "He shouted the morning." Explained: "Helping? I'd be asking for help, wouldn't I?"
Name TRIANGLE After much effort, "T-R-I-A-N-G-L-E (pause) no."	Write HE SHOUTED THE WARNING.
Spell TRIANGLE	Compute 85 - 27 = Patient first added, but incorrectly. Examiner then questioned patient about the minus sign. Then patient wanted to rework the problem. Subtracted, but incorrectly.
Name BABY	Compute 17 X 3 = Wrote "52". Examiner then gave 8x3. Patient responded "21".
Write CLOCK	Name KEY "A lock locker."
Name FORK	Demonstrate use of KEY
Read 7 SIX 2 "7" Patient told to read it all, then responded correctly.	Draw KEY
Read MGW "G W M"	Read PLACE LEFT HAND TO RIGHT EAR. "That's my right." Patient prompted repeatedly to read the item. Finally responded correctly.
Reading I "See the black fog (pause) dog."	Place LEFT HAND TO RIGHT EAR Right hand to right ear. Self-corrected.
Reading II "He is a fiendly animal, a famous winter (pause) wonder (pause) of dog shows. Wonder (pause) wonder."	Place LEFT HAND TO LEFT ELBOW "I don't have any." On questioning he tried and shook his head.

REITAN-KLØVE SENSORY-PERCEPTUAL EXAMINATION

(Instance indicated where stimulus was not perceived or was incorrectly perceived.)

TACTILE:

RH					LH		X		X	Both: RH					LH	X	X	X	X
RH					LF					Both: RH					LF		X	X	
LH	X	X		X	RF					LH	X	X	X	X	RF				

AUDITORY:

RE					LE	X	X	X	X	Both:	RE					LE	X	X	X	X

VISUAL:

						X		X								X	X	X	X	– (Above eye level)
RV					LV				X	Both: RV					LV	X	X	X	X	– (Eye level)
							X	X	X							X	X	X	X	– (Below eye level)

TACTILE FINGER RECOGNITION:

Right:	1					2					3					4					5					0 / 20
Left:	1			2	2	2			1		3		2		2	4	3	2	3	3	5	3	4	3	3	13 / 20

COMMENTS:

FINGER-TIP NUMBER WRITING PERCEPTION:

	4	6	3	5	3	5	4	6	6	5	4	3	5	4	6	3	6	3	5	4	
Right:				0			X	X		X		X					X		X		7 / 20
Left:	X									X				X			X		0		5 / 20

COMMENTS: YOUNG CHILDREN's system used for all Sensory-Perceptual Tests

VISUAL FIELDS:

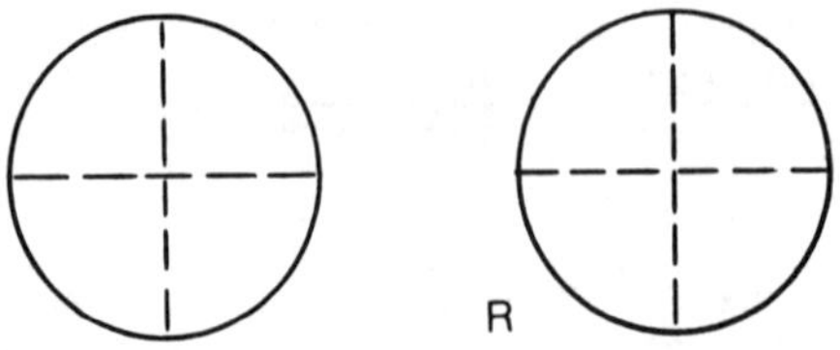

L R

FULL

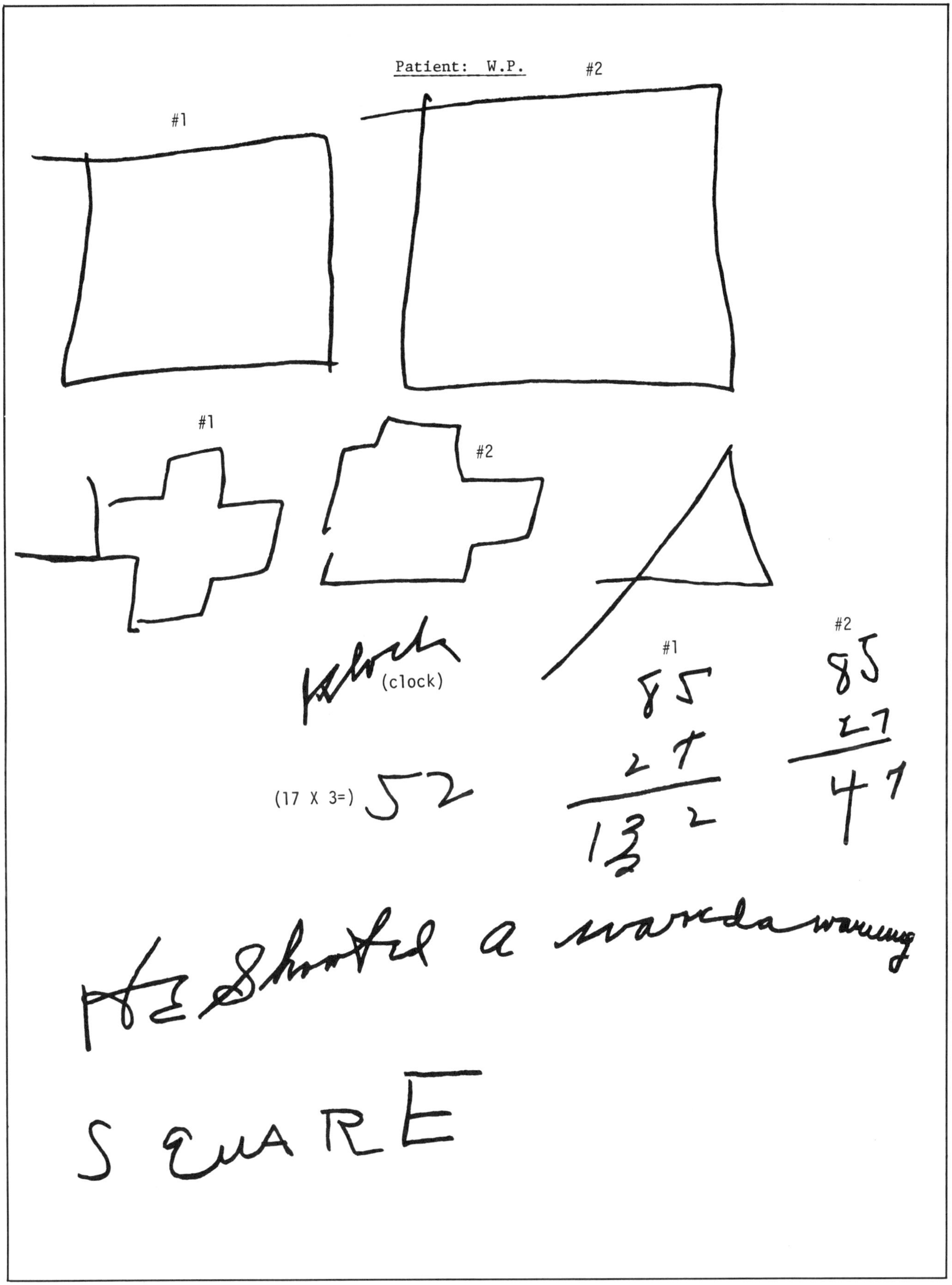
Patient: W.P.
#1
#2
#1
#2
(clock)
#1
#2
(17 X 3=)

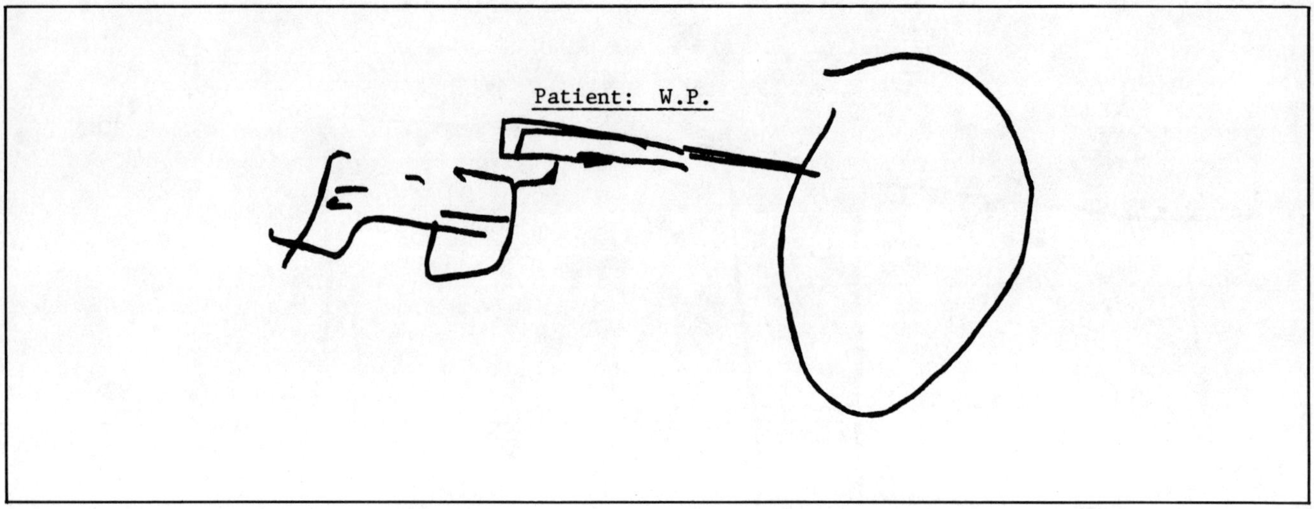

W.P. – A 69-year-old right-handed male engineer with a twelfth grade education.

Identification of brain-related deficits:

Reference to the Aphasia test form indicates that this man had a number of difficulties. He was able to name the square correctly, but when asked to spell the word, he began with a "c" rather than an "s." The patient knew that the "c" was wrong but was not able to make a correction. This is rather typical of dysphasic persons. He had spelling difficulty again when attempting to spell CROSS. He obviously confused the sequence of the letters and demonstrated typical aphasic spelling difficulties. He spelled TRIANGLE correctly although he did so with a great deal of effort and did not recognize that he had spelled the word correctly. The next mistake occurred on 7 SIX 2. The patient responded only to the first aspect of the stimulus configuration until he was told to read the entire thing. One could wonder whether this might represent a tendency to ignore the *right* side of the stimulus configuration, although such deficits rarely occur even in persons with severely destructive left cerebral lesions. (In contrast, ignoring the *left* side of a stimulus configuration occurs not uncommonly in persons with severely destructive right cerebral lesions.) His confusion of the sequence of the letters MGW also suggests that the patient had some clear difficulty with verbal material. This was made equally apparent in his difficulty with reading. The slurring of MASSACHUSETTS may possibly go beyond acceptable limits for peripheral dysarthria and raise a question of some degree of central dysarthria. However, "epistical" for EPISCOPAL is not particularly abnormal because it occurs in a number of control subjects. The patient had some difficulty in reading SEVEN having to count on his fingers in order to reach the correct word, but finally being able to say the word correctly. This probably represents a combination of dyslexia and dysnomia. When asked to repeat the sentence, "He shouted the warning," he said "morning" instead of "warning." He had clear difficulty in his explanation of the sentence, apparently not understanding the concept of danger nor clearly understanding what the sentence might mean. This response demonstrates the presence of auditory verbal dysgnosia. His naming deficit (dysnomia) was clearly demonstrated in his response when asked to name the key, calling the key "a lock locker." He had some difficulty in reading the sentence PLACE LEFT HAND TO RIGHT EAR and needed repeated instructions from the examiner, even to the point of helping him to begin reading the sentence. These difficulties probably represent a failure to understand instructions (auditory verbal dysgnosia) and reading difficulty (dyslexia). He showed evidence of mild right-left confusion, although he corrected himself. His response to the last item, concerned with putting his left hand to his left elbow was, "I don't have any." The verbal response was not exact, but the patient probably was trying to indicate that he recognized that it was impossible. It is clear from these responses that the patient has some definite organic language deficit.

In referring to the patient's drawing and writing, he added instead of subtracted in his first attempt to work out the problem 85 − 27 = ____. This occurs with left hemisphere lesions about four times as frequently as with right hemisphere lesions. His attempt to write the sentence, "He shouted the warning," is a perfectly characteristic example of dysgraphia. This is particularly clear in his attempt to write "warning." He became confused in forming the letters until he finally made almost a desperate effort and got the letters written fairly well. His confusion between writing and printing on the word SQUARE also is typical of difficulty in dealing with language symbols. Thus, the aphasia examination indicates the presence of spelling dyspraxia, dysnomia, dyslexia, possible visual letter dysgnosia, possible central dysarthria, auditory verbal dysgnosia, dyscalculia, and some degree of right-left confusion. These are all signs of left cerebral damage.

The patient also had very pronounced difficulty in copying simple spatial configurations. Probably, his drawings of the square were within normal limits, although he seemed to draw the first line somewhat long. His confusion in two attempts to draw the cross is quite typical of serious constructional dyspraxia of the type that is frequently seen with involvement of the middle to posterior part of the right cerebral hemisphere. The first line on the triangle also was entirely too long. Even though the patient did draw the shape of the triangle, he obviously had some difficulty with the spatial configuration. The same type of difficulty was clearly evident in the patient's attempt to draw the key. He tried to go into detail but obviously failed to represent the figure at all well. This was particularly true on the left side of the figure. Thus, constructional dyspraxia was clearly indicated by the patient's performances in addition to language difficulty.

The Sensory-perceptual Examination yielded overall evidence of much more serious damage of the right cerebral hemisphere than the left. The patient showed evidence of some degree of hypesthesia involving the left hand although the imperception phenomena with double simultaneous tactile stimulation involved only the left side. The patient apparently had a primary hearing loss involving the left ear because he was unable to respond to a stimulus on that side either with unilateral or bilateral stimulation. Although the patient's visual fields were full on the basis of confrontation testing, he showed a tendency to fail to respond to visual stimuli toward his left side. However, his failure to perceive stimuli on the left side was complete and absolute when competing stimuli were given on the right side.

This man had no difficulty in tactile finger recognition on his right hand but made 13 mistakes in 20 trials on his left hand. Finger-tip symbol writing was done because the patient was too confused to do finger-tip number writing. He made seven mistakes on his right hand and five mistakes on his left hand. Instead of interpreting this as necessarily showing bilateral cerebral damage in the parietal areas, the results may have been due to confusion on the part of the patient.

Interpretation of the results:

It is apparent that this man had clear language difficulties of the kind that occur with left cerebral damage. As shown in Table 12, such pronounced and widespread language deficits scarcely occur in persons with lesions involving only the right cerebral hemisphere. It is equally clear that the patient had evidence of pronounced constructional dyspraxia and that the Sensory-perceptual Examination consistently indicated that his right cerebral hemisphere was more seriously damaged than his left cerebral hemisphere. It is important to realize that aphasic symptoms as such, while they may definitely implicate the left cerebral hemisphere,do not permit a direct comparison with constructional dyspraxia as a basis for comparing the functional status of homologous areas within each cerebral hemisphere as is done with the Sensory-perceptual Examination. On the Sensory-perceptual Examination, when both sides were given an equal chance for response, the results indicated that this man's left cerebral hemisphere consistently performed fairly well, but evidence of impairment was present for the right cerebral hemisphere. Using these comparisons, based on essentially identical input into each cerebral hemisphere, we would postulate that the principal damage of this man's brain was in the right cerebral hemisphere, particularly involving the middle part. Results of this kind might very well be associated with neoplastic damage or with a stroke. However, because the test results provided positive evidence involving both cerebral hemispheres one might be more inclined to think of focal damage in each cerebral hemisphere and this, in turn, would incline one to postulate the presence of bilateral neoplasms. In addition, the patient's visual fields were full, and this again is a factor pointing toward tumor rather than CVA. If a vascular lesion had caused as many deficits as shown by this man in other respects, he almost certainly would have had impairment of his visual fields. Our interpretation of these results, therefore, would be that this man had a large tumor in the middle part of his right cerebral hemisphere. The area of involvement in the left cerebral hemisphere, however, would seem to be more discrete and delimited. The patient showed no evidence of tactile finger recognition losses (finger dysgnosia) on his right hand, a finding that would probably tend to clear his left parietal area. However, the presence of definite aphasia inescapably points toward left cerebral damage. Thus, the remaining area for this damage would principally fall in the left temporal lobe. It would appear from the overall findings that the patient had definite damage of his left temporal lobe and more extensive damage in the middle part of the right cerebral hemisphere. We were inclined to postulate the presence of metastatic carcinoma, considering the fact that primary tumors of the brain rarely occupy more than one contiguous location.

I learned the nature of the pathology of this man's brain at a brain-cutting session. The neuropathologist originally asked the neurosurgeon who had operated on this man to review his findings. He reviewed the clinical history, x-rays, and results of the examination together with histological examinations of the removed tissue. All of the findings pointed toward a large tumor in the middle part of the right cerebral hemisphere. The neuropathologist then asked about the neuropsychological findings and the types of conclusions that I had reached. I pointed out that we saw clear evidence of this large lesion in the right cerebral hemisphere but that I felt that there must be a lesion of the left temporal lobe as well, considering the evidence of aphasia in this right-handed man. As the neuropathologist inspected the brain, he noted the evidence of surgical intervention in the right cerebral hemisphere. He also noted that there was a rather extensive area in the left temporal lobe that was represented by softening and loss of cerebral cortical tissue. Exactly the reason for this left temporal lobe involvement was not identified, although the evidence of structural damage in that area was quite clear. The patient did not have a tumor involving the left temporal lobe, but the manifestations of aphasic deficits almost certainly were related to the softening and loss of cerebral cortex in that area.

If one is knowledgeable with respect to the types of deficits that almost certainly represent brain dysfunction, one can draw conclusions that represent the entire picture for the individual. The neurosurgeon had not been aware, until autopsy, that the left temporal lobe was also damaged. However, this damage was entirely clear and implied unequivocally by the language difficulties shown by this man on the Aphasia test. It is also interesting to note, however, that if the patient had not died, providing the opportunity for autopsy, we would not have had confirming evidence of the left temporal lobe damage.

Perhaps one could raise a question as to whether all of the deficits on the aphasia examination might not be attributed to a left cerebral lesion, presuming that the constructional dyspraxia might have been caused by involvement of the posterior part of the language area. However, the kinds of mistakes made by this man in dealing with spatial configurations are not typical of the drawing difficulties seen in persons with left cerebral damage. Instead, they clearly manifest confusion with respect to spatial relationships, a type of deficit that is much more common with right cerebral lesions. Secondly, the importance of the Sensory-perceptual Examination, in conjunction with the Aphasia test, is clearly indicated. The Sensory-perceptual Examination presented very clear evidence of striking damage to the right cerebral hemisphere. In this case one would expect the results of the remainder of the Halstead-Reitan Battery to show evidence of very serious and profound impairment and very possibly to provide additional evidence of neoplastic involvement (as contrasted with a stroke) through retention of a degree of motor functions in the left upper extremity.

W.P.

NEUROLOGICAL SUMMARY

Symptoms and Prior Findings:

For one year the patient had been increasingly forgetful and had difficulty walking.

Three months prior to admission had a seizure that principally consisted of turning of head and eyes to the right.

After some delay he was admitted to a local hospital where a cerebral angiogram suggested a tumor in the right cerebral hemisphere.

Admitted to our hospital for further evaluation and possible treatment.

Signs:

Physical neurological examination: Impaired ability to walk, some weakness and dyspraxia of left upper extremity, weakness of left upper eyelid and some droop of left side of mouth, dysstereognosis on the left, dressing dyspraxia and possibly some aphasia.

Diagnostic Tests:

EEG: Delta waves, Grade II, right Sylvian area.

Bilateral cerebral angiogram: Definite shift of the pericallosal vessel to the left under the falx and elevation of the right Sylvian vessels. Large tumor stain of the anterior portion of the right temporal lobe.

Neuropsychological examination: Eleven days after hospital admission and ten days before surgery.

Treatment:

Craniotomy 21 days after hospital admission with partial removal of a tumor in the right temporal area. The surgeon observed that there was extensive infiltration in the right temporal lobe and probably posteriorly to more of the right cerebral hemisphere.

Postoperative Course:

Mild improvement following surgery, but within two months he clearly was deteriorating, and he died 71 days after surgery.

Autopsy Findings:

Pronounced swelling of both cerebral hemispheres. Right hemisphere shifted to the left; right lateral ventricle had crossed the midline and was impinging on the left lateral ventricle. Dura mater thickened and inflamed in the area of the right temporal lobe and evidence of surgical tissue removal in this area was apparent. The carotid and cerebral supply systems had only minimal arteriosclerotic plaques. The dura mater had some adhesion to the left temporal lobe and there was some softening and loss of left temporal cortex. A large neoplasm extended through the entire right temporal area, invading the deep white matter and extending into the right pulvinar. Grossly, the tumor did not extend into the right parietal area, but it had displaced the parietal operculum upward. The histological diagnosis was glioblastoma multiforme.

REITAN-INDIANA APHASIA SCREENING TEST

Form for Adults and Older Children

Name: C.L. Age: 46 Date: _____ Examiner: _____

Copy SQUARE	Repeat TRIANGLE
Name SQUARE	Repeat MASSACHUSETTS
Spell SQUARE	Repeat METHODIST EPISCOPAL
Copy CROSS	Write SQUARE
Name CROSS "Not a star." (Examiner asked, Is it a circle?) "No. I've seen a red shape like (pause) Red Cross (pause) call this a cross?"	Read SEVEN
Spell CROSS	Repeat SEVEN
Copy TRIANGLE	Repeat/Explain HE SHOUTED THE WARNING.
Name TRIANGLE	Write HE SHOUTED THE WARNING.
Spell TRIANGLE	Compute 85 – 27 =
Name BABY	Compute 17 X 3 = Patient verbalized "17x2=34+17= (pause) 17x3 (pause) 3x7=21." Then wrote on table with fingers and finally said "51". Examiner gave 8x6 and patient responded "48".
Write CLOCK	Name KEY
Name FORK	Demonstrate use of KEY
Read 7 SIX 2	Draw KEY
Read MGW	Read PLACE LEFT HAND TO RIGHT EAR.
Reading I	Place LEFT HAND TO RIGHT EAR Right hand to right ear, then corrected.
Reading II	Place LEFT HAND TO LEFT ELBOW

REITAN-KLØVE SENSORY-PERCEPTUAL EXAMINATION

(Instance indicated where stimulus was not perceived or was incorrectly perceived.)

TACTILE:

RH					LH					Both: RH					LH			
RH					LF					Both: RH					LF			
LH					RF					LH					RF			

AUDITORY:

RE					LE	X	X	X	X	Both: RE					LE	X	X	X	X

VISUAL:

																			– (Above eye level)
RV					LV					Both: RV		X			LV				– (Eye level)
	X	X	X	X							X	X	X	X					– (Below eye level)

TACTILE FINGER RECOGNITION:

Right:	1					2					3					4					5					0 / 20
Left:	1					2					3					4					5					0 / 20

COMMENTS:

FINGER-TIP NUMBER WRITING PERCEPTION:

	4	6	3	5	3	5	4	6	6	5	4	3	5	4	6	3	6	3	5	4	
Right:																					0 / 20
Left:																					0 / 20

COMMENTS:

VISUAL FIELDS:

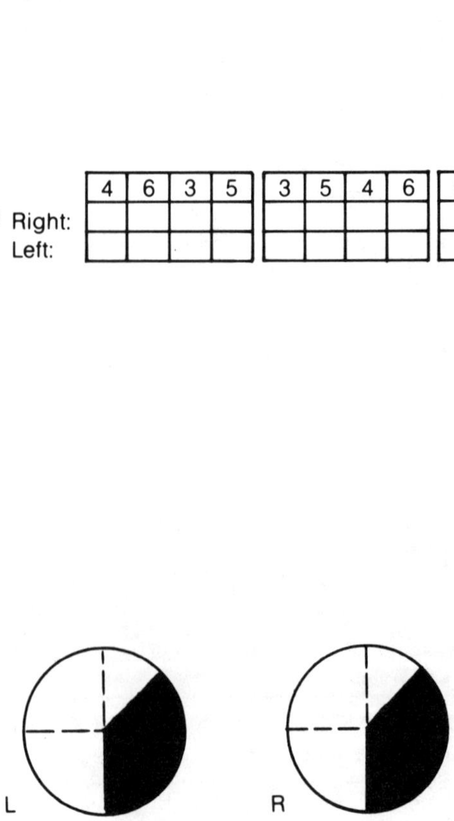

Principally a right homonymous lower quadrant defect.

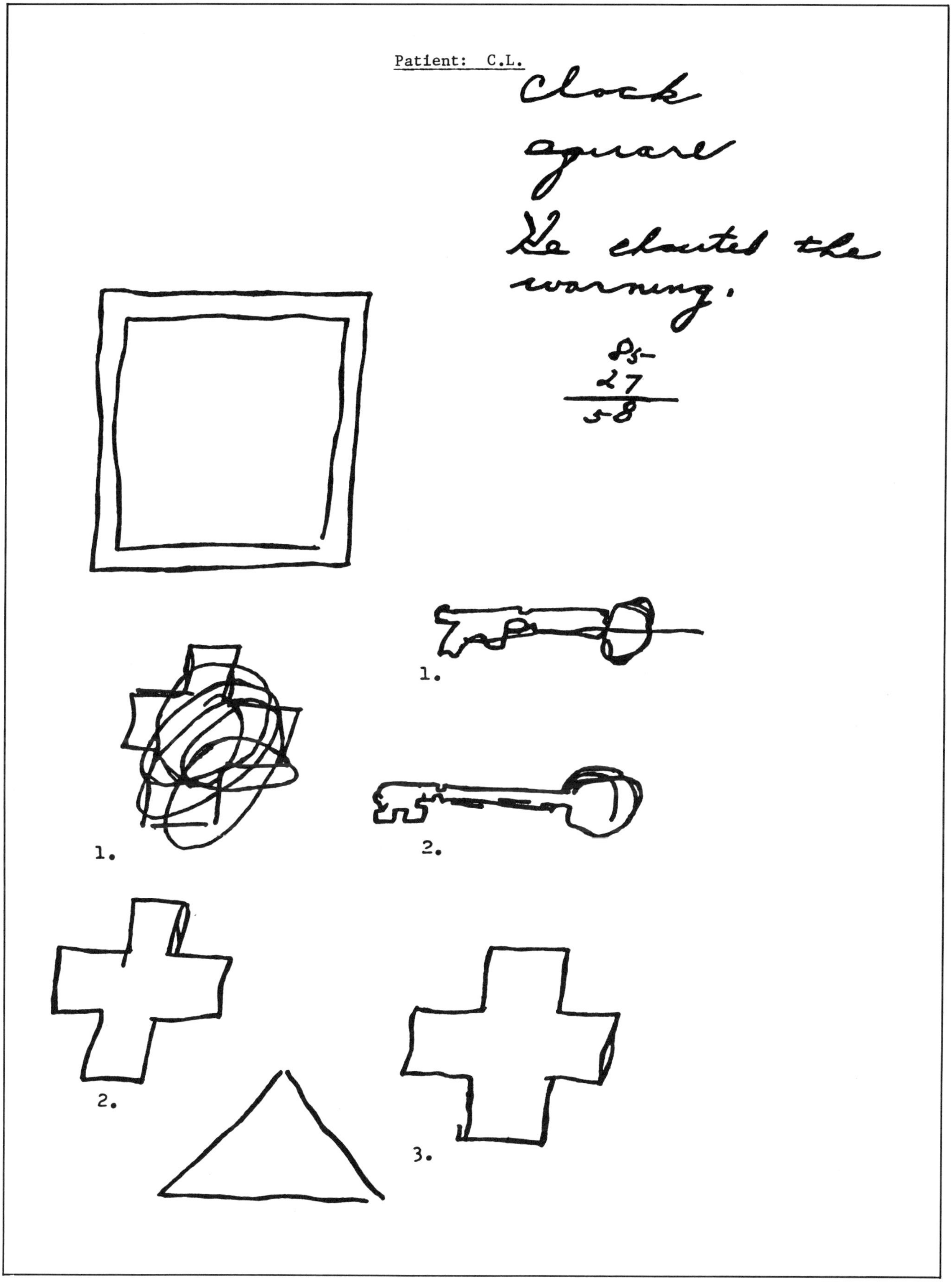
Patient: C.L.
Clock
85
27
58
1.
1.
2.
2.
3.

C.L. – A 46-year-old right-handed female homemaker with a twelfth grade education.

Identification of brain-related deficits:

This woman had relatively few difficulties with the verbal aspects of the Aphasia examination. However, she did have some difficulty in naming the cross. She indicated that it was not a star but was not able to make further progress in offering a name. The examiner prompted her to a certain extent, asking if it was a circle. She would not accept that name and was able, through association with Red Cross, to ask the examiner if it was a cross. For a high school graduate, this kind of confusion in terms of naming is probably pathological and indicative of left cerebral damage. There is strong reason to believe that she has a mild degree of dysnomia.

The patient was able to compute 85 − 27 correctly but she became rather confused in attempting to do 17 × 3 in her head. She was able to multiply 17 × 2 and then was going to add another 17. However, she appeared to become confused and attempted again to do 17 × 3. She said that 3 × 7 was 21 but then, in her head, she was not able to make additional progress. She proceeded to write the numbers on the table with her fingers and then came up with the correct answer. Even though she was able to do 8 × 6 correctly (very possibly on a rote basis), the confusion and difficulty she had with 17 × 3 may well qualify as an indication of mild dyscalculia. The patient also showed evidence of mild right-left confusion, even though she was able to correct her initial error.

Reference to the patient's writing and drawing indicates that she had some trouble with the drawing. This woman drew a double line for the cross. Sometimes we permit a patient to go ahead and do this if they have started (representing the width of the heavy black line used for the stimulus figure), even though we are interested only in the outside shape. She made three attempts to draw the cross. She became very frustrated and dissatisfied with her first drawing and, before the examiner was able to stop her, had scribbled all over the drawing. However, it is possible to see the drawing, and the distortion and asymmetrical placement of both the lateral and vertical extremities is quite clear. The bottom extremity is much wider than the top, and the extremity on the right is longer and not quite in the same plane as the extremity on the left. The patient was asked to draw the cross again and she made very similar mistakes. Finally, she did the task a third time and the drawing was fairly good. Nevertheless, the third drawing of the cross has one type of mistake that is rarely made by control subjects. She proceeded to draw the bottom line of the lower extremity a little too long and then started with the ascending vertical line. However, she changed her mind and went back to begin the vertical line on the left-hand side of the lower extremity a second time. This particular kind of mistake almost certainly is an indication of some difficulty in dealing with the spatial configuration and is of the type that is seen in persons with right cerebral damage.

The patient's first attempt in copying the key was poorly done and illustrated some deficiencies. The notches on the stem of the key, close to the teeth, were not symmetrical and the teeth also deviated strikingly from symmetry. It is difficult, sometimes, to determine whether the deficits in the drawing are actually indicative of right cerebral dysfunction or only poor artistic skill. The second drawing of the cross apparently was done with greater effort and care. However, the "nose" of the figure is rather typical of right cerebral dysfunction. Instead of creating the extension at the top of the figure, the patient apparently had some confusion with respect to the spatial relationships and has the "nose" out of place.

In reviewing this patient's test results, some observers in the past have raised a question with regard to the "h" in the sentence, "He shouted the warning." Very probably this is not a specific deficiency but instead represents an idiosyncratic type of writing response. Thus, while the aphasia examination was performed satisfactorily in the main, the patient did show evidence of mild dysnomia, mild dyscalculia, mild right-left confusion, and mild constructional dyspraxia.

Results of the Sensory-perceptual Examination also showed certain deficiencies. The test for auditory imperception was precluded by the fact that this woman apparently had a primary hearing loss of her left ear. The visual test showed positive findings inasmuch as the patient was not able to appreciate a visual stimulus in the lower part of the right visual field for each eye. The deficit showed up on both unilateral and bilateral simultaneous stimulation. In confrontation testing of the visual fields, the results were definitely abnormal, showing a homonymous loss on the right side in the lower quadrant. This type of deficit would imply the presence of a lesion of the left cerebral hemisphere, perhaps principally in the left parietal area but possibly involving the left temporal lobe as well.

Interpretation of the results:

This woman did not have a great deal of difficulty, but the overall results definitely are not within the normal range. In other words, the types of problems that she had are suggestive of cerebral damage. The mild dysnomia, dyscalculia, and right-left confusion would point toward left cerebral damage. It is difficult to be specific on the basis of these symptoms with respect to localization. However, the fact that the patient had only a partial homonymous visual field loss on the right side suggests that the lesion probably was not exceptionally large. Thus, one could think of a rather discrete lesion in the temporo-parietal area of the left cerebral hemisphere. One would be somewhat reluctant to postulate involvement of the parietal lobes to any major extent because the patient had absolutely no difficulty on either hand in finger localization or finger-tip number writing.

The remaining question concerns the evidence of constructional dyspraxia. It is debatable as to whether one would postulate a specific lesion in the right cerebral hemisphere on the basis of the patient's drawings. Even though she had no difficulty on tactile finger recognition or finger-tip number writing perception, her drawings were mildly deficient. Such a deficit could possibly have been represented by a lesion in the posterior part of the right temporal lobe, but a conservative interpretation probably would call for this as a question rather than as a conclusion.

A cerebral angiogram showed evidence of a left posterior temporal-occipital mass and a right inferior mediotemporal mass. We would postulate that these lesions, representing metastatic carcinoma, were relatively well encapsulated and quite discrete in terms of their overall effects on the brain. The deficits shown by this woman are not as severe as usually seen in persons with bilateral metastatic tumors.

C.L.

NEUROLOGICAL SUMMARY

Symptoms:

Patient had left simple mastectomy 10 months prior to admission. Diagnosis was cystosarcoma phyllodes.
Blurring of vision and severe headaches for 3 months. Also had hallucinatory visual experiences.
Syncopal attacks without clonic or tonic movements, 2 months.
Carotid angiogram done at home town hospital showed displacement of the left anterior cerebral artery.
Received three x-ray therapy treatments and then stopped because of nausea and vomiting.

Signs:

Bilateral papilledema.
Right homonymous lower quadrant visual field defect.

Diagnostic tests:

Routine laboratory tests: Normal.
Bone marrow showed malignant cells.
EEG: Delta Grade II, bilateral temporal. Dysrhythmia Grade II, generalized.
X-ray: Tumor, right lower lung. Angiogram shows shift, left to right. Left posterior temporal-occipital mass. Right inferior medial temporal mass.

Treatment:

Patient given x-ray therapy with some improvement.

Diagnosis:

Cystosarcoma phyllodes with metastases to lung and cerebrum (temporal lobes bilaterally).

REITAN-INDIANA APHASIA SCREENING TEST

Form for Adults and Older Children

Name: A.C. Age: 61 Date: ______ Examiner: ______

Copy SQUARE	Repeat TRIANGLE
Name SQUARE "Paste board"	Repeat MASSACHUSETTS
Spell SQUARE "S-Q-U-E-L-E"	Repeat METHODIST EPISCOPAL "Methodist apisopal."
Copy CROSS	Write SQUARE
Name CROSS	Read SEVEN
Spell CROSS "C-L-O-R-S (pause) double C"	Repeat SEVEN
Copy TRIANGLE	Repeat/Explain HE SHOUTED THE WARNING. Explained meaning of sentence poorly.
Name TRIANGLE "Cross"	Write HE SHOUTED THE WARNING.
Spell TRIANGLE "T-R-A-I-N-G-S"	Compute 85 − 27 = At first patient asked if he was to "add or what?"
Name BABY	Compute 17 X 3 = Patient unable to work problem; then examiner gave 6x2. Patient still very confused.
Write CLOCK	Name KEY
Name FORK	Demonstrate use of KEY
Read 7 SIX 2 "6-2 (pause) 6 and 2 (pause) 6 and 2." Examiner pointed to 7, then responded correctly.	Draw KEY
Read MGW	Read PLACE LEFT HAND TO RIGHT EAR.
Reading I "See the black clock."	Place LEFT HAND TO RIGHT EAR Placed right hand to right ear.
Reading II "He is a friendly animal, a former winner of your dog shows."	Place LEFT HAND TO LEFT ELBOW Tried to place left hand to left elbow, then left hand to right elbow after repetition of instructions.

REITAN-KLØVE SENSORY-PERCEPTUAL EXAMINATION

(Instance indicated where stimulus was not perceived or was incorrectly perceived.)

TACTILE:

RH					LH					Both: RH	X				LH				
RH					LF					Both: RH					LF				
LH					RF					LH					RF				

AUDITORY:

RE					LE					Both: RE					LE				

VISUAL:

																				– (Above eye level)
RV					LV					Both: RV					LV					– (Eye level)
																X	X			– (Below eye level)

TACTILE FINGER RECOGNITION:

Right:	1			1		2					3	2			4	4	3		3	3	5					6/20
Left:	1				1	2		3			3	4		2	2	4	3	3	3		5					8/20

COMMENTS:

FINGER-TIP NUMBER WRITING PERCEPTION:

	4	6	3	5	3	5	4	6	6	5	4	3	5	4	6	3	6	3	5	4	
Right:	5	3							2		3	5	3	5			3				8 / 20
Left:	5						3	4	3		6	5		3	4	5	3		4	6	12 / 20

COMMENTS:

VISUAL FIELDS:

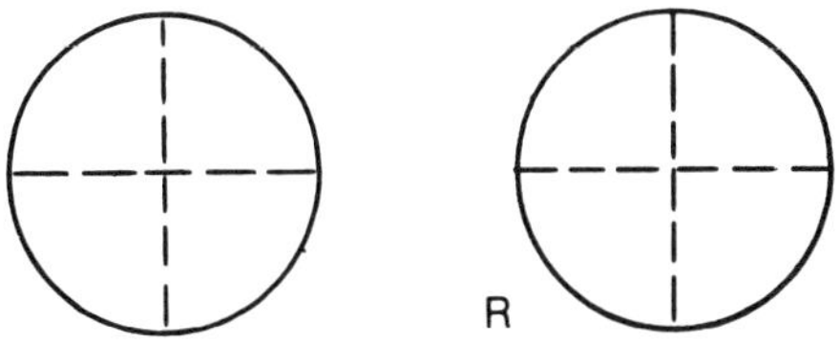

L R

FULL

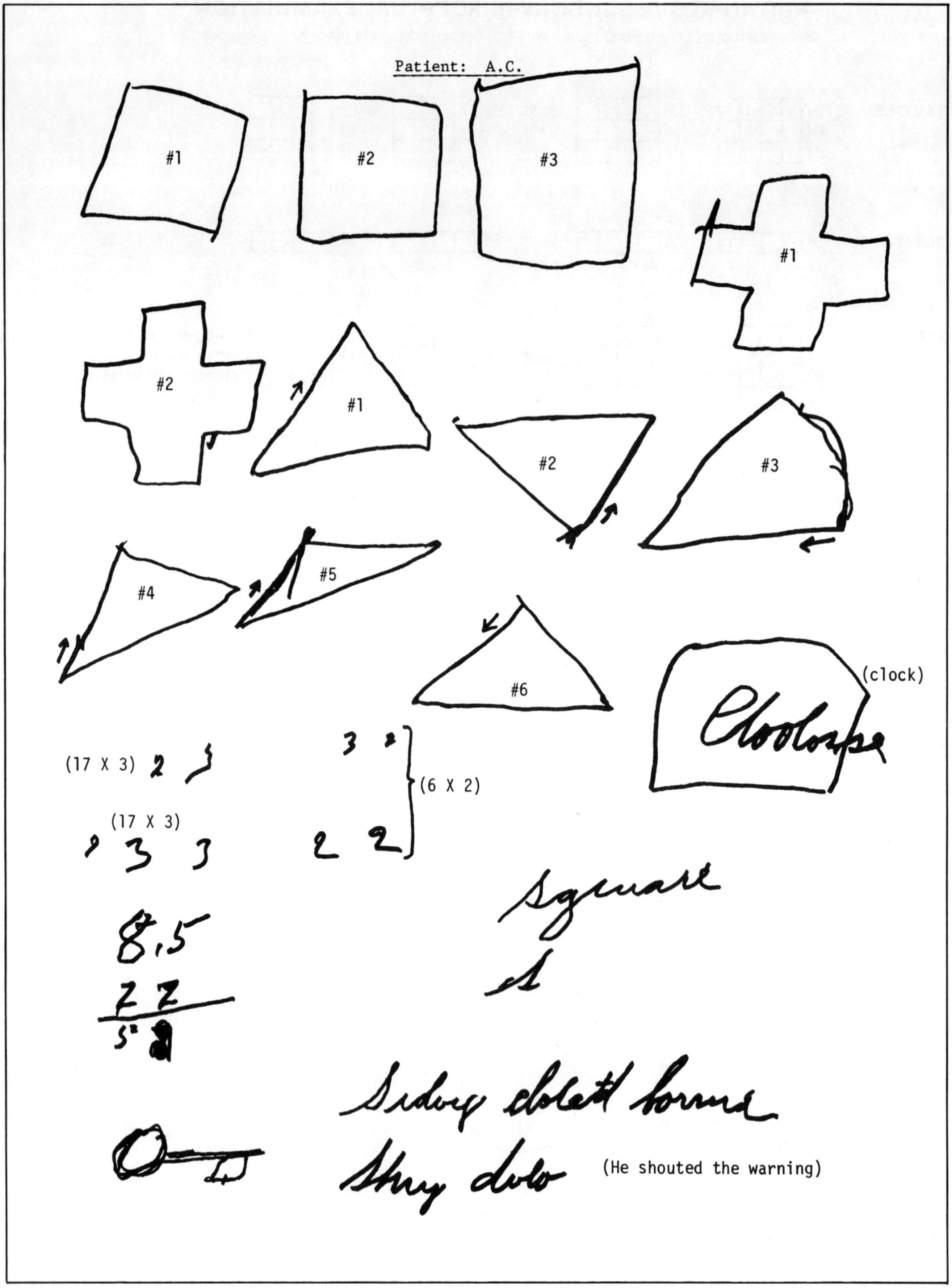
Patient: A.C.
#1
#2
#3
#1
#2
#1
#2
#3
#4
#5
#6
(clock)
(17 X 3)
(17 X 3)
(6 X 2)
(He shouted the warning)

A.C. – A 61-year-old right-handed male saw operator with a fifth grade education.

Identification of brain-related deficits:

Considering the fact that this man had only a fifth grade education, evaluation of his performances must take into consideration the possibility that he has never developed language and verbal communicational skills to a very high level. However, reference to the Aphasia test form quickly indicates that the patient showed deficits that go beyond educational deficiency and are quite characteristic of left cerebral damage. The only name he could give for the square was "pasteboard." He began spelling the word "square" correctly but lost his ability to relate the letters to the sound of the word. Although he named the cross correctly, he also demonstrated definite confusion between appropriate letters and the sound of the word during his atttempt at spelling. He showed a verbal perseverative tendency in his naming of the triangle as a "cross." He showed further spelling difficulty typical of left hemisphere damage in his attempt to spell the word "triangle." The next error occurred on the 7 SIX 2 item. In this case, however, he showed a definite tendency to ignore the left side of the stimulus configuration until the examiner pointed to the 7. Then the patient responded correctly. It is difficult to interpret this response as an indication of language difficulty. Instead, it appears very much as if it were a genuine failure to perceive the 7 (even though the patient's visual fields were full), and thus is an indication of right cerebral dysfunction. Confusion in reading was demonstrated on both reading items. The first item, in which the patient substituted the word "clock" for the word "dog," probably represents another instance of verbal perseveration because the patient had previously been exposed to the clock and had attempted to write the word. This type of verbal perseveration, however, is a manifestation of left cerebral damage. It is difficult to be sure that this man had central dysarthria. His mistake in enunciation involved the word "Episcopal," but the error was more in line with a slurring of the word rather than a loss of the appropriate sounds.

It is sometimes difficult to evaluate the explanation of the sentence, "He shouted the warning." A notation indicated that the patient explained the meaning of the sentence poorly, but it would have been more helpful to have had an actual quotation of his verbalization. Thus, whether the poor explanation of the sentence merely represents generalized cognitive impairment and confusion, or actually indicates the presence of auditory verbal dysgnosia, is difficult to judge. Even though it is often difficult to record the complete verbalizations of patients, it is definitely worthwhile trying to write down as much as possible so that a judgment of the specific nature of the deficiency can be made.

This man was definitely impaired in his ability to do arithmetical computations. However, it is possible that the problems included formally in this test were too difficult for a man with only a fifth grade education. However, when he asked if he was to "add or what?" on the 85 − 27 problem, it is clear that the patient had some confusion with regard to arithmetical processes and this constitutes evidence of dyscalculia. Almost certainly this man would normally have known the meaning of the minus sign. It is possible that 17 × 3 was too difficult for him; the examiner was quite correct in giving a simpler problem. As will be noted on the page showing the patient's written efforts, he was grossly confused even with respect to this problem. Thus, it seems quite definite that this man did demonstrate dyscalculia. On the last two items of the test the patient showed evidence of right-left confusion and may also have shown some degree of auditory verbal dysgnosia. The evidence of right-left confusion was shown when the patient placed his right hand to his right ear. Even though he responded correctly on the last item, the examiner repeated the instructions, probably because the patient asked to hear the instructions again, and then the patient confused the right and left sides. It is possible that this was another manifestation of right-left confusion, although it may also have represented confusion in comprehension through the auditory avenue of the verbal instructions.

Reference to the patient's writing and drawing indicates that he had a number of problems. The examiner had him draw the figures a number of times because he undoubtedly was having problems with them. The most significant deficiency probably related to the second triangle. In this case the patient became quite confused and drew the figure upside down. He also had great difficulty closing the third triangle. These drawings were not as bad as one might expect from a person having a clinically obvious lesion of the right cerebral hemisphere, and they might be explained partially by the patient's poor educational level, but in all probability they represent a degree of constructional dyspraxia.

It is not uncommon for persons with left cerebral lesions to attempt to respond to the instruction to write the name for the clock by drawing a picture of the clock. This patient began to draw the outside of the figure and probably was stopped in the process by the examiner after the outside line had been drawn. He was then asked to write the name and his obvious confusion, probably both with respect to spelling and writing, was apparent. Even when he had the printed letters SQUARE directly before him, he showed some degree of confusion in his writing. Inspection of the writing itself would suggest that this man probably has never developed much skill in writing. However, he still seemed to have some particular difficulty in forming individual letters (dysgraphia) as well as in spelling (spelling dyspraxia). This was particularly apparent in his attempt to write the sentence, "He shouted the warning."

Finally, although the patient drew the key very poorly in terms of detail, it is clear that he had turned the key in the wrong direction. Many people are inclined to postulate that an error of this type is a definite sign of brain damage. However, we have reviewed thousands of cases and the frequency with which the key is drawn in the wrong direction is just as common among controls as among brain-damaged persons. Thus, drawing the key in the "wrong" direction cannot be used as a specific sign of cerebral disease or damage. While "reversals" of this type are interpreted by many judges, perhaps on the basis of "scientific hearsay," as definite evidence of cerebral damage, one must remember the need for empirical verification of hypotheses and resist the tendency to presume that one's interpretation must be valid merely because it came to mind. Examples of this kind emphasize the importance of studying every individual case in this manual quite carefully in order to gain an understanding of the types of deficits that actually do represent impaired brain functions as contrasted with the types of deviations in performance that are not directly related to pathological involvement of the brain.

In summary, in spite of his limited education, this man showed evidence of dysnomia, spelling dyspraxia, dyslexia, possible mild central dysarthria, possible auditory verbal dysgnosia, dyscalculia, dysgraphia, and right-left confusion. These signs point definitely toward damage of the left cerebral hemisphere. In addition, the patient showed a distinct tendency in one instance to fail to respond to the left side of a stimulus configuration and showed evidence of constructional dyspraxia. These findings point toward right cerebral damage.

Results on the Sensory-perceptual Examination also yielded a number of positive findings. The patient did not show any significant tendency toward sensory imperception except on visual stimulation. While the one error in tactile stimulation on the right side probably should be noted, it is difficult to count a single error as being significant. However, the patient made two errors in the left lower quadrant with double simultaneous visual stimulation. This finding probably does point toward some mild degree of right cerebral dysfunction. The patient had a good deal of difficulty in both tactile finger recognition and finger-tip number writing perception. While the errors were nearly evenly distributed in tactile finger recognition, the total of 12 errors on the left hand and only 8 errors on the right hand in finger-tip number writing perception probably does have some lateralizing significance. In fact, the frequency of errors on both sides probably must be considered as pointing toward impaired function of both cerebral hemispheres, even though the results lean in the direction of more serious imvolvement of the right cerebral hemisphere than the left. Thus, results from the Sensory-perceptual Examination also point toward bilateral involvement but suggest that the right cerebral hemisphere is somewhat more dysfunctional.

Interpretation of the results:

The findings from both the Aphasia Screening Test and the Sensory-perceptual Examination point toward bilateral cerebral involvement. It would be difficult to discern which cerebral hemisphere was more severely involved. There is no doubt, however, that the aphasic symptoms implicate the left cerebral hemisphere and the evidence of constructional dyspraxia, a tendency to ignore the left side of a stimulus configuration, and the sensory-perceptual deficits all combine to implicate the right cerebral hemisphere. Consideration could be given to the prospect that involvement of only one hemisphere or the other could be responsible for these results. However, there seems to be no way to support such a hypotheseis.

It is difficult to be specific with regard to the area of involvement. However, the fact that the visual fields were full in spite of the indications of serious damage to both cerebral hemispheres would tend to argue in favor of neoplastic involvement rather than a vascular lesion. Since evidence is present for bilateral cerebral damage, a postulate of neoplastic involvement would require consideration of metastatic carcinoma of the brain to account for lesions of both hemispheres. Thus, these results definitely point toward serious damage of the cerebral hemispheres of a pathological nature that definitely would require neurological (medical and perhaps surgical) evaluation, if the patient had not already received such attention.

A review of the medical and neurological history for this man indicates that he was operated on for a malignant tumor in the left fronto-parietal area six days after our examination was done. This lesion was a metastasis from a lung carcinoma. Even though bilateral cerebral angiography had been done, only evidence of the left cerebral lesion was noted. Involvement of the right cerebral hemisphere was not diagnosed by neurological tests, although it is not uncommon for cerebral metastases to be multiple, involving both cerebral hemispheres. It would seem entirely likely that the conclusion from the Aphasia Screening Test and the Sensory-perceptual Examination of right as well as left cerebral damage was quite accurate.

A.C.

NEUROLOGICAL SUMMARY

Symptoms:

Nine months before hospital admission the patient's family noticed that he did not converse readily, did not initiate conversation, was sometimes irrelevant in his responses, and was more argumentative than usual. Five months before admission he was warned by his supervisor regarding unsatisfactory work and three months later he was dismissed because he was so forgetful. His general efficiency continued to deteriorate and his memory grew worse. Motor problems became apparent consisting of unsteadiness of gait and loss of motor control especially in his right hand. He lost 25 pounds during the month before admission.

Signs:

Upon hospital admission the patient was generally confused and was not oriented for place or time. He was thought to have possible dysphasia, a slight right facial palsy, and a slight weakness of the right upper extremity. No evidence of papilledema.

Diagnostic Tests:

Chest x-ray: Mass lesion of left upper lobe, measuring 3 × c.5 × 5.5 centimeters, compatible with bronchogenic carcinoma.
Bilateral carotid angiogram: Shift of anterior cerebral artery to the right and some shifting and straightening of the candelabra vessels on the left side.
Pneumoencephalogram: Definite shift of the third and lateral ventricles to the right with the left lateral ventricle being pushed beneath the falx.
EEG: Delta waves, Grade I, and dysrhythmia, Grade II, maximally in the left fronto-temporal area.
Neuropsychological examination done six days before surgery.

Treatment:

Left fronto-temporo-parietal craniotomy with evacuation of cyst and partial removal of a tumor from the left fronto-parietal area.

Postoperative Course:

Gradual improvement over five weeks before discharge, but severe impairment including dysphasia and right hemiplegia.

Diagnosis:

Metastatic bronchogenic carcinoma of the left fronto-parietal area and left upper lung carcinoma.

REITAN-INDIANA APHASIA SCREENING TEST

Form for Adults and Older Children

Name: W.M. Age: 44 Date: ______ Examiner: ______

Copy SQUARE	Repeat TRIANGLE
Name SQUARE	Repeat MASSACHUSETTS
Spell SQUARE "S-Q-U-A-I-R"	Repeat METHODIST EPISCOPAL
Copy CROSS	Write SQUARE
Name CROSS	Read SEVEN
Spell CROSS	Repeat SEVEN
Copy TRIANGLE	Repeat/Explain HE SHOUTED THE WARNING.
Name TRIANGLE	Write HE SHOUTED THE WARNING.
Spell TRIANGLE	Compute 85 – 27 =
Name BABY	Compute 17 X 3 =
Write CLOCK	Name KEY
Name FORK	Demonstrate use of KEY
Read 7 SIX 2 "7 S-I-X 2"	Draw KEY
Read MGW	Read PLACE LEFT HAND TO RIGHT EAR.
Reading I	Place LEFT HAND TO RIGHT EAR Left hand to left ear then corrected spontaneously.
Reading II "He is a friendly animal, a __mous winner of dog shows." Examiner questioned, then patient read again the same way.	Place LEFT HAND TO LEFT ELBOW

REITAN-KLØVE SENSORY-PERCEPTUAL EXAMINATION

(Instance indicated where stimulus was not perceived or was incorrectly perceived.)

TACTILE:

RH					LH					Both: RH					LH			
RH					LF					Both: RH					LF			
LH					RF					LH					RF			

AUDITORY:

RE					LE					Both: RE					LE			X

VISUAL:

						X	X	X	X										– (Above eye level)
RV					LV	X	X	X	X	Both: RV					LV				– (Eye level)
						X	X	X	X										– (Below eye level)

TACTILE FINGER RECOGNITION:

Right:	1					2					3	X	X	X	X	4					5					4 / 20
Left:	1					2					3	X	X		X	4	X	X	X	X	5	X		X	X	10 / 20

COMMENTS:

FINGER-TIP NUMBER WRITING PERCEPTION:

	4	6	3	5	3	5	4	6	6	5	4	3	5	4	6	3	6	3	5	4	
Right:			X		X			X					X		X			X			6 / 20
Left:		X					X			X	X						X				5 / 20

COMMENTS:

VISUAL FIELDS:

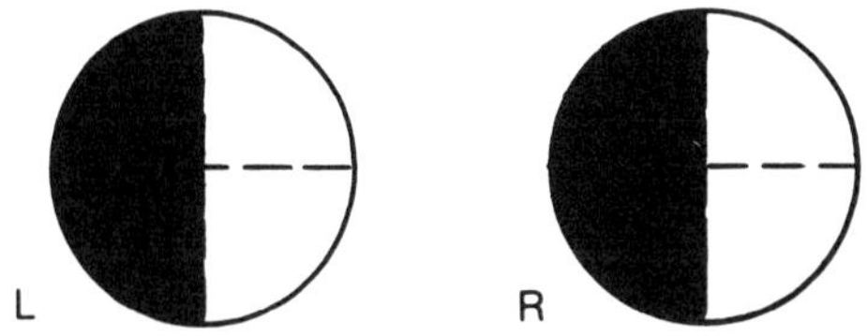

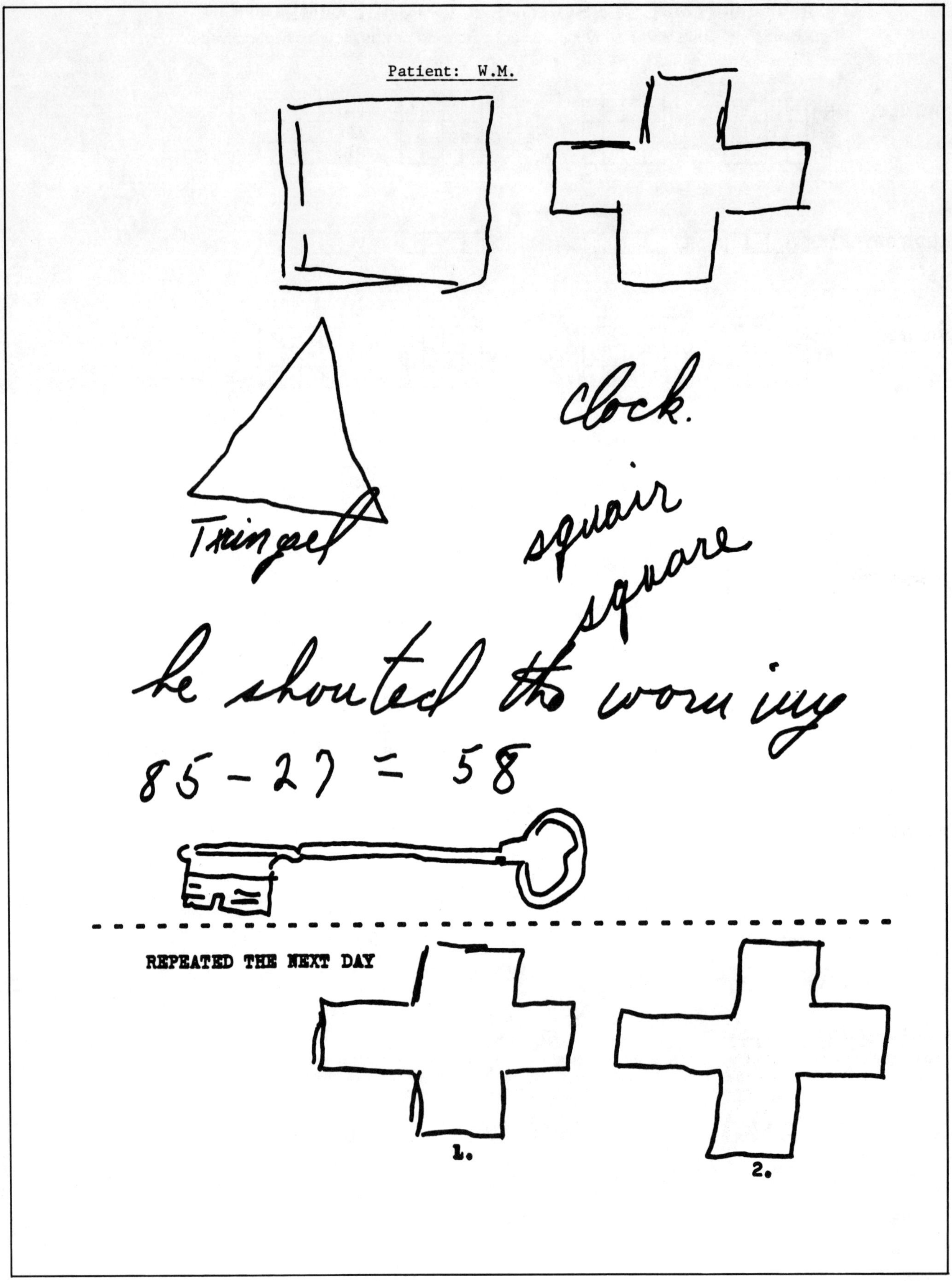
Patient: W.M.
clock.
Tringel
squair
square
he shouted the worn ing
85 - 27 = 58
REPEATED THE NEXT DAY
1.
2.

W.M. – A 44-year-old right-handed male salesman with fourteen years of education.

Identification of brain-related deficits:

The form for the Aphasia test indicates that this man had only a few difficulties on the verbal part of the examination. He spelled SQUARE as "squair." This is an unusal type of spelling error even for persons with poor educational backgrounds. Although this man had two years of college, and one would expect him to be able to spell this word, one cannot count on correct spelling in every instance even from persons at this educational level. However, this particular spelling is definitely unusual and probably related to left cerebral dysfunction. A more common error in spelling SQUARE is "squar," not infrequently made by persons with limited education.

The patient read 7 SIX 2 as "7 S-I-X 2," naming each letter individually. Reading of the letters rather than reading the word is a sign of left cerebral dysfunction in many instances. Most persons with normal brains are able to recognize that this item is represented by three numbers, with the middle number being in the form of a written word. Persons with left cerebral dysfunction frequently fail to recognize that SIX is a number just as are the 7 and 2. Thus, this item turns out often to be an excellent stimulus for identification of minimal difficulties in reading.

Although the patient read the first reading item correctly, he made a strange type of mistake with the second item. He read this item as follows, "He is a friendly animal, a mous winner of dog shows." The examiner questioned the patient, asking him to read it again and be sure that he got it right. He read the item again in exactly the same way. This may be an instance in which the patient, for some reason, failed to recognize the "fa" at the beginning of the word "famous," thus manifesting a tendency to ignore the left side of the word. However, right cerebral lesions are rarely manifested in this particular way. Instead, they relate to he entire spatial configuration represented by the stimulus rather than certain letters within the overall configuration. Thus, it is difficult to interpret this particular error. Finally, the patient showed evidence of mild right-left confusion when asked to place his left hand to his right ear. He corrected this error spontaneously, but it still should be noted as a possible indication of left cerebral dysfunction.

The patient's writing and drawing show some distinct abnormalities. Considering the drawings first, the double line for the square probably represented only the patient's beginning attempt to draw the inside frame of the heavy line and did not represent a deficit. It is apparent that the patient did not keep his pencil on the paper continuously in his attempt to draw the cross, but this examination was done years ago when we did not hold as strictly to this rule. Thus, the square, cross, and triangle seemed to be within normal limits. However, the cross was repeated when the patient was finishing the examination the next day. These figures were drawn on separate pieces of paper but, for purposes of the present communication, were appended to the bottom of the page. It is apparent that these crosses are abnormal. The lateral extremity on the left side extends too far and definitely distorts the spatial configuration. These drawings give evidence of a mild constructional dyspraxia. However, the drawing of the key, on the first day of the examination, definitely showed evidence of constructional dyspraxia typical of right hemisphere damage. It is important to realize that the overall configuration may look fairly good, but specific deficits place the end result in the category of an abnormal performance. An important indicator in this example relates to the notches on the stem of the key. Sometimes the notches are not in the drawing at all, and this is not particularly uncommon with control or with brain-damaged subjects. However, when the notches do not oppose each other, in a mirror-image fashion, one may begin to think about right cerebral damage. In this instance the notches toward the handle of the key were not symmetrical nor were the notches toward the teeth. Thus, although not grossly impaired, this aspect of the drawing would be a possible sign of right cerebral damage. The lack of symmetry of the teeth of the key, with those on the right side being wider than those of the left, probably also has this kind of implication. However, probably the most significant sign in the drawing relates to the "nose" of the key. This man did not manage to draw the nose in a proper spatial position with relation to the rest of the key. In terms of the overall configuration, therefore, this key is quite characteristic of those drawn by persons with right cerebral lesions. Failure to complete the inside of the handle may possibly be of some significance, but this type of error tends to occur with many control as well as brain-damaged subjects.

There were additional indications of deficit. Although it is not part of our standard procedure, it was fortunate that the examiner in this instance asked the patient to write the word TRIANGLE. This man wrote the "T" correctly but then had some difficulty in getting started with the "r." This kind of difficulty is seen in persons with a mild tendency toward dysgraphia. He proceeded to spell the word incorrectly, deviating from the phonics involved. It is not unusual, in persons with low educational levels, for a Y to be used instead of an I, but this man left out the A and wrote "gel" instead of "gle." Both of these responses would be quite unusual for a man of this educational level and these errors probably do represent a mild indication of dysgraphia and spelling dyspraxia. Secondly, when the patient was shown the word SQUARE and the stimulus was directly in front of him, he still wrote the word "squair." This is almost certainly a sign of left cerebral dysfunction. When asked to do the task again, the patient was able to perform correctly. This correct performance, however, does not excuse the original error.

Thus, this man showed evidence of bilateral deficiencies on the Aphasia test. These were rather subtle but nevertheless quite real. They included spelling dyspraxia, mild dyslexia, mild right-left confusion, and mild dysgraphia. Often judges respond to this patient's writing of the sentence, "He shouted the warning," as if there were deficiencies of a left hemisphere type. Reference is sometimes made to "the" and especially to "warning." However, if one traces through the letters one finds that they are all there, that there are no extra marks, and that the deviations (for example, failure to drop the line after the "a" in warning) are of the type that are frequently seen among control subjects. As noted before, it is important to become familiar with the idiosyncracies that occur among individuals with respect to performances in writing. One can develop such familiarity by use of standard stimulus material, as is done in the Aphasia Screening Test.

The Sensory-perceptual Examination showed evidence of deficiencies that implicate the right cerebral hemisphere particularly. This man had relatively little difficulty on the tactile and auditory parts of the test involving double simultaneous stimulation. However, in one instance he failed to report the stimulus to his left ear when it was given bilaterally. Visual testing was not done because this man clearly had a deficiency toward his left side. In confrontation testing of the visual fields, he showed evidence of a definite left homonymous hemianopsia. This sign inescapably implicates the visual system behind the optic crossing on the right side.

The patient had distinct difficulty in tactile finger recognition involving fingers three, four and five of the left hand. Undoubtedly this represents a pathological manifestation. In addition, however, he was completely unable to identify the third finger of the right hand. This also is distinctly a pathological condition and would suggest the possiblity of a rather small and discrete lesion of the left cerebral hemisphere. Finger-tip number writing perception was not particularly helpful in that the patient made mistakes on both sides. One could postulate that this may be due to the difficulty of the task, but is is possible that it also represents bilateral cerebral damage.

In total, the test results point toward evidence of specific deficits involving the left cerebral hemisphere as well as other specific deficits that involve the right cerebral hemisphere.

Interpretation of the test results:

Probably the most serious lesion is in the right cerebral hemisphere, especially considering results from the Sensory-perceptual Examination. The patient had considerably more difficulty on his left hand than his right hand in tactile finger recognition and also had definite evidence of a left homonymous hemianopsia. These findings were complemented by evidence of mild though definite constructional dyspraxia. The presence of tactile-perceptual deficits and constructional dyspraxia were helpful in indicating that the right cerebral hemisphere was involved, because the left homonymous hemianopsia conceivably could have been due to a lesion interrupting the visual pathway between the optic crossing and the right lateral geniculate body. Thus, the combination of deficits requires us to postulate that this man has a lesion in the posterior part of the right cerebral hemisphere. However, the positive indications of a left cerebral lesion cannot be ignored. These included the mild but definite manifestations of aphasic deficits as well as definite finger dysgnosia of the third finger of the right hand.

The test results related quite closely to the neurological diagnosis of the patient. He had a metastatic melanoma in the posterior part of the right cerebral hemisphere. No lesion was demonstrated with bilateral cerebral angiography that involved the left cerebral hemisphere. However, the patient had evidence of metastases in many parts of his body and it is entirely possible that he had a small lesion in his left cerebral hemisphere that was not revealed by cerebral angiography. While some persons who have reviewed the results for this man have tended to overlook the mild indications of aphasia, or attribute them to a lifelong condition of difficulty in dealing with language symbols, the ability to recognize that they were brain-related manifestations of language impairment complemented by tactile agnosia of the right third finger, was a great advantage in drawing confident conclusions about brain-behavior relationships. As noted, these findings strongly point toward some kind of lesion, probably small in size, in the left temporo-parietal area. Without having discerned evidence of involvement of the left as well as right cerebral hemisphere there would have been no way to distinguish the findings from expected results with a primary glioma.

W.M.

NEUROLOGICAL SUMMARY

Symptoms:

Patient had severe frontal headaches of increasing severity for 3 weeks. He has bumped into things on the left for several weeks.
Malignant melanoma removed 10 months before admission.
Right axillary nodes, positive 4 months after surgical removal of tumor.

Signs:

Left homonymous hemianopsia.
Hypesthesia, right ulnar area.

Diagnostic Tests:

EEG: Delta Grade III, right parietal area.
X-ray: Metastatic lesion, upper left chest area.
Angiogram: Metastatic lesion, right posterior parietal-occipital area.

Treatment:

Headaches improved. Because of multiple lesions, the patient was discharged with no further treatment. Surgical removal of the tumor was not attempted and histological verification of the lesion was not possible.

Diagnosis:

Probable metastatic melanoma, right posterior parietal-occipital area.

CEREBRAL VASCULAR DISEASE

Introduction

The prior section indicated that aphasic and sensory-perceptual disorders occur frequently among patients with intrinsic tumors. The nature of the symptoms and deficits are related to the cerebral hemisphere that is principally involved. However, among patients with metastatic carcinoma it is possible that both cerebral hemispheres may be damaged even though neurological diagnostic evidence (physical neurological examination, EEG, and contrast studies) may point toward damage of only one cerebral hemisphere.

Cerebral vascular lesions generally are accompanied by symptoms similar to those seen with patients having intrinsic tumors. Frequently sensory-perceptual deficits are more profound in patients with strokes, although patients with intrinsic tumors may sometimes show very serious lateralized losses as well. It is important to judge the severity of higher-level losses (language losses and impairment in being able to copy spatial configurations) with losses involving sensory-perceptual and motor functions. The particular tests included in this manual do not assess adequacy of motor functions. However, this is important in terms of the differentiation between strokes and intrinsic tumors. Customarily motor losses, as well as sensory-perceptual deficits, are more profound in patients with strokes (Hom and Reitan, 1982). Patients with generalized cerebral vascular disease frequently show some deficits that involve both cerebral hemispheres, although they may be relatively mild in nature. In many instances, of course, it is not possible to differentiate with confidence focal vascular as compared with neoplastic lesions on the basis of the Aphasia Screening Test and the Sensory-perceptual Examination. History information, especially relating to sudden onset, may be of value in this respect, but even patients with intrinsic tumors sometimes show evidence of sudden onset or precipitous exacerbation of symptoms.

REITAN-INDIANA APHASIA SCREENING TEST

Form for Adults and Older Children

Name: W.F. Age: 55 Date: ______ Examiner: ______

Copy SQUARE Could not do on first day, second day-see.	Repeat TRIANGLE "Triango", then responded correctly.
Name SQUARE "1-2-3-4-evens, a 7-8 octer, same uh one."	Repeat MASSACHUSETTS "Massachussa"
Spell SQUARE "Q (pause) something like that (pause) empty"	Repeat METHODIST EPISCOPAL "Too much. Menosanist (pause) Echmenispal."
Copy CROSS Could not do on first day, second day-see.	Write SQUARE "Two weeks now, I can't think. S-Q-U-A-R-E (pause) quare." Patient couldn't do.
Name CROSS "Even (pause) like a 1-2-3-4 (pause) I know what it is but I can't."	Read SEVEN "Sevun"
Spell CROSS "Red course (pause) yah (pause) I guess not."	Repeat SEVEN
Copy TRIANGLE Could not do on first day, second day-see.	Repeat/Explain HE SHOUTED THE WARNING Repeated correctly. Explained: "Say the quar (pause) I should do em call em."
Name TRIANGLE "Tra (pause) tragul, triangul"	Write HE SHOUTED THE WARNING. Could not do.
Spell TRIANGLE Patient had difficulty understanding what to do, but responded correctly.	Compute 85 – 27 = Examiner wrote problem, patient verbalized, "Off empty (pause) take away" then wrote "222".
Name BABY "Baby?"	Compute 17 X 3 = Patient verbalized "2 x 5 = 12, I mean 7, 1."
Write CLOCK Patient said that he couldn't write.	Name KEY
Name FORK	Demonstrate use of KEY Patient verbalized, "Keep this key", then wanted to put test booklet in door.
Read 7 SIX 2 "7 x 2, or 7 six 2"	Draw KEY Could not do.
Read MGW "M-gick-oh in the movie", then responded correctly.	Read PLACE LEFT HAND TO RIGHT EAR. "Place after half each uh hand place back your hand to right ear."
Reading I "See those black dog."	Place LEFT HAND TO RIGHT EAR When patient asked for left hand, pointed to right hand then responded correctly.
Reading II "Heech his shew finley adimal, famous winter of the dog shows."	Place LEFT HAND TO LEFT ELBOW Left hand to right elbow.

REITAN-KLØVE SENSORY-PERCEPTUAL EXAMINATION

(Instance indicated where stimulus was not perceived or was incorrectly perceived.)

TACTILE:

RH					LH					Both: RH	X	X	X	X	LH				
RH					LF					Both: RH	X	X	X	X	LF				
LH					RF					LH					RF				

AUDITORY:

RE					LE					Both: RE	X	X		X	LE				

VISUAL:

																				– (Above eye level)
RV					LV					Both: RV					LV					– (Eye level)
														X						– (Below eye level)

TACTILE FINGER RECOGNITION:

	1				2				3				4				5				could not / do
Right:																					
Left:														2	3						2 / 20

COMMENTS: Not given with right hand. Patient could not answer correctly.

FINGER-TIP NUMBER WRITING PERCEPTION:

	4	6	3	5	3	5	4	6	6	5	4	3	5	4	6	3	6	3	5	4	could not / do
Right:																					
Left:		4	X					X	X	4	X						4				7 / 20

COMMENTS: Not given with right hand. Patient could not answer correctly.

VISUAL FIELDS:

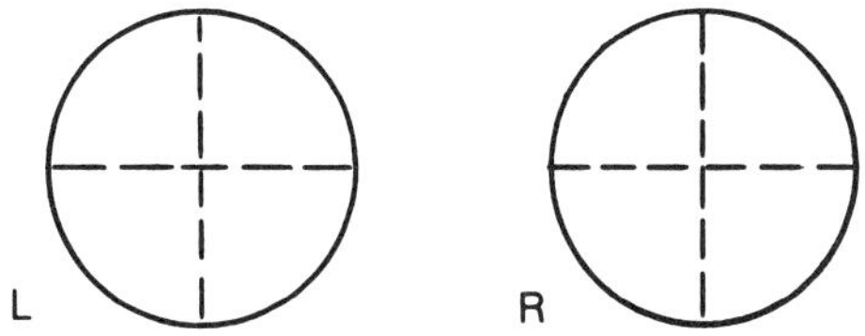

FULL

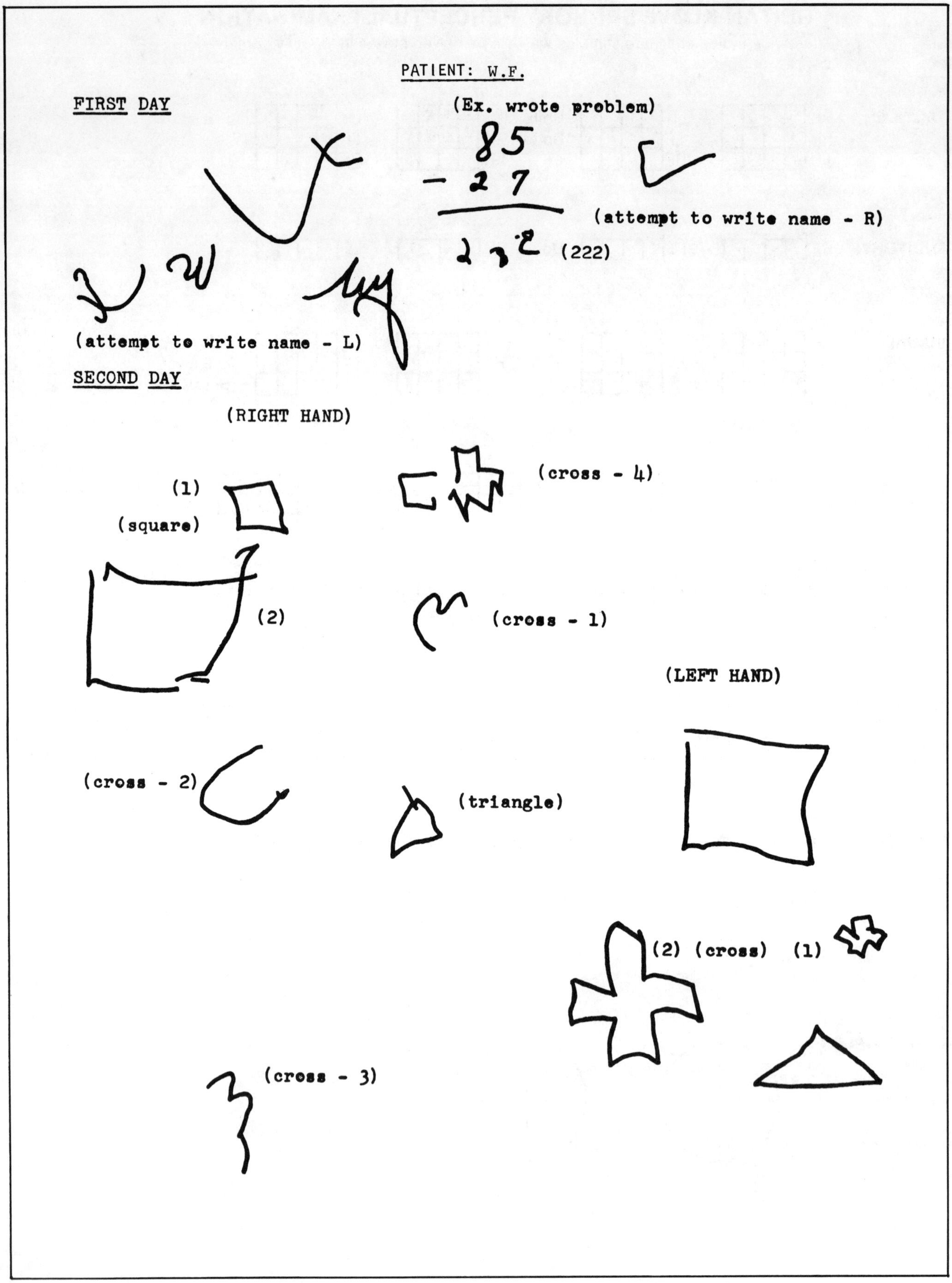
PATIENT: W.F.
FIRST DAY
(Ex. wrote problem)
85
- 27
(222)
(attempt to write name - R)
(attempt to write name - L)
SECOND DAY
(RIGHT HAND)
(1)
(square)
(cross - 4)
(2)
(cross - 1)
(LEFT HAND)
(cross - 2)
(triangle)
(2) (cross) (1)
(cross - 3)

W.F. – A 55-year-old right-handed male painter with an eighth grade education.

Identification of brain-related deficits:

The recording form for the Aphasia Test obviously indicates that this man had a great number of aphasic difficulties. He was examined over the course of two days and because of his severe impairment some tasks were attempted with the left hand to see if there was any improvement over his right (preferred) performances.

There is no doubt that this man shows brain-related deficits. Careful review of his actual responses will give the reader some insight and understanding of the types of responses made by seriously aphasic persons. The patient's attempt to name the cross was quite typical. He showed a perseverative counting response and then indicated that he knew what the figure was but was not able to name it. Persons with dysnomia frequently do indicate that they actually know the name of the figure even though they are not able to say the word. In the patient's attempt to spell the word "cross" he was able to say "red course," but his comment "I guess not" either referred to his inability to spell or his recognition that he had not said the name correctly. When asked to spell TRIANGLE the patient actually was able to spell the word although he demonstrated evidence of auditory verbal dysgnosia in his difficulty in understanding the instructions. In responding to the letters MGW the patient gave some evidence of his insight by commenting "in the movie." He obviously was thinking of the initials for Metro Goldwyn Mayer, although he confused the W with the M. His difficulty in reading items 1 and 2 undoubtedly was influenced by both reading and naming deficits. While reading is largely a receptive kind of function and naming is expressive, most aphasic patients have both expressive and receptive deficits, sometimes demonstrated, as in this instance, in the single performance. As noted previously, even in the simplest task it is necessary to use receptive (registration) functions, central processing, and expressive (response) functions.

The patient's impairment in pronouncing words after the examiner was demonstrated quite clearly and serves as a rather typical example of central dysarthria. In other responses it is possible to discern some degree of understanding even in responses that appear, on first glance, to show nothing but confusion. For example, in attempting to explain the sentence "He shouted the warning," the patient responded in part by saying, "I should do em call em." He apparently was trying to indicate that he recognized that there was a problem or perhaps danger, and that he should call someone. With respect to arithmetic complications, however, it is difficult to discern that the patient had any understanding of what was involved.

When the patient was asked to demonstrate the use of the key, he showed evidence of a very concrete response. It was not possible for him to show how a key would be used without having an actual object of some kind to use in the procedure. In this case, he wanted to put the test booklet, showing the picture of the key, in a door in order to demonstrate how the key would be used. In instances of this kind it is possible to observe the extreme degree of concreteness in behavior that is sometimes shown in persons with serious aphasia. On the other hand, in general, aphasic patients do not show evidence of more impairment in the area of abstraction and reasoning abilities on non-verbal tasks, such as the Category Test, than do patients with comparable brain lesions but without impairment of language functions (Reitan, 1960). The remaining items show further illustrations of serious and pronounced dyslexia and evidence of right-left confusion.

The patient's attempts at writing and drawing further illustrated his severe deficits. On the first day he was scarcely able to make any progress. He was so limited in his language capabilities that he was not even able to write his name. This is highly unusual. Most people retain some ability in such an overly practiced task as writing one's own name. On the second day of the examination the patient was able to make a little more progress than on the first day. Comparisons of his performances with his two hands suggests that he probably did somewhat better with his left hand (across from what probably was his better cerebral hemisphere) than with his right hand, even though he was right-handed. This may, of course, have been due in part to impairment of motor functions. We learned from results with the rest of the Halstead-Reitan Battery that the patient was markedly impaired in motor functions with the right upper extremity, although this information would not have been directly available, unless specifically recorded, from the Aphasia Test and the Sensory-perceptual Examination. It does not appear, however, that the patient's entire problem of drawing simple spatial configurations can be explained by a motor deficit of the right upper extremity. The kinds of difficulties shown by this man in his attempts to copy the square and the cross are quite typical of persons with seriously destructive damage in the posterior part of the left cerebral hemisphere. Of course, the extensive nature of other aphasic symptoms suggests that the lesion is, in fact, fairly widespread in the left cerebral hemisphere.

The results of the Sensory-perceptual Examination were quite helpful in providing a comparison of the two cerebral hemispheres. The patient showed evidence of pronounced impairment of perception of a tactile stimulus presented to his right hand when it was given in competition either with a stimulus to the left hand or the left face. It is somewhat unusual that the patient did not demonstrate the deficit when his right face was in competition with his left hand. Retention of ability to respond to the right face may possibly be related to the specific area of involvement in this case or perhaps to the general finding that the face is somewhat more sensitive than the hand and therefore competes better. The patient demonstrated right-sided imperception with auditory stimulation, but the one error in 12 trials with visual stimulation probably cannot be counted as a significant finding. We should note that the patient's visual fields did not show any evidence of loss on confrontation testing and this finding is much more suggestive of a neoplastic than vascular lesion when considered with relation to the pronounced aphasic deficits shown by the patient.

It was not possible to administer the test for tactile finger recognition or finger-tip number writing perception on the right side because the patient had no idea of the correct responses. However, this finding of hemihypesthesia, in its own right, clearly points toward left cerebral damage. It is not surprising that this patient had some difficulty in tactile finger recognition with his left hand. In fact, one would probably have predicted that he would make more than two mistakes in 20 trials. He also performed perhaps better with his left hand on the test of finger-tip number writing perception than one might have expected, making errors in 7 out of 20 trials. These results suggest that the right cerebral hemisphere was not seriously damaged on a structural basis and suggest that the patient probably does not have bilateral focal damage.

Interpretation of the results:

This patient performed so poorly that it would be possible to conclude that he shows evidence of positive results on all of the types of deficits measured by the Aphasia test. The symptoms would include dysnomia, spelling dyspraxia, dysgraphia, visual letter dysgnosia, possible visual form dysgnosia, dyslexia, central dysarthria, auditory verbal dysgnosia, dyscalculia, ideokinetic dyspraxia, constructional dyspraxia, and right-left confusion.

A question would exist as to whether the impairment in figure drawing was a function of posterior involvement of the left cerebral hemisphere or might be related to focal damage of the right cerebral hemisphere. First, the type of difficulty in drawing the cross (particularly see the fourth attempt) is quite typical of the kind of distortion of the figure that is seen with posterior left hemisphere damage. In addition, results of the Sensory-perceptual Examination were very helpful in this regard. The results point definitely toward structural damage of the left cerebral hemisphere but do not present enough evidence of impairment of the right cerebral hemisphere to conclude there is an independent focal lesion on the right side. In all probability, however, this man would show evidence of generalized impairment of cerebral cortical functions on the entire Halstead-Reitan Battery.

It would be difficult to differentiate from these results the possiblity of a stroke versus a rapidly growing intrinsic tumor. Both could cause very serious deficits. However, neoplastic lesions are frequently associated with less striking specific sensory-perceptual and motor difficulties than occur with strokes. In this case, the absence of a homonymous visual field deficit causes the interpretation to lean in the direction of a tumor. The striking left-sided tactual losses are more in line with a stroke. Motor measures from the rest of the Halstead-Reitan Battery indicated that the patient could not do the Finger Tapping Test at all with his right hand and had very minimal grip strength on that side. The Aphasia Test and Sensory-perceptual Examination suffer from not providing measures of motor function (although the impairment was obvious in this case). If one had knowledge of the fact that this man had very striking and serious right-sided motor deficiencies (not being able to finger tap at all), this knowledge would be an advantage in estimating that the lesion was possibly vascular in nature.

With respect to localization, one would have to postulate extensive involvement in the left cerebral hemisphere. While anterior frontal lesions often do not show very much in the way of deficit, the striking expressive and receptive difficulties shown by this man, including left cerebral impairment in dealing with spatial configurations, probably implies involvement in the distribution of the left middle and posterior cerebral arteries. As will be noted from the neurological summary, the medical diagnosis expressed this same conclusion.

W.F.

NEUROLOGICAL SUMMARY

Symptoms:

Sudden onset of confusion, numbness of right hand and arm, and speech difficulties that occurred 2 days before admission.

Signs:

Almost a complete loss of tactile sensitivity of right arm and marked decrease of sensitivity of right leg.
Right central facial paresis.
Hyperactive muscle stretch reflexes on the right and severe weakness of right upper extremity.
Pronounced aphasia, right-left disorientation, facetious behavior.
Fundoscopic evidence of arteriosclerotic changes.

Diagnostic Tests:

CSF: Within normal limits.
EEG: Delta, Grade I, left parieto-occipital area. EEG improved 7 days later.
Bilateral carotid angiograms: A gap in filling of the left cerebral vessels suggestive of an arteriosclerotic plaque.
Glucose tolerance test: Suggestive of borderline diabetes.
Neuropsychological testing done 11 dyas after hospital admission and 3 days before discharge.

Hospital Course:

Progressive improvement.

Diagnosis:

Cerebral infarction, distribution of left posterior and middle cerebral arteries; generalized arteriosclerosis, mild diabetes mellitus.

REITAN-INDIANA APHASIA SCREENING TEST

PATIENT: C.S.

Copy SQUARE	Repeat TRIANGLE Speech slurred.
Name SQUARE "Cube"	Repeat MASSACHUSETTS Speech slurred.
Spell SQUARE	Repeat METHODIST EPISCOPAL Speech slurred.
Copy CROSS	Write SQUARE
Name CROSS	Read SEVEN
Spell CROSS	Repeat SEVEN
Copy TRIANGLE	Repeat/Explain HE SHOUTED THE WARNING.
Name TRIANGLE	Write HE SHOUTED THE WARNING.
Spell TRIANGLE	Compute 85 – 27 = Answered "58" quickly before writing down problem.
Name BABY	Compute 17 X 3 = Answered "51" quickly before writing down problem.
Write CLOCK	Name KEY
Name FORK	Demonstrate use of KEY
Read 7 SIX 2 Performed slowly but correctly.	Draw KEY
Read MGW	Read PLACE LEFT HAND TO RIGHT EAR.
Reading I	Place LEFT HAND TO RIGHT EAR
Reading II	Place LEFT HAND TO LEFT ELBOW

REITAN-KLØVE SENSORY-PERCEPTUAL EXAMINATION

(Instance indicated where stimulus was not perceived or was incorrectly perceived.)

TACTILE:

RH					LH	X	X	X	X
RH					LF	X			
LH	X	X	X	X	RF				

Both: RH					LH	X	X	X	X
Both: RH	X				LF			X	
LH	X	X	X	X	RF				

AUDITORY:

RE					LE	X	X	X	X
Both: RE					LE	X	X	X	X

VISUAL:

RV					LV		X		
RV					LV		X		
RV					LV				

Both: RV					LV	X				– (Above eye level)
Both: RV					LV	X	X			– (Eye level)
Both: RV					LV	X				– (Below eye level)

TACTILE FINGER RECOGNITION:

	1				2				3				4				5				
Right:	X				X			X		X				X		X	X				7/20
Left:	X	X	X	X	X	X	X	X	X	X	X	X	X	X	X	X	X	X	X	X	20/20

COMMENTS:

FINGER-TIP NUMBER WRITING PERCEPTION:

	4	6	3	5	3	5	4	6	6	5	4	3	5	4	6	3	6	3	5	4	
Right:	X					X		X	X					X	X		X				7/20
Left:	X	X	X	X	X	X	X	X	X	X	X	X	X	X	X	X	X	X	X	X	20/20

COMMENTS:

VISUAL FIELDS: 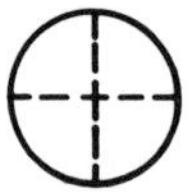 L 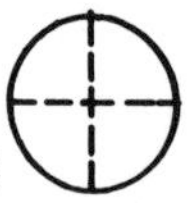 R FULL

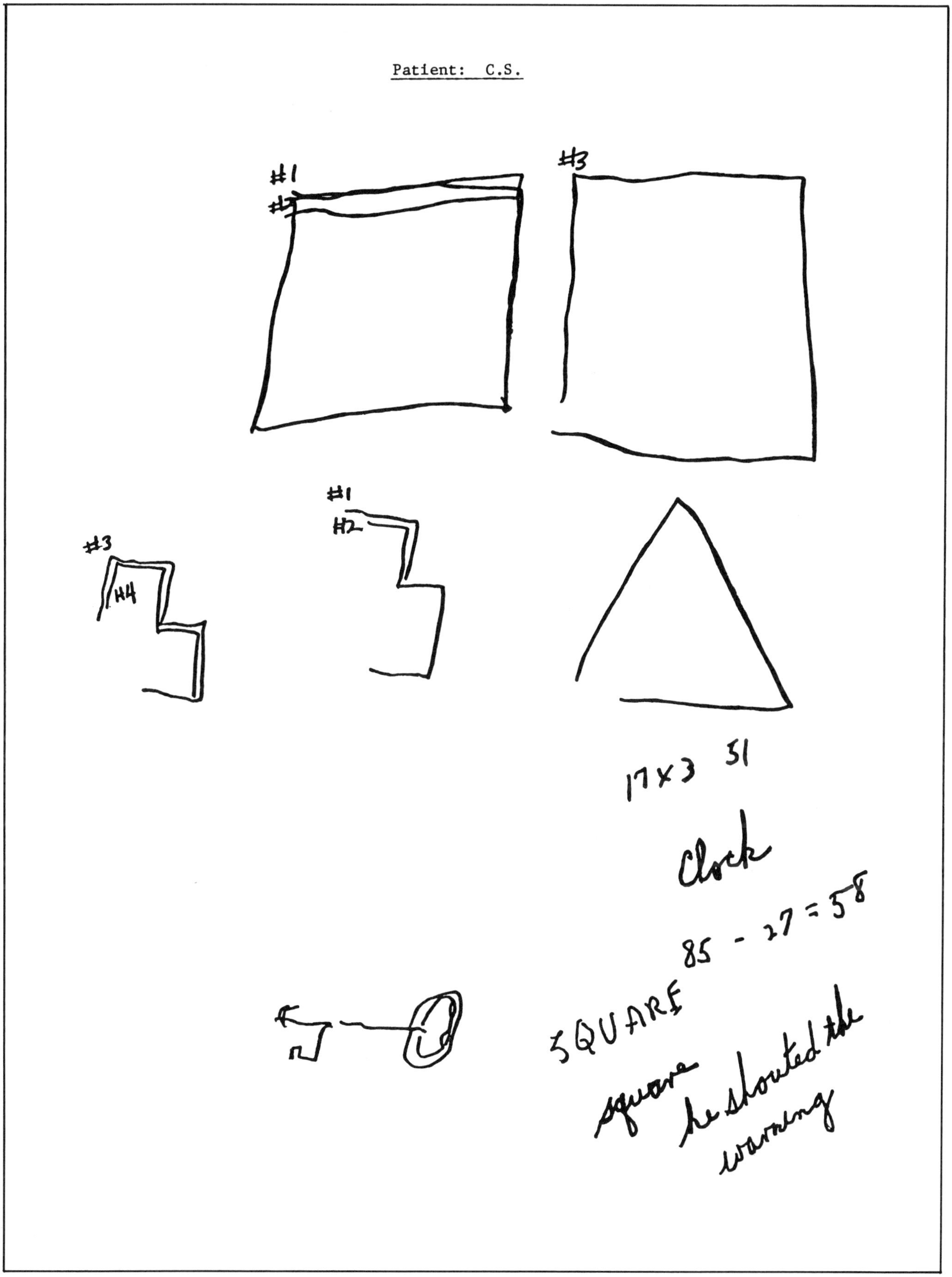
Patient: C.S.
#1
#2
#3
#3
#4
#1
#2
17 x 3 51
Clock
85 - 27 = 58
SQUARE
square
he shouted the warning

C.S. – A 70-year-old right-handed man with 20 years of education.

Identification of brain-related deficits:

The recording form for the Aphasia Screening Test indicates that this man had essentially no difficulties. He named the SQUARE as a "cube" which is an unusual response but not one characteristic of persons with language deficits. Considering the drawings done by this man, one might postulate that he did not perceive the square correctly and that he called it a "cube" because of visual form recognition (receptive) difficulties, but in any case this response is not common in patients with either left or right cerebral damage. The slurred speech shown by the subject in repeating words is sometimes seen in patients with cerebral damage that affects muscles on one side of the body (including muscles necessary for speech) to a greater extent than the other. However, there is no reason at all to believe from the test results that the patient had any significant dysphasia.

Reference to the subject's writing and drawings indicates that he had striking difficulties in dealing with simple spatial configurations. The patient began the first square two times and had a little difficulty in getting parallel lines drawn. The third attempt went a little better, but the patient made a mistake in drawing the third line (descending on the right side) too long then having a problem with respect to closing the figure. His difficulty with the cross was quite apparent. The patient began one cross but became confused and wanted to start again. He used the initial lines as a guide and made a little further progress but still became confused and did not know how to proceed. He continued with further attempts as shown in drawings 3 and 4. He made a little more progress than he had before but still reached a point at which he did not know which way to turn. His difficulty with the triangle also was apparent in that he did not quite seem to know how to close the figure on the left side. Finally, although the key was not done in any detail, the patient just did not have the appreciation of spatial relationships necessary to complete the figure. Thus, the deficit shown by this man in dealing with simple spatial configurations contrasted sharply with his adequate verbal abilities. On the basis of these findings one would postulate that the right cerebral hemisphere was severely deficient in contrast to the left.

Similar findings were shown on the Sensory-perceptual Examination. The patient had a marked hypesthesia involving the left side (particularly the left hand). It is not surprising, under these circumstances, that he was not able to respond on the left side with double simultaneous tactile stimulation. The patient showed a similar type of deficit with auditory stimulation. He did not respond to any of the individual stimuli to the left ear nor to stimuli to the left ear when given simultaneously with stimuli to the right ear. The patient also had a little difficulty in unilateral perception of visual stimulation toward his left side and showed only a small increase in number of errors on the left with double simultaneous visual stimulation. While these results did not demonstrate more deficits on the left side with double than with unilateral simultaneous stimulation, the deficiencies on the left side, in their own right undoubtedly reflect impairment of right cerebral functions.

The patient had a little difficulty in tactile finger recognition and finger-tip number writing perception on the right hand, but he was unable to perform these tasks at all with his left hand. Thus, results on the Sensory-perceptual Examination clearly support the findings from the Aphasia test in pointing toward serious destructive damage of the right cerebral hemisphere. Considering the severity of the deficit in dealing with simple spatial relationships, we would postulate that the middle and posterior part of the right cerebral hemisphere has been particularly damaged.

It is important to recognize that the Aphasia Screening Test and Sensory-perceptual Examination reflect only rather simple and specific types of abilities. In a case of this type it would be of great interest to know about the general as well as the specific deficits associated with cerebral damage. Emphasis in recent years, probably stemming from study of patients with disconnection of the cerebral hemispheres, has almost led to the supposition that all aspects of brain functions are totally represented by the specialized functions of the left and right cerebral hemispheres. This distinctly is not the case. In fact, the general neuropsychological correlates of brain functions are probably the most important abilities, in terms of meeting the complex needs of effective living. Additional testing of this man revealed that he had a Verbal IQ of 136. His excellent verbal abilities, in turn, led his physician (a neurological surgeon) to feel that he was an extremely bright person and, if only his left hemiplegia could somehow be cured, the person would be restored to a normal level. We must note in this respect, however, that his Impairment Index was 0.9 and his score on the Category Test was 130 errors. For those familiar with the Halstead-Reitan Battery, the importance of a complete neuropsychological examination in cases of this kind, for practical considerations related, for example, to rehabilitation and the ability to deal with complex everyday problems, becomes entirely obvious.

Interpretation of the results:

The findings show no positive evidence of damage or dysfunction of the left cerebral hemisphere but relate almost entirely to evidence of right cerebral damage. Thus, this situation clearly is one of a focal lesion involving the right cerebral hemisphere. The impairment is profound, considering the very severe losses in ability to deal with simple spatial configurations. Undoubtedly, this impairment is of very real practical significance. The contrast between the two cerebral hemispheres, in its own right, is almost certain to demonstrate itself in a striking way in everyday situations.

A question would exist as to whether the lesion is vascular or neoplastic, based on the evaluation of the test results alone. It would be helpful to have specific information regarding motor capabilities on the left side of the body as would be available in the Halstead-Reitan Battery. Perhaps the severe nature of sensory losses, including left hypesthesia, would incline the inference toward a vascular lesion, but with a vascular lesion one would also have expected a left homonymous visual field loss. As indicated in the Neurological Summary, the patient had suffered a stroke involving the right cerebral hemisphere just more than three years before the present examination.

C.S.

NEUROLOGICAL SUMMARY

Symptoms and History:

This 70-year-old man had retired from a position 17 years before as a high-ranking naval officer because of mild heart disease. He continued to work in a very responsible managerial position for 14 years until he had a severe stroke involving his right middle cerebral artery. Neuropsychological examination was done three years after the stroke.

Signs:

Right hemiplegia, right hemihypesthesia, slurred speech.

Diagnosis:

Cerebral thrombosis; right middle cerebral artery.

REITAN-INDIANA APHASIA SCREENING TEST

PATIENT: J.B.

Copy SQUARE	Repeat TRIANGLE
Name SQUARE	Repeat MASSACHUSETTS
Spell SQUARE	Repeat METHODIST EPISCOPAL
Copy CROSS	Write SQUARE
Name CROSS "Plus sign, isn't exactly a cross."	Read SEVEN
Spell CROSS	Repeat SEVEN
Copy TRIANGLE	Repeat/Explain HE SHOUTED THE WARNING.
Name TRIANGLE	Write HE SHOUTED THE WARNING.
Spell TRIANGLE	Compute 85 – 27 =
Name BABY	Compute 17 X 3 =
Write CLOCK	Name KEY
Name FORK	Demonstrate use of KEY
Read 7 SIX 2 "6" Then responded correctly.	Draw KEY
Read MGW	Read PLACE LEFT HAND TO RIGHT EAR.
Reading I	Place LEFT HAND TO RIGHT EAR Couldn't get left hand to right ear, but tried.
Reading II	Place LEFT HAND TO LEFT ELBOW

REITAN-KLØVE SENSORY-PERCEPTUAL EXAMINATION

(Instance indicated where stimulus was not perceived or was incorrectly perceived.)

TACTILE:

RH					LH	X	X	X		Both: RH					LH X X X
RH					LF					Both: RH					LF X X X
LH	X				RF					LH	X	X	X	X	RF

AUDITORY: RE ☐☐☐☐ LE ☐☐☐☐ Both: RE ☐☐☐☐ LE ☐☐☐☐

VISUAL:

RV					LV	X	X	X	X
RV					LV	X	X	X	X
RV					LV	X	X	X	X

Both: RV (crossed out) LV (crossed out) – (Above eye level) – (Eye level) – (Below eye level)

TACTILE FINGER RECOGNITION:

	1	2	3	4	5	
Right:						0 / 20
Left:	_ _ X _	_ _ _ X		X _ X _	X X X X	8 / 20

COMMENTS:

FINGER-TIP NUMBER WRITING PERCEPTION:

	4	6	3	5	3	5	4	6	6	5	4	3	5	4	6	3	6	3	5	4	
Right:			2		6	4						2			2						5 / 20
Left:																					can do / not

COMMENTS: Patient could feel stimulus being administered on the left hand but could not distinguish numbers. None correct.

VISUAL FIELDS:

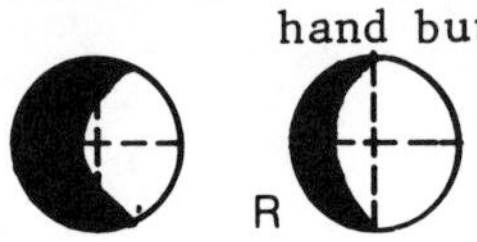

L R

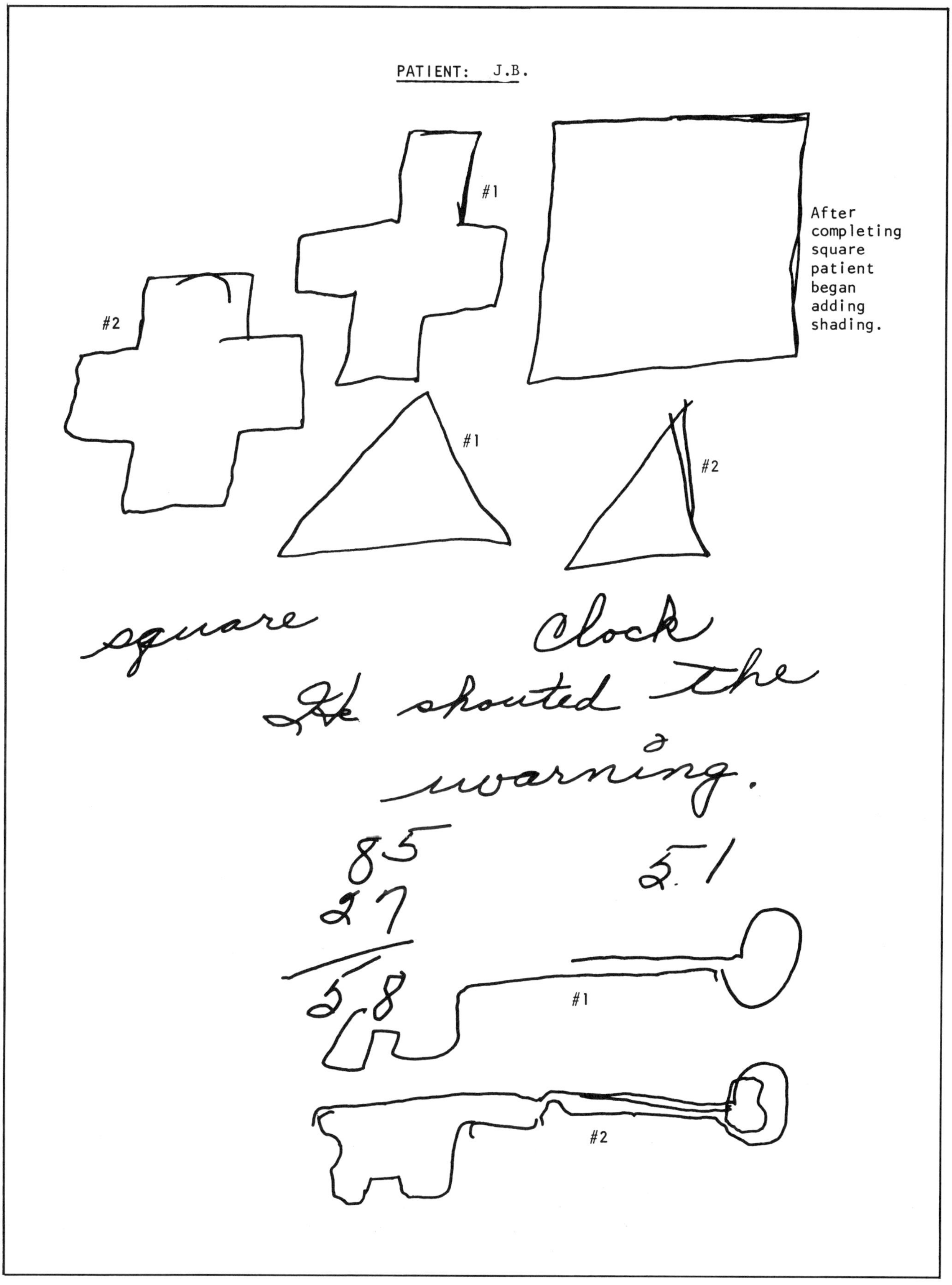
PATIENT: J.B.
#1
#2
After completing square patient began adding shading.
#1
#2
square
clock
He shouted the warning.
85
27
58
5.1
#1
#2

J.B. – A 29-year-old right-handed female homemaker with a twelfth grade education.

Identification of brain-related deficits:

The Aphasia test form indicates that this woman had few difficulties with the verbal items. In naming the cross, she indicated that it was a plus sign which is possibly a correct response. She said that it wasn't exactly a cross, very possibly thinking in terms of a Christian cross rather than other types of crosses. Her response to the item 7 SIX 2 is a little difficult to understand because she responded only with the word six. However, she went on to read the item correctly. She had no other difficulties. These particular responses are certainly not sufficient to draw any conclusion with respect to the presence of dysphasia nor of left hemisphere dysfunction.

The patient's writing and drawings show evidence of adequate writing but definite difficulty with the drawings. The square was reasonably adequate, but the patient had definite difficulty with the cross. Inspection shows that imbalance of the upper and lower extremities is quite apparent on the first drawing and there was an overlapping of lines in the right upper quadrant in the second drawing. She had even more difficulty with her drawing of the key. It is important that the person who interprets the test results know the sequence in which the items were performed, so that a judgment can be made regarding what was on the paper at the time any particular performance was attempted. For example, the patient had already written the first arithmetic problem (85 − 27) before she began drawing the first key. Thus, it is clear that she did not allow herself sufficient space for completion of the key. This manifestation, in its own right, clearly indicates that the patient had a significant problem in dealing with spatial relationships. She attempted to draw the key again and made mistakes of the kind that are clearly characteristic of right cerebral dysfunction. The notches on the stem fall toward the middle of the stem rather than toward the handle and the teeth. In addition, the line extending below the stem just before the teeth of the key clearly represents some kind of mistake with regard to spatial relationships. Finally, the details of the handle and teeth of the key are not in proper symmetry. Thus, in this instance, the key lends definite support to the mistakes made in drawing the cross and are quite characteristic of right cerebral dysfunction and the presence of constructional dyspraxia.

Results on the Sensory-perceptual Examination also point strongly toward right cerebral damage. The patient showed some degree of hypesthesia involving her left hand, but evidence of imperception on the left side with double simultaneous tactile stimulation was much more pronounced. Even though she had no difficulty with auditory stimulation, the results of tactile testing were quite distinct and definite in implicating the right hemisphere. It was not possible to do the visual test because the patient had a distinct homonymous visual field limitation on the left side for each eye. Of course, this visual field limitation, in its own right, added another significant and striking point of evidence with respect to right cerebral damage. The patient had no difficulty in tactile finger recognition on her right hand but made eight mistakes in total on her left hand. While she made some mistakes in finger-tip number writing perception on her right hand, she was not able to do the test at all with her left hand. Thus, the results on this measure lean strongly toward damage of the right cerebral hemisphere also. It should be noted that the mistakes with the right hand tended to be in the direction of numbers that involved circular strokes rather than sharp angles. Answering "four" for "five" represents a serious mistake but confusion between the other numbers is less serious. In total, the significant brain-related difficulties almost entirely involved the right cerebral hemisphere. The patient made a mistake in the "w" when writing the word WARNING. It is hard to explain this mistake in the context of the other test results, but considered by itself it probably does not have special significance for left cerebral dysfunction.

Interpretation of the results:

The aphasia examination failed to yield any indication, except possibly for the "w" in "warning," to implicate the left cerebral hemisphere. However, definite evidence of constructional dyspraxia, as demonstrated particularly in the drawing of the cross and the key, point toward right cerebral damage. The Sensory-perceptual Examination also pointed definitely toward right cerebral damage. The five mistakes in finger-tip number writing on the right hand were not sufficient to suggest structural damage of the left cerebral hemisphere, but the evidence of hypesthesia of the left hand, a homonymous left visual field loss, tactile imperception, and tactile finger recognition and finger-tip number writing perception impairment on the left side all point toward a significant lesion involving the middle part of the right cerebral hemisphere.

Specific deficits of the kind shown by this patient would be sufficient to raise a question regarding the presence of a medically significant brain lesion. However, it would be difficult to differentiate between an intrinsic tumor and a vascular accident. Considering the patient's age, a vascular accident probably would not be the usual kind of stroke or cerebral thrombosis but, instead, would probably be a manifestation of a vascular anomaly. If this were a vascular anomaly, we would postulate that the patient has either undergone surgical repair (resulting in the pronounced and definite deficits seen in the test results) or that the lesion had already bled, causing specific damage of the cerebral cortex and the underlying white matter.

A review of the neurological summary for this patient indicates that she had undergone surgery for repair of a large arteriovenous malformation of the right middle cerebral artery, particularly involving the right fronto-temporo-parietal area, 23 days before neuropsychological examination. The patient had evidence of intracranial bleeding before the surgery was performed and it is possible that the deficits, at least in part, are a result of the bleeding rather than residual manifestations of the surgical procedures.

J.B.

NEUROLOGICAL SUMMARY

Symptoms:

This patient developed a severe left-sided headache and was perspiring, weak, nauseated and shortly had a seizure involving the right arm and leg. She was hospitalized almost immediately and a lumbar puncture showed grossly bloody cerebrospinal fluid. A few hours later she had another seizure that lasted about one minute. During the first week of hospitalization the patient had several more seizures and was hardly responsive to environmental stimuli.

Signs:

Upon initial examination the patient was unresponsive except to pain.
She showed an extensor toe sign on the left.
Left eye deviated to the left.
No spontaneous movements of the left arm and only weak movements of the left leg.

Diagnostic Tests:

Bilateral carotid angiograms: Various abnormalities that suggested the presence of a large arteriovenous malformation of the right cerebral hemisphere.

Neuropsychological testing done 23 days after surgical repair of right fronto-temporo-parietal arteriovenous malformation.

Treatment:

Eight days after admission a large right fronto-temporo-parietal arteriovenous malformation was removed as well as a large hematoma overlying the malformation. The brain was swollen and the dura mater, therefore, was left open and the bone flap was not replaced.

Hospital Course:

The patient tolerated the operation well, started to improve promptly, and made steady progress in movement and use of her left extremities. Twenty-four days after the operation (one day before neuropsychological testing), a right cerebral angiogram showed no evidence of any remaining vascular anomaly.

REITAN-INDIANA APHASIA SCREENING TEST

PATIENT: W.E.

Copy SQUARE	Repeat TRIANGLE
Name SQUARE	Repeat MASSACHUSETTS
Spell SQUARE	Repeat METHODIST EPISCOPAL
Copy CROSS	Write SQUARE
Name CROSS	Read SEVEN
Spell CROSS	Repeat SEVEN
Copy TRIANGLE	Repeat/Explain HE SHOUTED THE WARNING.
Name TRIANGLE	Write HE SHOUTED THE WARNING.
Spell TRIANGLE	Compute 85 – 27 =
Name BABY	Compute 17 X 3 = Patient wrote "81" then examiner gave 13 x 4 and patient wrote "52".
Write CLOCK	Name KEY
Name FORK	Demonstrate use of KEY
Read 7 SIX 2 "Six (pause) 7 SIX 2"	Draw KEY
Read MGW	Read PLACE LEFT HAND TO RIGHT EAR.
Reading I	Place LEFT HAND TO RIGHT EAR
Reading II	Place LEFT HAND TO LEFT ELBOW

REITAN-KLØVE SENSORY-PERCEPTUAL EXAMINATION

(Instance indicated where stimulus was not perceived or was incorrectly perceived.)

TACTILE:

RH					LH					Both: RH	X				LH				
RH					LF					Both: RH					LF				
LH					RF					LH					RF				

AUDITORY:

RE					LE					Both: RE					LE				

VISUAL:

																				– (Above eye level)
RV					LV					Both: RV					LV					– (Eye level)
																				– (Below eye level)

TACTILE FINGER RECOGNITION:

Right:	1					2					3					4					5					0 / 20
Left:	1					2					3	4				4		3		5	5					3 / 20

COMMENTS:

FINGER-TIP NUMBER WRITING PERCEPTION:

	4	6	3	5	3	5	4	6	6	5	4	3	5	4	6	3	6	3	5	4	
Right:		3						3									0				3 / 20
Left:																					0 / 20

COMMENTS:

VISUAL FIELDS:

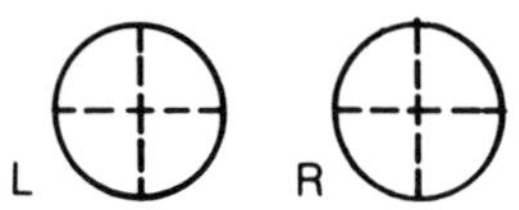

FULL

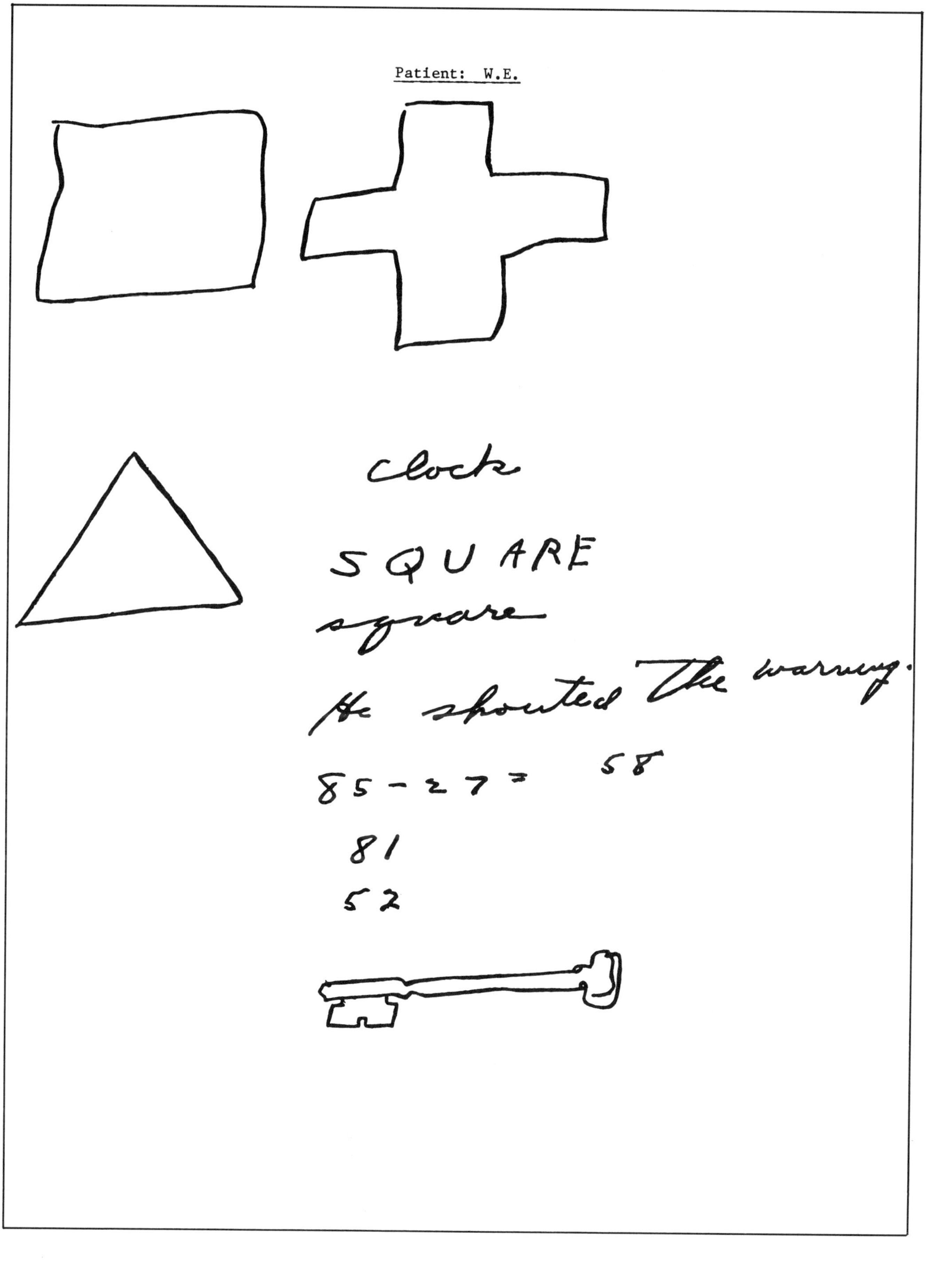
Patient: W.E.
clock
SQUARE
square
He shouted the warning.
85 - 27 = 58
81
52

W.E. – A 63-year-old right-handed male business executive with a twelfth grade education.

Identification of brain-related deficits:

This man showed very few deficits. The form for the Aphasia Screening Test indicates that all responses were basically correct except for 17 × 3. Referring to the patient's writing and drawings, his cross appears to be a little distorted, but is not clearly beyond normal limits. The key almost falls in the same category. However, the handle of the key is unusual and possibly even bizarre, suggesting that the patient had difficulty with the notches of the stem as well as with the handle itself. There may also have been some difficulty with the notches toward the teeth of the key. The drawings probably can be considered to be outside of the normal range, but they are close to being acceptable.

The Sensory-perceptual Examination showed the presence of mild deficits that do go beyond normal limits. The patient made one mistake with double simultaneous stimulation of the two hands, failing to report the stimulus to the right hand in one instance. This, considered by itself, could not be classified as a necessarily abnormal response. However, the patient made no mistakes in tactile finger recognition with his right hand but three mistakes with his left hand. The fact that he made no mistakes with his right hand identifies his ability to perform this test satisfactorily in terms of the attentional requirements. Thus, the three mistakes with the left hand take on added significance. The same type of interpretation applies to finger-tip number writing perception. The patient made no mistakes with his left hand but three mistakes with his right hand. These combined results have no lateralizing significance but point toward abnormalities of response that are mild in nature and implicate both cerebral hemispheres. Thus, results from the Sensory-perceptual Examination, interpreted as signs of cerebral dysfunction, suggest that this man has some generalized impairment.

Interpretation of the results:

As is true for many persons who do not have specific structural cerebral lesions, this man showed relatively little in the way of positive deficits. Medically, he had evidence of hypertensive encephalopathy, a condition that often does not impair IQ values but may have a significant impairing effect on general measures of cerebral functioning. In fact, reference to the complete set of test results indicated that this man had a Full-Scale Wechsler IQ of 124 but made 122 errors on the Category Test. The deficits shown on the Aphasia Test and the Sensory-perceptual Examination, based on a sign approach in a person with probable diffuse cerebral involvement, fail to identify the really significant deficits. This case serves as an excellent example to caution the reader that the tests being reviewed in this manual are particularly sensitive to focal, structural lesions.

W.E.

NEUROLOGICAL SUMMARY

Symptoms:

This 63-year-old man had been treated with variable success for essential hypertension for several years. He complained of occasional feelings of general weakness and unsteadiness on his feet and episodes of mild weakness on his right side. Every one or two months he had an episode of blurred vision of his left eye lasting about five minutes.

Signs:

None.

Diagnostic Tests:

None.

Diagnosis:

Essential hypertension.

TRAUMATIC BRAIN INJURIES, PARKINSON'S DISEASE, MULTIPLE SCLEROSIS, ALZHEIMER'S DISEASE, AND ENCEPHALITIS

The following cases include persons with traumatic brain injuries, Parkinson's disease, multiple sclerosis, Alzheimer's disease, and encephalitis.

REITAN-INDIANA APHASIA SCREENING TEST

Form for Adults and Older Children

Name: R.S. Age: 26 Date: ______ Examiner: ______

Copy SQUARE	Repeat TRIANGLE "Triango"
Name SQUARE "Triangle (pause) no (pause) rectangle." Examiner had to tell him "square".	Repeat MASSACHUSETTS "Massachusess"
Spell SQUARE	Repeat METHODIST EPISCOPAL
Copy CROSS	Write SQUARE
Name CROSS "A regular triangle." Examiner questioned, then patient responded,"An American cross".	Read SEVEN
Spell CROSS	Repeat SEVEN
Copy TRIANGLE	Repeat/Explain HE SHOUTED THE WARNING. Patient repeated correctly, then explained: "He shout the warning at seven, whatever it was".
Name TRIANGLE	Write HE SHOUTED THE WARNING.
Spell TRIANGLE	Compute 85 – 27 =
Name BABY	Compute 17 X 3 =
Write CLOCK	Name KEY
Name FORK	Demonstrate use of KEY Patient could not respond correctly without using a pencil as a key.
Read 7 SIX 2	Draw KEY
Read MGW "M-G-1-2 (pause) 1-2,1-2, W, well W, whatever it is."	Read PLACE LEFT HAND TO RIGHT EAR.
Reading I	Place LEFT HAND TO RIGHT EAR
Reading II	Place LEFT HAND TO LEFT ELBOW

REITAN-KLØVE SENSORY-PERCEPTUAL EXAMINATION

(Instance indicated where stimulus was not perceived or was incorrectly perceived.)

TACTILE:

RH		LH		Both: RH		LH	
RH		LF		Both: RH		LF	
LH		RF		LH		RF	

AUDITORY: RE | LE | Both: RE | LE

VISUAL:

								– (Above eye level)
RV		LV		Both: RV		LV		– (Eye level)
								– (Below eye level)

TACTILE FINGER RECOGNITION:

Right:	1	2	3	4	5	0 / 20
Left:	1	2	3	4	5	0 / 20

COMMENTS:

FINGER-TIP NUMBER WRITING PERCEPTION:

	4	6	3	5	3	5	4	6	6	5	4	3	5	4	6	3	6	3	5	4	
Right:																					0 / 20
Left:																					0 / 20

COMMENTS:

VISUAL FIELDS:

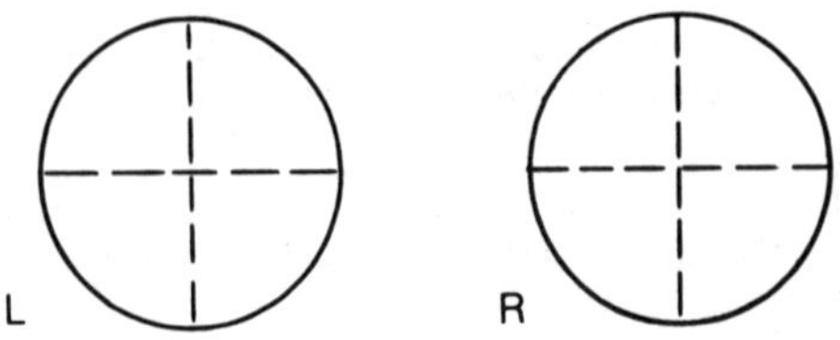

L R

FULL

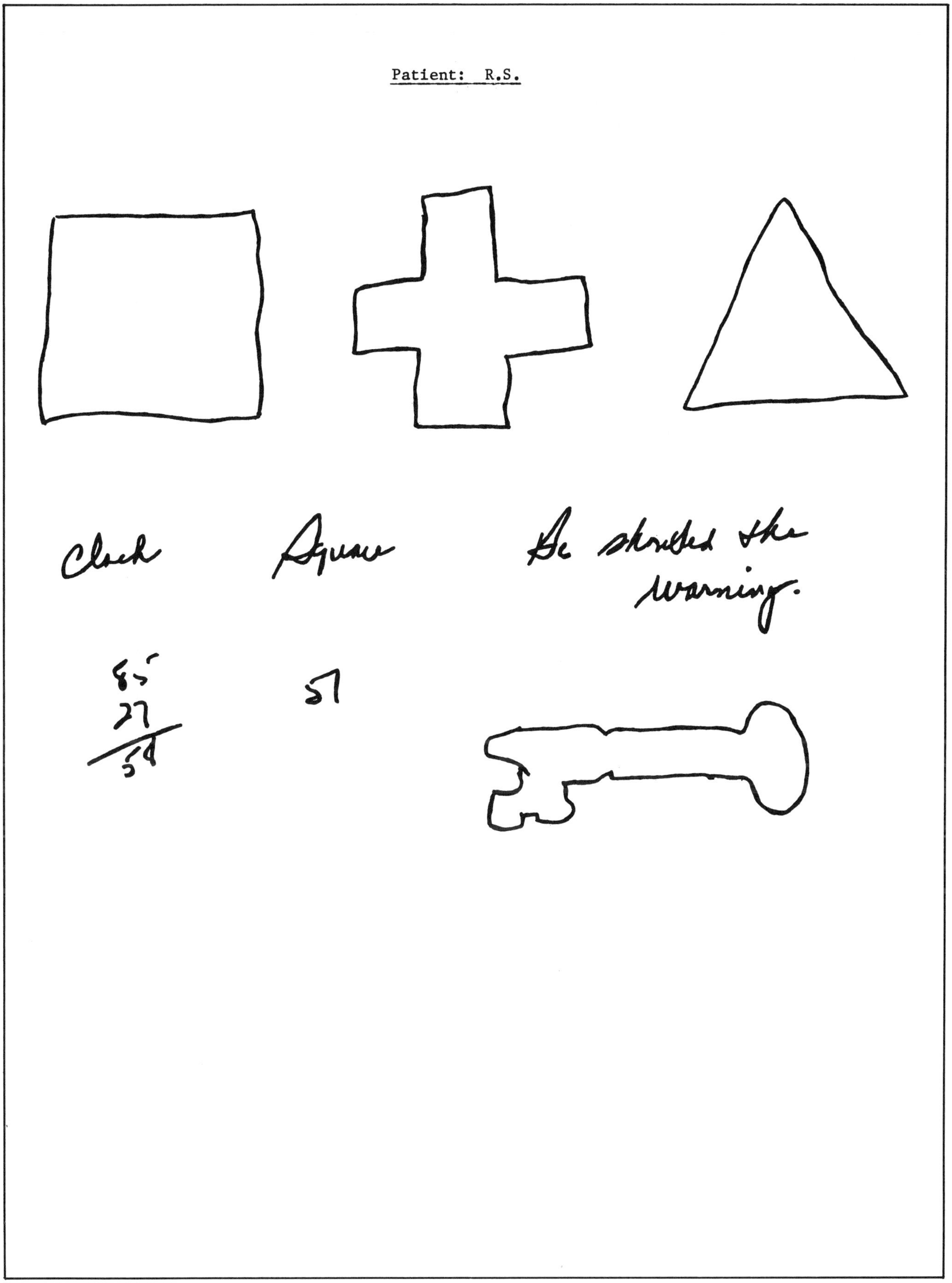
Patient: R.S.

R.S. – A 26-year-old right-handed salesman with 18 years of education.

Identification of brain-related deficits:

The form for the Aphasia test indicates that this man was able to perform a number of things quite satisfactorily but, nevertheless, he did made some mistakes that clearly point toward left cerebral damage. His naming difficulty (dysnomia) was clearly apparent when he was asked to give the name of the square. He was not able to name the figure correctly, first saying "triangle," recognizing that he had given the wrong response, and then saying "rectangle." He had similar difficulty when asked to name the cross. He called it a "a regular triangle" and, when questioned by the examiner if he couldn't think of a better name, he said "an American cross." He was able to spell various words and name other figures. It is apparent from his writing that he has had a good educational background and he showed no deficiencies of any kind in his writing. However, he made mistakes even on very simple items. For example, when asked to read MGW he encountered great difficulties. He read "M-G-1-2 – 1-2, 1-2,W, well, W, whatever it is." This is not a matter of stuttering or stammering. It is a failure to be able to respond correctly, in much the same manner as the patient's difficulty in naming the square and the cross. His repetitions of TRIANGLE, MASSACHUSETTS, and METHODIST EPISCOPAL were within normal limits except for a little slurring. He was able to repeat the sentence HE SHOUTED THE WARNING without difficulty, but when asked to explain its meaning he offered an explanation that did not make sense. In this case it is difficult to conclude that the response represents an auditory verbal dysgnosia. It is possible that the expressive limitations of this man were principally responsible for his difficulty. When asked to demonstrate the use of a key, he was not able to connect the idea with the act until he had a pencil to use as a prop. This difficulty demonstrates the presence of ideokinetic dyspraxia. He performed arithmetic problems quickly and without hesitation, as was true for other items for which no entries were made.

The patient showed no deficiencies in his writing. However, his drawings were not within normal limits. Perhaps the cross would be considered normal, but the lateral extremity on the right side is out of balance with that on the left side. Considered by itself, however, one would probably have to accept the drawing of the cross as being within normal limits. However, the patient did have some difficulties with the key. The stem is entirely too wide, but this is not the critical problem. The problem suggesting brain dysfunction (and probably some degree of right cerebral dysfunction) involves the teeth of the key, where symmetry definitely was lost.

This man showed no evidence of difficulty in any respect on any aspect of the Sensory-perceptual Examination.

Interpretation of the results for R.S.:

The naming difficulties of this man clearly implicate the left cerebral hemisphere. It is possible that his difficulty with language was related to dysnomia. This could have been true even with respect to naming the W in MGW and in the verbalization that was needed to explain HE SHOUTED THE WARNING. However, the patient definitely had quite a concrete attitude as demonstrated by his need for a pencil to substitute for a key when he was demonstrating the use of a key. There is no doubt that the left cerebral hemisphere is principally involved, although the drawing of the key might also suggest some right cerebral impairment. The complete absence of any deficits on the Sensory-perceptual Examination, in the context of the other positive signs, is definitely of significance. Sensory-perceptual deficits occur less frequently with traumatic injuries than with either vascular or neoplastic lesions. Thus, in this sense, the results are entirely compatible with a traumatic injury of the left cerebral hemisphere. The indications of right cerebral impairment were not sufficient to postulate a structural lesion in the right cerebral hemisphere, but it is not at all uncommon in persons who sustain traumatic injuries to have major damage on one side and some additional indications of impairment on the other side. In a case of this kind, however, it would be most important to have a complete neuropsychological assessment in order to understand the overall strengths and weaknesses of the patient.

As indicated in the neurological summary, this man was in a motorcycle accident 12 days before our examination and carotid angiography revealed an area of contusion in the left frontal area. Very probably the failure to find any evidence of sensory-perceptual loss related to the fact that the lesion was anterior in location and very probably did not involve the parietal areas. In addition, however, as noted above, deficits on the Sensory-perceptual Examination frequently are not very prominent in instances of craniocerebral trauma.

R.S.

NEUROLOGICAL SUMMARY

Symptoms:

For several months prior to hospitalization patient had experienced headaches of increasing frequency especially on the left side. He also reported having a "strange feeling" which he couldn't describe. Sometimes he had involuntary and purposeless movements of the right arm. Ten days before hospitalization he fell while riding a motorcycle, struck his head, and was dysphasic when regaining consciousness a few minutes later. He was admitted for observation and evaluation, but 10 days later was transferred to a Medical Center for a more definitive evaluation after cerebral angiography revealed a left cerebral abnormality. By this time his dysphasia appeared to have cleared.

Signs:

Possible mild dysphasia.
Possible mild impairment of purposeful movements of right upper extremity.

Diagostic Tests:

EEG: Left frontal focus suggestive of a destructive lesion, possibly a neoplasm.
Echoencephalography: Possible mild shift from left to right.
Radioisotopic brain scan: Definite left frontal uptake.
Pneumoencephalogram: Depression of left frontal horn and shift from left to right.
Prior cerebral angiogram: Left frontal abnormality.
All of these findings pointed toward a laterally positioned mass in the left frontal area.
Neuropsychological examination done four days before cranitomy.

Treatment:

Craniotomy with removal of left frontal intracerebral hematoma.

REITAN-INDIANA APHASIA SCREENING TEST

PATIENT: F.C.

Copy SQUARE	Repeat TRIANGLE
Name SQUARE	Repeat MASSACHUSETTS
Spell SQUARE "S-Q-U-A-R"	Repeat METHODIST EPISCOPAL
Copy CROSS	Write SQUARE
Name CROSS	Read SEVEN
Spell CROSS	Repeat SEVEN
Copy TRIANGLE	Repeat/Explain HE SHOUTED THE WARNING.
Name TRIANGLE	Write HE SHOUTED THE WARNING.
Spell TRIANGLE	Compute 85 – 27 =
Name BABY	Compute 17 X 3 =
Write CLOCK	Name KEY
Name FORK	Demonstrate use of KEY
Read 7 SIX 2	Draw KEY
Read MGW	Read PLACE LEFT HAND TO RIGHT EAR.
Reading I	Place LEFT HAND TO RIGHT EAR
Reading II	Place LEFT HAND TO LEFT ELBOW

REITAN-KLØVE SENSORY-PERCEPTUAL EXAMINATION

(Instance indicated where stimulus was not perceived or was incorrectly perceived.)

TACTILE:	RH		LH		Both: RH		LH	
	RH		LF		Both: RH		LF	
	LH		RF		LH		RF	
AUDITORY:	RE		LE		Both: RE		LE	
VISUAL:	RV		LV		Both: RV		LV	– (Above eye level) – (Eye level) – (Below eye level)

TACTILE FINGER RECOGNITION:

	1	2	3	4	5	
Right:		X X _ X	X X X X	X X X X		11/20
Left:						0/20

COMMENTS:

FINGER-TIP NUMBER WRITING PERCEPTION:

	4	6	3	5	3	5	4	6	6	5	4	3	5	4	6	3	6	3	5	4	
Right:					X				X	X		X	X			X			X		7/20
Left:								X								X					2/20

COMMENTS:

VISUAL FIELDS:

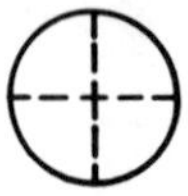
L

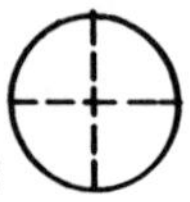
R

FULL

Patient: F.C.

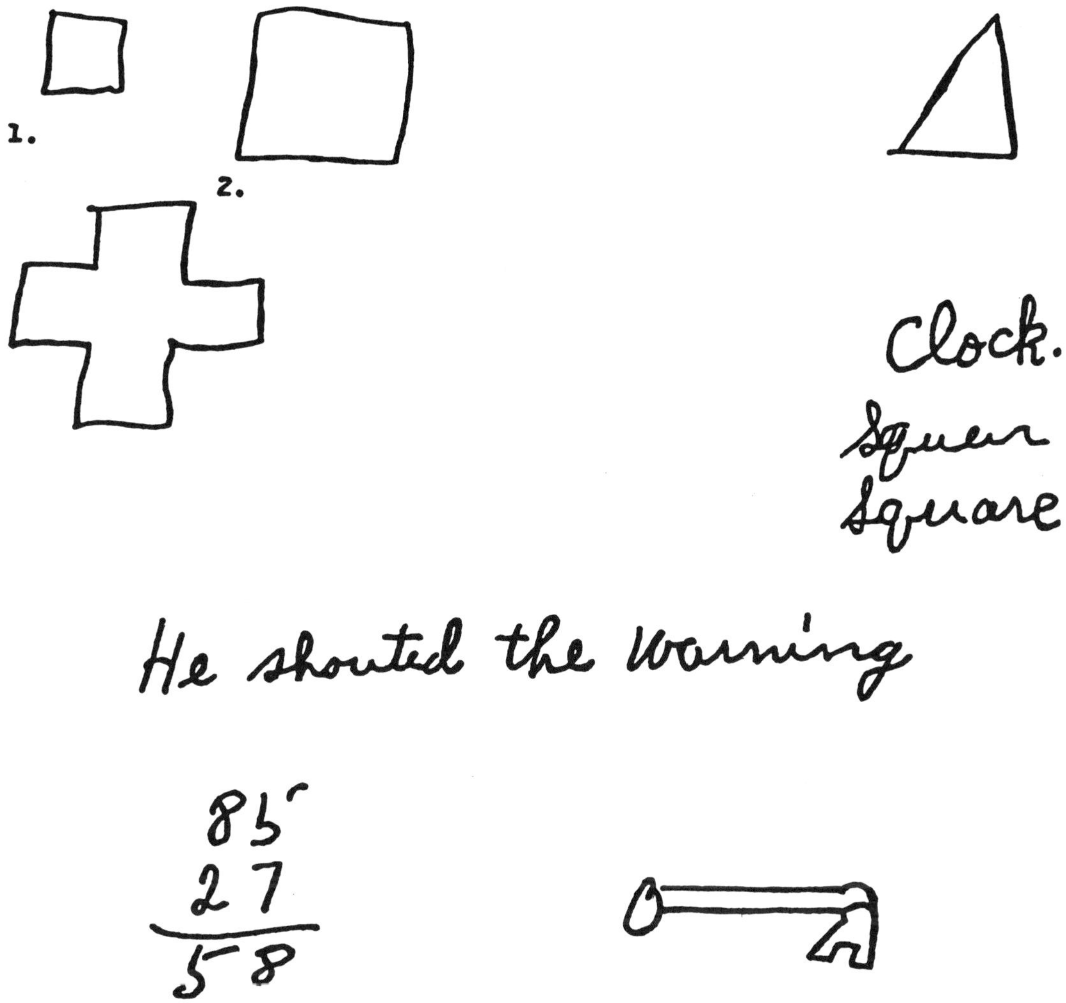

F.C. – A 62-year-old right-handed male painter with a tenth grade education.

Identification of brain-related deficits:

As shown on the Aphasia test form, this man had essentially no difficulty in dealing with the verbal items of the test. His only error was in spelling SQUARE, leaving off the E. This mistake is not uncommon for persons with a rather limited educational background.

The writing and drawings were essentially within normal limits. The patient did appear to have a little difficulty in forming the Q in his writing of SQUARE and, again, ommitted the E at the end of the word. When he was asked to repeat his writing of SQUARE, and be sure to get it right, he wrote the Q with a little more facility and did not omit the E. Aside from this error there were no other deficiencies. His drawing of the figures was within normal limits, even though the key lacked detail and was facing the wrong direction. Thus, one could not conclude that this man had any significant deficits on the Aphasia test.

Results on the Sensory-perceptual Examination did not reveal evidence of any tendency toward sensory imperception. However, the patient had a great deal of difficulty on fingers two, three, and four on his right hand in tactile finger recognition. This is particularly significant because he made no errors in all 20 trials with his left hand. He also had considerably more difficulty in finger-tip number writing perception on his right hand than his left hand. The fact that more errors occurred in the easier task (tactile finger recognition) than the more difficult task (finger-tip number writing perception) probably lends additional validity to the significance of the errors in tactile finger recognition. We extended the Sensory-perceptual Examination with this patient by also writing numbers on his left and right thighs. He had no difficulty recognizing the numbers on his left thigh but was significantly impaired on his right thigh. Thus, even though the patient was able to perceive even light touch on his right side, he had a good deal of difficulty interpreting the significance of symbolic material on that side. It should be noted that these deficits were distinct but quite circumscribed in terms of content, thereby very possibly corresponding to a definite cerebral lesion with distinctly delimited biological effects.

Interpretation of the deficits:

This patient had only certain tactile-perceptual difficulties on the right side and did not show significant evidence of aphasia. He may have had mild difficulty in processing certain aspects of verbal information (as noted in his writing of SQUARE), but in general his language performances and simple drawings were within normal limits. A question would exist as to what kind of lesion would be responsible for the pronounced tactile-perceptual deficits on the right side of the body that could still permit his left cerebral hemisphere to function in a relatively unimpaired way with respect to language and verbal tasks. The lesion would, in all probability, be located principally in the parietal area (because of the tactile-perceptual deficits) and be relatively discrete in terms of its effects. Secondly, the lesion would have to be relatively static and chronic in nature. Of course, additional information from the entire Halstead-Reitan Battery might well be useful in the overall assessment as might also be true of history information and results of neurological diagnostic procedures.

As indicated in the neurological summary, this man did show evidence of generalized cortical atrophy together with evidence of some type of irritative lesion in the middle part of the left cerebral hemisphere. Very probably this lesion represented scar tissue formation from a head injury sustained many years before. It was also of interest that this man showed evidence of a right hemiparesis and Jacksonian seizures particularly involving the right upper extremity.

F.C.

NEUROLOGICAL SUMMARY

Symptoms:

Right hemiparesis, starting suddenly at night four years before present hospitalization. Patient cried out and was found on floor unconscious. Hemiparesis lasted 8-12 hours, and he was amnestic during that time. "Black out" four months after, accompanied by drawing of feet and toes and followed by weakness of right arm. Scattered seizures after that. Struck head during an epileptic attack seven months before hospitalization and received a bruise; 1-5 attacks per day since that have begun to focus in seizures involving the right upper extremity.

Signs:

Neurological examination normal.

Diagnositc Tests:

CSF: OP 180 mm Protein 85 mgm %.
Normal skull films.
Normal carotid angiograms bilaterally.
Normal encephalogram.
EEG: Grade I dysrhythmia, left Sylvian area.
Diffuse cerebral atrophy.

Course:

Stable condition. Anti-epileptic medication adjusted before discharge from hospital.

Diagnosis:

Cortical atrophy, with convulsions due to irritation of left motor area of brain.

Addendum:

Head injury at age 19 years; unconscious 6 hours, headache 3 days.

REITAN-INDIANA APHASIA SCREENING TEST

PATIENT: G.P.

Copy SQUARE First attempt carelessly done.	Repeat TRIANGLE
Name SQUARE	Repeat MASSACHUSETTS "Massaschusess"
Spell SQUARE	Repeat METHODIST EPISCOPAL "Methodist episistixal"
Copy CROSS	Write SQUARE
Name CROSS	Read SEVEN
Spell CROSS	Repeat SEVEN
Copy TRIANGLE	Repeat/Explain HE SHOUTED THE WARNING.
Name TRIANGLE "Rectangle"	Write HE SHOUTED THE WARNING.
Spell TRIANGLE	Compute 85 – 27 =
Name BABY	Compute 17 X 3 = Wrote "42". Examiner gave 13x3 and patient responded correctly.
Write CLOCK	Name KEY
Name FORK	Demonstrate use of KEY
Read 7 SIX 2	Draw KEY
Read MGW	Read PLACE LEFT HAND TO RIGHT EAR.
Reading I	Place LEFT HAND TO RIGHT EAR
Reading II "Here is a friendly animal, a famous winner of dog shows."	Place LEFT HAND TO LEFT ELBOW

REITAN-KLØVE SENSORY-PERCEPTUAL EXAMINATION

(Instance indicated where stimulus was not perceived or was incorrectly perceived.)

TACTILE: RH | LH | Both: RH | LH
RH | LF | Both: RH | LF
LH | RF | LH | RF

AUDITORY: RE | LE | Both: RE | LE

VISUAL: RV | LV | Both: RV | LV – (Above eye level) – (Eye level) – (Below eye level)

TACTILE FINGER RECOGNITION:

	1	2	3	4	5	
Right:			2	3 3		3/20
Left:				3 3		2/20

COMMENTS:

FINGER-TIP NUMBER WRITING PERCEPTION:

	4 6 3 5	3 5 4 6	6 5 4 3	5 4 6 3	6 3 5 4	
Right:						0/20
Left:				_ _ 3 _		1/20

COMMENTS:

VISUAL FIELDS: 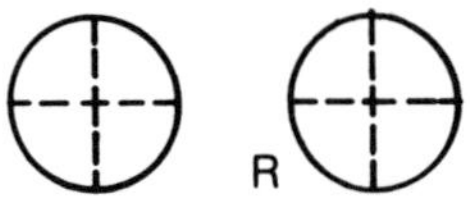 L R FULL

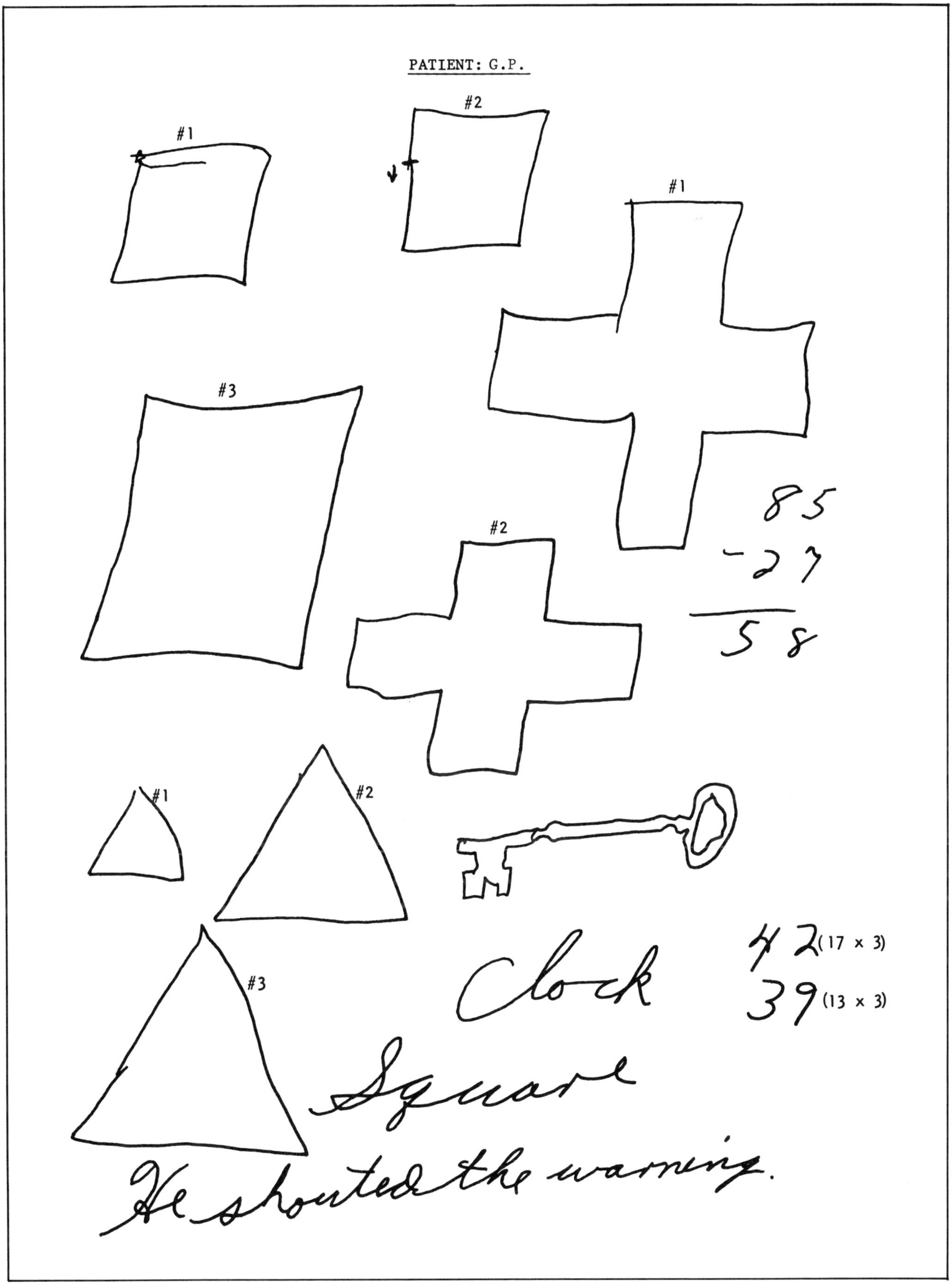
PATIENT: G.P.
#1
#2
#1
#3
#2
85
-27
58
#1
#2
#3
Clock
42 (17 x 3)
39 (13 x 3)
Square
He shouted the warning.

G.P. – A 33-year-old right-handed male farmer with an eighth grade education.

Identification of brain-related deficits:

This patient did not have many aphasic deficits, but nevertheless he did make some mistakes that are distinctly abnormal and indicative of impaired brain functions. When asked to give the name of the triangle he responded "rectangle." One might consider this error to be within the range of normal variation for a person with only an eighth grade education, although it is suggestive of possible left hemisphere damage. On the second reading item the patient read "here" instead of "he." Again one might consider this to be a reflection of the patient's limited education. However, in repeating METHODIST EPISCOPAL the patient made a significant mistake on EPISCOPAL. This error probably provided a basis for answering the question that existed regarding the two previous errors. It would definitely appear that this man has mild brain-related impairment of language functions, even though his deficits may not be sufficient to merit classification as having definite dysphasia. In spite of the foregoing errors, we would postulate that the error in multiplication of 17 × 3 probably is attributable to the patient's limited educational background and is not necessarily a reflection of cerebral damage.

The patient's writing and drawings were also only mildly deviant. Writing of this type is fairly characteristic of a person with limited educational background but the patient made no mistakes. However, the drawings deviate just a little beyond normal expectancy. The first square, as indicated by the examiner, was drawn rather carelessly and was difficult to judge. However, the patient had some definite difficulties with the shape of the second square. He began the figure on the left side drawing a vertical line in a downward direction. His next line was too long and he also made the third line rather long, finally having to come back across the top and draw another descending vertical line in order to complete the figure. Errors of this kind, even though the subject ends up with a fairly adequate looking figure, indicate the presence of some degree of difficulty with spatial relationships. The first cross drawn by the subject was somewhat out of balance, with the lateral extension on the left being somewhat larger and elongated. Although the overall figure looks fairly good, again one can discern a degree of mild difficulty in dealing with spatial configuration. Finally, the key demonstrates additional difficulties. The wavy and uneven lines are not necessarily characteristic of impaired brain functions. However, the imbalance and loss of symmetry in the teeth of the key are probably brain-related. Thus, one would conclude that this patient has at least mild impairment of brain functions as shown by his attempts to draw simple spatial configurations. Whether one calls this by a technical term such as constructional dyspraxia may actually be an unimportant consideration. The important point is to be able to recognize brain-related difficulties, even though they may be quite mild in nature and perhaps not merit the use of a specific technical term.

The Sensory-perceptual Examination yielded few indications of deficit. This man had no difficulties in perceiving either unilateral or bilateral simultaneous sensory stimuli. He did make three mistakes in tactile finger recognition on his right hand and two mistakes on his left hand. These results show no significant lateralizing effect, but the mistakes should not have happened and give a further suggestion of mild impairment of brain functions. The patient made only one mistake in the total of 40 trials in finger-tip number writing perception. This good performance indicates that the patient had the ability to pay attention to stimulus material and that he should have been able to do the tests of tactile finger recognition somewhat more adequately than he did. This finding reinforces the conclusion of mild finger dysgnosia involving both hands.

Interpretation of the test results:

As noted in the neurological summary, this man sustained two serious insults in the form of a severe electric shock 14 years before the present examination and a penetrating wound of the left side of the head 11 years before the examination. Since the man currently was 33 years of age, these insults occurred at approximately the ages of 19 and 22. It is apparent, therefore, that his brain injury was long-standing in nature and there should have been stabilization of brain functions and some degree of recovery from the initial deficits.

The mild difficulties with language performances and the difficulty with drawing of figures very probably do represent residual impairment from these previous injuries. This may also be true of the mild finger dysgnosia. It should be noted, however, that when an insult to the brain occurs, and the biological condition becomes relatively chronic and static in nature, coupled with a sufficient lapse of time for spontaneous recovery of initial impairment, the Aphasia examination may show relatively few residual deficits. In a case of this kind one cannot expect the "sign" approach to provide a very comprehensive assessment of the patient. In fact, the reader should be aware that in many instances of prior cerebral insult the Aphasia test and the Sensory-perceptual Examination miss many of the significant deficits of the patient and fail to provide an assessment that does justice to brain-behavior relationships. In a case of this kind higher-level aspects of brain functions may be seriously and significantly impaired even though the Aphasia test and the Sensory-perceptual Examination show only mild deficits.

G.P.

NEUROLOGICAL SUMMARY

History and Symptoms:

Patient had a severe electric shock while working as an electrician 14 years before current hospital admission, had to be cut from the live electrical wires, and was unconscious for several minutes. Eleven years before admission he suffered a gunshot wound entering his left eye and head, with bullet fragments still lodged in his left cerebral hemisphere. He has had major motor seizures from this injury. He has been anxious and depressed and was hospitalized 5 months before current admission for an overdose of barbiturates, apparently in a suicide attempt. Current admission was to the Psychiatry service because of the patient's emotional disturbance and several attempts over the past two years to seduce his 10-year-old daughter.

Signs:

Neurological examination within normal limits.
Artificial left eye.

Diagnosis:

Gunshot wound of the left eye and head; post-traumatic epilepsy; sociopathic personality, sexual deviate.

REITAN-INDIANA APHASIA SCREENING TEST

PATIENT: L.P.

Copy SQUARE	Repeat TRIANGLE
Name SQUARE	Repeat MASSACHUSETTS
Spell SQUARE	Repeat METHODIST EPISCOPAL
Copy CROSS After first attempt patient commented that it was too small.	Write SQUARE
Name CROSS	Read SEVEN
Spell CROSS	Repeat SEVEN
Copy TRIANGLE	Repeat/Explain HE SHOUTED THE WARNING.
Name TRIANGLE	Write HE SHOUTED THE WARNING.
Spell TRIANGLE	Compute 85 – 27 =
Name BABY	Compute 17 X 3 = Wrote "41". Examiner then gave 15 x 3 and patient responded correctly.
Write CLOCK	Name KEY
Name FORK	Demonstrate use of KEY
Read 7 SIX 2	Draw KEY
Read MGW	Read PLACE LEFT HAND TO RIGHT EAR.
Reading I	Place LEFT HAND TO RIGHT EAR
Reading II	Place LEFT HAND TO LEFT ELBOW

REITAN-KLØVE SENSORY-PERCEPTUAL EXAMINATION

(Instance indicated where stimulus was not perceived or was incorrectly perceived.)

TACTILE: RH, RH, LH; LH, LF, RF; Both: RH, Both: RH, LH; LH, LF, RF

AUDITORY: RE; LE; Both: RE; LE

VISUAL: RV; LV; Both: RV; LV – (Above eye level) – (Eye level) – (Below eye level)

TACTILE FINGER RECOGNITION:

	1	2	3	4	5	
Right:				3		1/20
Left:						0/20

COMMENTS:

FINGER-TIP NUMBER WRITING PERCEPTION:

	4	6	3	5	3	5	4	6	6	5	4	3	5	4	6	3	6	3	5	4	
Right:			2	4																	2/20
Left:				3			5														2/20

COMMENTS:

VISUAL FIELDS:

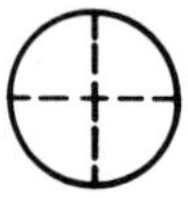

L

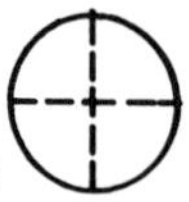

R

FULL

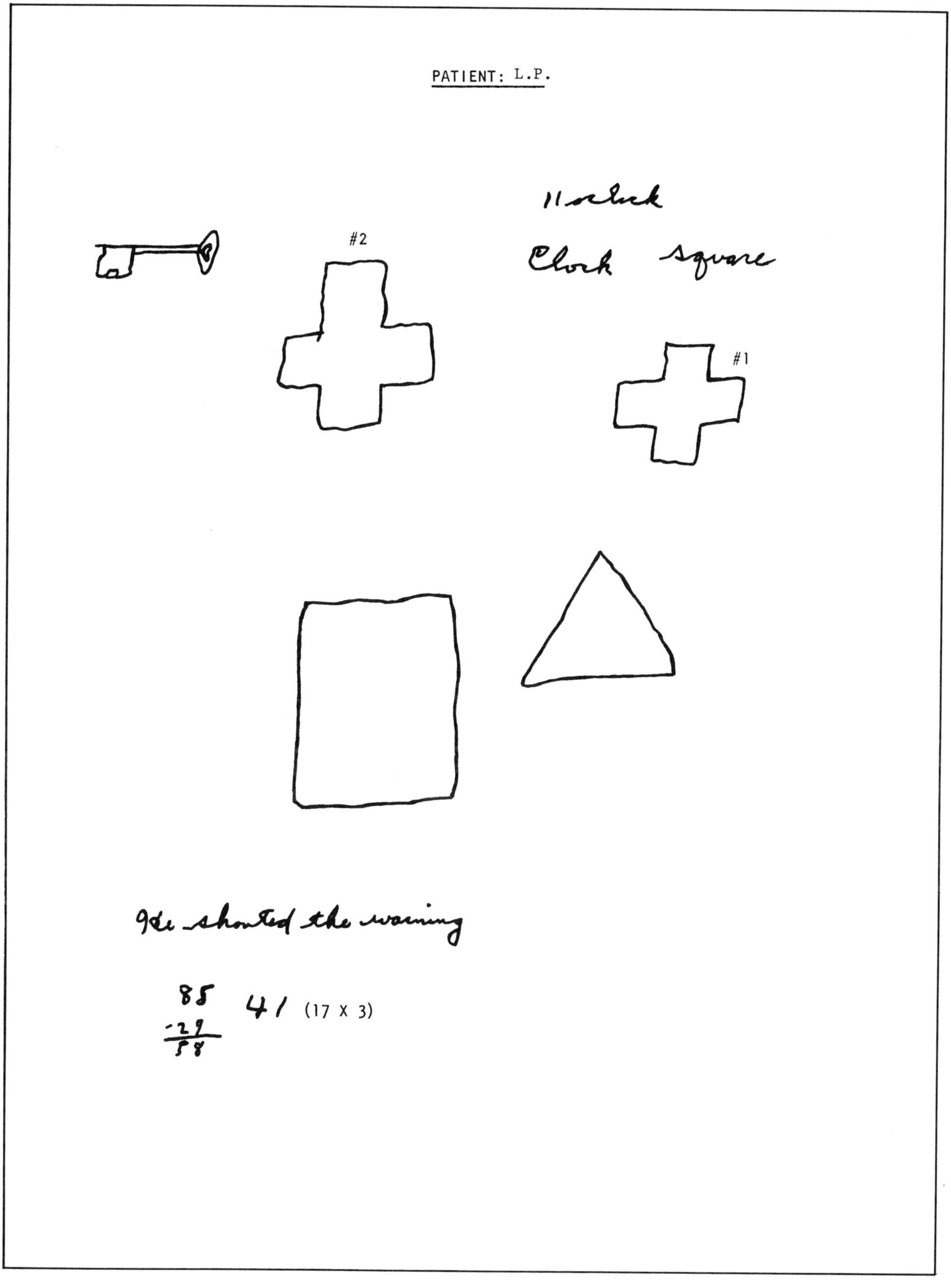
PATIENT: L.P.
11 oclock
Clock square
#2
#1
He shouted the warning
85
-29
58
41 (17 X 3)

L.P. – A 40-year-old right-handed male hydrotherapist with a tenth grade education.

Identification of brain-related deficits:

The form for the Aphasia test indicates that this patient had no particular difficulties on any of the items dealing with verbal material. Reference to his writing and drawings, however, did yield some positive findings. His writing was entirely satisfactory in terms of its symbolic communicational content. His mistake on 17 × 3 is probably of no significance with respect to impaired brain functions. Thus, the difficulties relate to the drawings.

The first cross is probably within normal limits, although a mild tremor is apparent. The drawing of the second cross demonstrates the tremor more obviously and also deviates mildly from normal expectancy, especially regarding the left lateral extremity. The drawing of the key is rather simplified, making it difficult to judge whether or not the patient had special problems in dealing with spatial relationships. It does seem likely, however, particularly considering the "nose" of the key, that this man did have a mild problem in this area. Again, however, one might not elect to apply the term constructional dyspraxia but instead merely to identify that the patient had a little difficulty, that appeared to be brain-related, in dealing with spatial relationships and configurations.

The tremor demonstrated in this case is seen most often in instances of nervous system diseases that impair motor functions. One would raise a question almost immediately, in this instance, of possible Parkinson's disease. Two factors contribute to this. One is the tremor and the second is the tendency toward micrographia. Many patients with a tremor will make a deliberate effort to write rather small letters in order to achieve better motor control. Patients with multiple sclerosis may also demonstrate a tremor but, on the Aphasia test, do not as frequently write in small letters.

The patient had practically no difficulty on the Sensory-perceptual Examination. He made one mistake on the right hand in tactile finger recognition and two mistakes on each hand in finger-tip number writing perception. These errors must be considered to fall within normal limits.

Interpretation of the test results:

There is relatively little to interpret in this case because of the paucity of positive findings. One could speculate regarding the possible presence of Parkinson's disease on the basis of the tremor, the mild deviation from normality in the shape of the cross and the key, and the relatively small handwriting. It must be recognized, however, that the Aphasia test and the Sensory-perceptual Examination do not constitute an adequate neuropsychological examination. In fact, in more detailed testing, this man was found to have a Full-Scale Wechsler IQ of 106, but nevertheless, made 91 errors on the Category Test and had significant deficits on other neuropsychological tests as well. This is a rather typical example of Parkinson's disease as far as the Aphasia test and Sensory-perceptual Examination is concerned, indicating quite clearly that these tests do not measure the significant brain-related deficits in this and many other conditions (Reitan & Boll, 1971).

L.P.

NEUROLOGICAL SUMMARY

History and Symptoms:

Fourteen years prior to admission, at age 27, the patient had encephalitis and was comatose for several months and hospitalized for one year. Patient had a long history of vagrancy, irregular employment, and emotional instability. He first noted onset of tremor of left extremities 10 years before current admission. Right chemopallidectomy was performed 22 months before current admission with improvement of rigidity on the left side but little if any change in the tremor. However, his facial expression and gait became almost normal. Tremor of the right upper extremity began about one year ago.

Signs:

Mask-like facies; frequent eye blinking; inadequate convergence of eyes.
Oscillatory tremor of all extremities, more pronounced on left side.
Cogwheel rigidity bilaterally but more pronounced on left side.

Diagnostic Tests:

Skull x-rays: Normal.
EEG: Dysrhythmia, Grade I, generalized.
Neuropsychological examination done 22 months after right chemopallidectomy and 10 days before left chemopallidectomy.

Treatment:

A left chemopallidectomy was attempted but the patient had a series of major motor seizures. A series of complications ensued and the patient died 49 days following surgery.

Diagnosis:

Post-encephalitic Parkinson's disease, confirmed by autopsy and histopathologic findings.

REITAN-INDIANA APHASIA SCREENING TEST

Form for Adults and Older Children

Name: G.D. Age: 55 Date: ______ Examiner: ______

Copy SQUARE	Repeat TRIANGLE
Name SQUARE	Repeat MASSACHUSETTS "Massachusess"
Spell SQUARE "S-Q-U-A-I-E"	Repeat METHODIST EPISCOPAL "Methodit episcobal"
Copy CROSS Patient repeatedly lifted pencil from paper because of tremor.	Write SQUARE
Name CROSS	Read SEVEN
Spell CROSS	Repeat SEVEN
Copy TRIANGLE	Repeat/Explain HE SHOUTED THE WARNING.
Name TRIANGLE "Rectangle"	Write HE SHOUTED THE WARNING. Patient says she hasn't written for years.
Spell TRIANGLE "T-R-I-A-N-G-L-E-R"	Compute 85 - 27 = Couldn't do. Patient said minus sign was a "t". Examiner gave 15-9 and still couldn't do.
Name BABY	Compute 17 X 3 = Couldn't do. Examiner gave 8 x 5 and still couldn't do.
Write CLOCK	Name KEY
Name FORK	Demonstrate use of KEY
Read 7 SIX 2 "6-7-6-6-2"	Draw KEY
Read MGW	Read PLACE LEFT HAND TO RIGHT EAR.
Reading I	Place LEFT HAND TO RIGHT EAR
Reading II Stumbling performance.	Place LEFT HAND TO LEFT ELBOW

REITAN-KLØVE SENSORY-PERCEPTUAL EXAMINATION

(Instance indicated where stimulus was not perceived or was incorrectly perceived.)

TACTILE:

										Both:									
RH					LH					Both: RH				X	LH				
RH					LF					Both: RH	X	X	X	X	LF				
LH					RF					LH		X	X		RF				

AUDITORY:

RE					LE					Both: RE					LE	X	X	X	X

VISUAL:

																				– (Above eye level)
RV					LV					Both: RV			X		LV					– (Eye level)
													X							– (Below eye level)

TACTILE FINGER RECOGNITION:

Right:	1					2					3	4	2		2	4	3	3	3	3	5	4	4	4	4
Left:	1					2					3					4					5				

11 / 20 (can do / not)

COMMENTS: Patient could not do with left hand.

FINGER-TIP NUMBER WRITING PERCEPTION:

	4	6	3	5	3	5	4	6	6	5	4	3	5	4	6	3	6	3	5	4
Right:		X	2		2			X	3							2		X		X
Left:																				

8 / 20 (can do / not)

COMMENTS: Not attempted with left hand because of tremor.

VISUAL FIELDS:

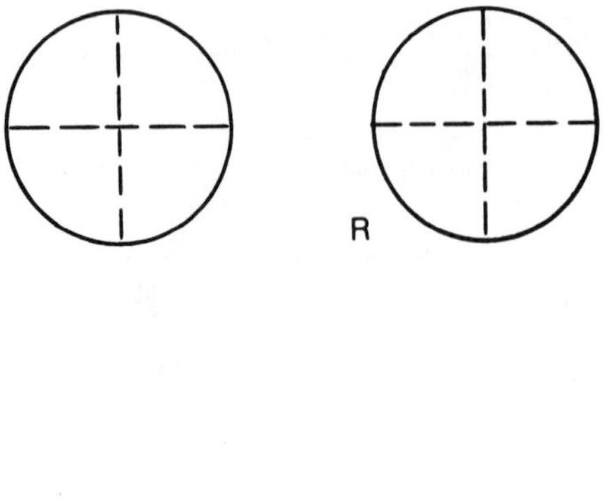

L R

FULL

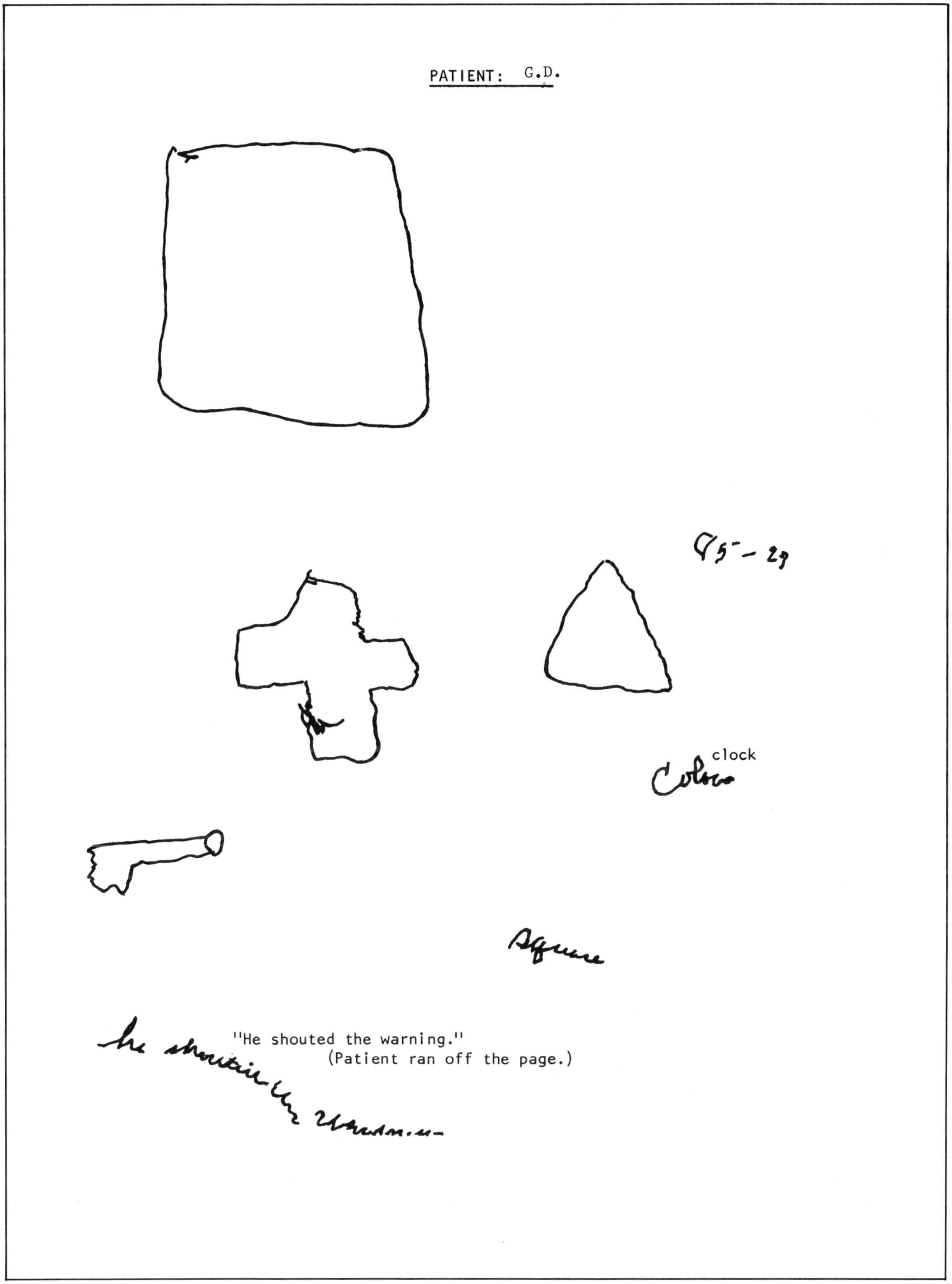
PATIENT: G.D.
clock
"He shouted the warning."
(Patient ran off the page.)

G.D. – A 55-year-old right-handed female homemaker with a fourth grade education.

Identification of brain-related deficits:

Considering the fact that this woman completed only four grades in school, it will be necessary to bear in mind the possiblity that deficiencies in performance may be a reflection of limited educational background. However, reference to the form for the Aphasia test indicates almost immediately that her problems reflect more than a limited education. She shows definite deficits of the kind that are associated with left cerebral damage. For example, in her attempt to spell SQUARE she used an "i" instead of an "r." She also misnamed the TRIANGLE as a "rectangle," a mistake that does not often happen among normal subjects and probably is reflective of a naming deficit. Her spelling of TRIANGLE, with an "r" added incorrectly at the end, is another manifestation of left cerebral dysfunction. Her response to the item 7 SIX 2 probably represents dysnomia. She said "six" instead of "2" and had some difficulty correcting herself. Her stumbling effort in the second reading item could well have been due to limited education and her enunciation of MASSACHUSETTS was within normal limits. However, her repetition of METHODIST was not satisfactory although substitution of a "b" sound instead of the "p" sound for EPISCOPAL is satisfactory. The patient was seriously limited in her ability to perform simple arithmetic problems, apparently failing even to recognize the symbolic significance of a minus sign. This deficit probably goes beyond expectation for a person with only a fourth grade education and may very well constitute a sign of at least mild dyscalculia. These deficits definitely seem to be brain-related and point toward impairment of cerebral cortical function, particularly involving the left cerebral hemisphere.

The patient's attempts at writing and drawing showed definite deficiencies. First, it is obvious that the patient has a definite motor problem that involves both fine and more gross motor control. Over and beyond these problems, however, it is clear that the patient also has a significant problem in dealing with spatial relationships. This was not particularly apparent from her drawings of the square or triangle, but she definitely lost symmetry in the extensions of the cross. Her key was so primitive in its nature that it is difficult to judge what kind of difficulties she may have had.

It is sometimes useful to assess the ability of the patient to write and to make numbers legibly in contrast to the drawing attempts. This woman had sufficient motor control to be able to write 85 − 27 legibly and to write the word SQUARE. Being able to do these things, she should have had the ability, in terms of motor control, to have drawn a better cross and key. Therefore, we would conclude that this woman showed evidence of constructional dyspraxia.

The patient indicated that she had not written for years because of her motor problem. However, we would also judge that her motor problem probably was not entirely responsible for her difficulty in writing the sentence HE SHOUTED THE WARNING. Although she ran off the page, she seemed to lose ability to form letters properly when writing the word WARNING, as is quite typical for persons with dysgraphia.

It would appear, therefore, that this patient demonstrated evidence of spelling dyspraxia, dysnomia, central dysarthria, dyscalculia, dysgraphia, and constructional dyspraxia.

The Sensory-perceptual Examination also showed positive findings. This woman had a distinct tendency to fail to perceive a tactile stimulus to the right hand while it was given in competition, particularly with the left face. However, she also showed a tendency to fail to perceive a stimulus to the left hand when it was in competition with the right face. This tendency to fail to perceive a stimulus to either hand, when in competition with the face, is a sign of generalized deterioration of cerebral function. Although this woman had more difficulty on the right side than the left in terms of tactile stimulation, the overall results would point toward impairment of both cerebral hemispheres. With auditory stimulation, however, the patient showed marked imperception on the left side. She had a tendency toward mild difficulty on the right side with visual stimulation.

It was difficult to evaluate the results of testing for tactile finger recognition and finger-tip number writing perception, except that the patient was clearly impaired. Her tremor of the left upper extremity was so pronounced that the tests could not be carried out reliably. However, the patient made more mistakes on the right hand than should normally have occurred, indicating the presence of finger dysgnosia.

Interpretation of the test results:

These results are quite typical for a patient with fairly advanced Parkinson's disease. The evidence of motor dysfunction (dyskinesia) is perfectly apparent. The patient demonstrated problems in fine motor control as well as gross motor control and also showed a definite tendency toward micrographia. Over and beyond this, the test results point toward involvement of both cerebral hemispheres. Although the neuropathology of Parkinson's disease consists mainly of neuronal degradation in the substantia nigra and hyaline inclusion bodies (Lewy bodies) in many cells of the pars compacta, the brains of many Parkinson patients with clinically apparent dementia also have neurofibrillary tangles and senile plaques that are essentially similar to those seen in Alzheimer's disease (Oppenheimer, 1976). It is not surprising, therefore, that the results of the Aphasia test and Sensory-perceptual Examination may also indicate in many cases of Parkinson's disease that deficits characteristic of involvement of the cerebral cortex are also present.

G.D.

NEUROLOGICAL SUMMARY

History and Symptoms:

Patient had a history of influenza in 1918, at 13 years of age, followed by "sleeping sickness." At age 41 she first noticed twitchings of her right fingers which progressed and was diagnosed as Parkinson's disease. In 1949 the patient had a left pre-motor cortical undercutting but said that this provided no relief from her movement disorder. A left chemopallidectomy was performed when the patient was 53 years of age, resulting in great relief of the tremor on her right side but residual weakness was still present. Currently complained of movement disorder principally on the left side.

Signs:

Mask-like facies.
Marked resting tremor on the left side with typical pill-rolling movements of the left hand.
Speech difficult to understand because of tremor of lips and tongue.
Shuffling gait with dragging of right foot.

Diagnostic Tests:

Skull films: Surgical defect of left fronto-parietal area.
EEG: Probably normal but numerous muscle and movement artifacts.
Neuropsychological examination performed 5 days before right chemothalamotomy for relief of movement disorder.

Treatment:

Chemothalamotomy on the right side with disappearance of left-sided tremor.

Diagnosis:

Parkinson's disease, probably post-encephalitic, with prior surgical alleviation of pronounced movement disorder on the right side and current improvement post-operative of dyskinesia on left side.

REITAN-INDIANA APHASIA SCREENING TEST

PATIENT: W.V.

NOTE: Patient had difficulty using pencil due to poor motor control.

Copy SQUARE	Repeat TRIANGLE
Name SQUARE	Repeat MASSACHUSETTS
Spell SQUARE	Repeat METHODIST EPISCOPAL
Copy CROSS	Write SQUARE
Name CROSS	Read SEVEN
Spell CROSS	Repeat SEVEN "Sever" then responded correctly.
Copy TRIANGLE	Repeat/Explain HE SHOUTED THE WARNING.
Name TRIANGLE	Write HE SHOUTED THE WARNING.
Spell TRIANGLE	Compute 85 − 27 =
Name BABY	Compute 17 X 3 = Patient verbalized "42" then "51".
Write CLOCK	Name KEY
Name FORK	Demonstrate use of KEY
Read 7 SIX 2 "S-I-X"(pause)"7 S-I-X 2." Examiner asked to repeat, then responded correctly.	Draw KEY
Read MGW	Read PLACE LEFT HAND TO RIGHT EAR.
Reading I	Place LEFT HAND TO RIGHT EAR
Reading II	Place LEFT HAND TO LEFT ELBOW

REITAN-KLØVE SENSORY-PERCEPTUAL EXAMINATION

(Instance indicated where stimulus was not perceived or was incorrectly perceived.)

TACTILE:

RH					LH					Both: RH					LH			
RH					LF					Both: RH					LF			
LH					RF					LH					RF			

AUDITORY:

RE					LE					Both: RE				X	LE	X	X		

VISUAL:

																			– (Above eye level)
RV					LV					Both: RV					LV				– (Eye level)
																			– (Below eye level)

TACTILE FINGER RECOGNITION:

Right:	1					2					3					4					5					0 / 20
Left:	1					2					3					4					5					0 / 20

COMMENTS:

FINGER-TIP NUMBER WRITING PERCEPTION:

	4	6	3	5	3	5	4	6	6	5	4	3	5	4	6	3	6	3	5	4	
Right:	X	X	X	X	X	X	X			X	X	X	X	X		X	X	X	X	X	17 / 20
Left:		X			X					X			X	X			X	X			7 / 20

COMMENTS:

VISUAL FIELDS: 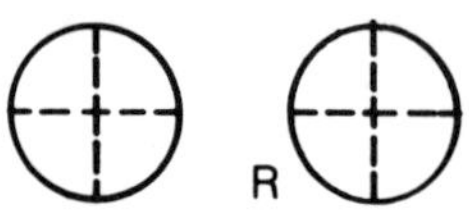 FULL

L R

Patient: W.V.

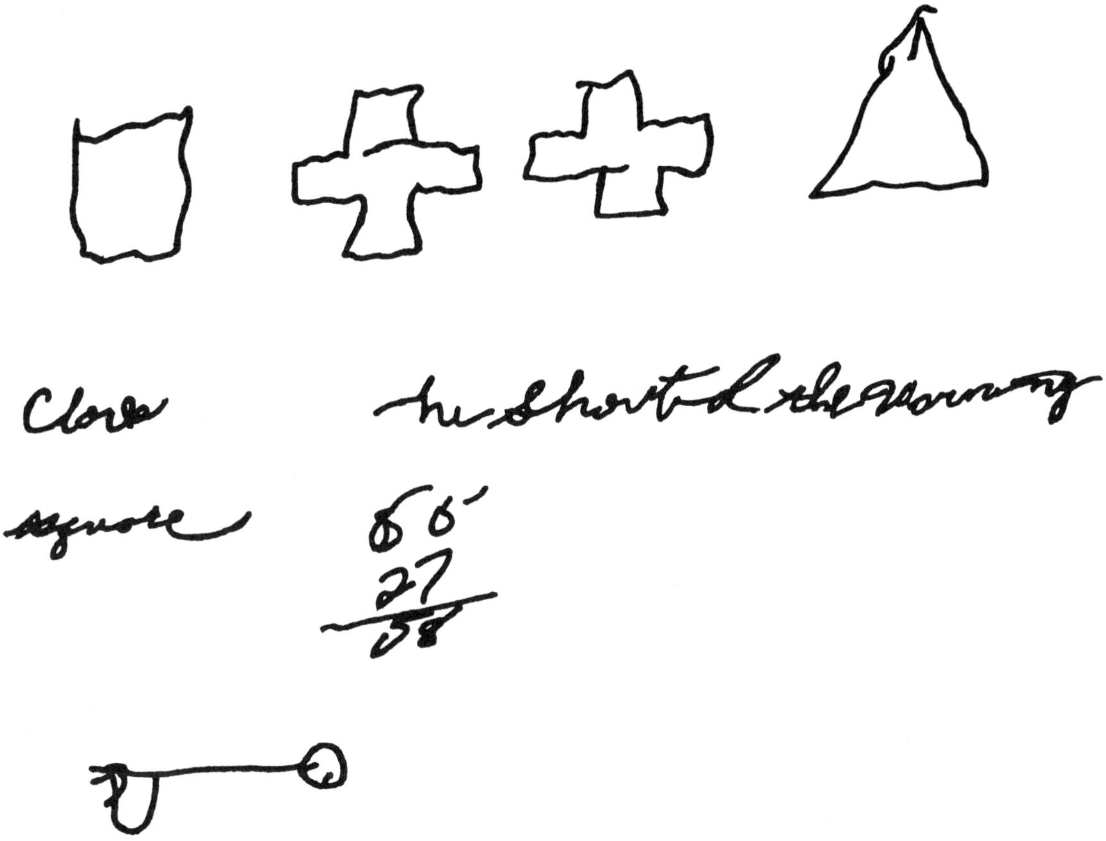

W.V. – A 32-year-old right-handed male painter with a sixth grade education.

Identification of brain-related deficits:

The form for the Aphasia examination does not reveal very many difficulties. However, some responses were quite unusual and worthy of note. For example, in responding to a request to read 7 SIX 2 the patient merely said the letters S-I-X. Next he spontaneously said "7 S-I-X 2." He was asked to look at the item again and to be sure that he got it right and he finally responded correctly. A failure to note that the letters SIX represent a number is not uncommon in patients with mild left cerebral dysfunction.

The next mistake occurred when the patient was asked to read SEVEN. He responded, "sever" and then corrected himself. One might postulate that the mistake may have been due to a loss of visual acuity, but the patient's self-correction tends to suggest that it was a mistake validly representing left cerebral dysfunction.

The patient's confusion in doing 17 × 3 in his head may well have been related to his rather limited educational background. He made a mistake on his first trial and then corrected himself. Corrections on this item, especially among persons with limited educational backgrounds, are less reliable as an indication of brain damage than is true of many of the simpler tasks in this test.

The patient's writing and drawings show evidence of some abnormalities. The writing seems to represent both problems in motor control and a limited educational background. However, if one traces the letters through, there does not seem to be any extra lines or marks, each letter is recognizable and the overall effort seems to be basically within normal limits. While evidence of motor control problems are obvious in the patient's attempts to copy the figures, the distortion of the spatial configuration, especially of the second cross, and the overlapping line in both attempts at drawing the cross, point toward a definite problem in dealing with simple spatial configurations. Thus, we would count both of the crosses as contributing evidence of constructional dyspraxia. The patient drew a very simplistic version of the key. His confusion at the end represented by the teeth (left side) probably also demonstrates the presence of constructional dyspraxia, although it is difficult to know exactly what the patient was trying to do.

The Sensory-perceptual Examination yielded evidence of scattered errors. These occurred particularly with double simultaneous auditory stimulation. In two instances, with stimulation on both sides, the patient failed to perceive the stimulus to the left ear and in one instance failed to perceive the stimulus to the right ear. In other words, the patient failed to perceive stimulation to both ears in three of four trials, a rather unusual performance and probably indicative of some kind of cerebral pathology. However, the patient had no difficulty with tactile stimulation or visual stimulation. On the test for tactile finger recognition he made no mistakes on either hand. Nevertheless, he made quite a number of mistakes in finger-tip number writing perception, missing 17 of 20 trials on his right hand and 7 of 20 trials on his left hand. Obviously there is a difference between the performances with the two hands, definitely implicating the left cerebral hemisphere more than the right.

Interpretation of the results:

Although most items were done correctly and without error, the mistakes made by this man definitely deviate from normal expectancy. Misreading 7 SIX 2 and SEVEN point toward left cerebral damage whereas difficulty with the cross and perhaps the key points toward right cerebral damage. Auditory imperception suggests that bilateral damage may be present as does finger-tip number writing perception, even though the latter test pointed toward more left than right cerebral damage. These scattered and limited findings raise a question regarding terminology – should the patient be called aphasic? Should he be identified as having contructional dyspraxia? Answers to these questions will be debatable in many individual instances, even though the errors are definitely beyond the normal range. The important point is that regardless of whether or not the deficits are reported by name, one can still use the abnormal responses of the patient as signs of cerebral damage. A conclusion definitely would not be reached in this case that pointed toward unilateral cerebral damage. Instead, the overall results point toward involvement of both cerebral hemispheres. Perhaps the left cerebral hemisphere may be somewhat more involved than the right, but this question is essentially academic in consideration of the definite but mild impairment of both hemispheres.

This patient had a diagnosis of multiple sclerosis and the test results are quite typical for this condition. When positive findings occur in patients with multiple sclerosis, they tend to be relatively scattered on both the Aphasia examination and the Sensory-perceptual Examination. In other words, some tasks may be done quite successfully and without any hint of error whereas others show evidence of definite abnormalities. Usually the overall configuration of positive findings points toward involvement of both cerebral hemispheres. Again, it is necessary to note that a complete neuropsychological examination would provide more information regarding strengths and weaknesses among adaptive abilities in patients with multiple sclerosis.

W.V.

NEUROLOGICAL SUMMARY

Symptoms:

Ten days prior to admission patient awoke with smoky, hazy vision in the right eye. This became worse so he could barely perceive light with the right eye. Patient had a similar episode of loss of vision on left 5 years previously.

Signs:

Serious impairment of vision in the right eye. Only light-dark changes and gross movements could be detected.
Left eye, 20/35 vision.
Right pupil slightly dilated and reacted sluggishly.
10 degree central scotoma, left eye.
Neurological examination otherwise normal.

Diagnostic Tests:

CSF: Protein 45.
Gold curve flat.
Serology negative.
EEG: Normal.

Treatment:

Vision improved without treatment.

Diagnosis:

Retrobulbar neuritis, right.
Multiple sclerosis suspected.

Symptoms:

Two years later patient was again hospitalized because of progressive weakness and numbness of both lower extremities, 5 day's duration. The day of admission he developed difficulty using his right hand. Neuropsychological testing done during this hospitalization.

Signs:

Neurological examination: Temporal pallor of discs.
Bilateral mild weakness, both lower extremities.
Vague sensory loss below T4.
Nystagmus.
Mild dysmetria, right upper extremity.
Adiachokinesis, right upper extremity.

Diagnostic Tests:

EEG: Normal.
X-rays: Spine and skull films normal.

Treatment:

Treated with cortisone and physical therapy and improved.

Diagnosis:

Multiple sclerosis.

REITAN-INDIANA APHASIA SCREENING TEST

PATIENT: W.L.

Copy SQUARE	Repeat TRIANGLE
Name SQUARE	Repeat MASSACHUSETTS
Spell SQUARE	Repeat METHODIST EPISCOPAL
Copy CROSS	Write SQUARE
Name CROSS	Read SEVEN
Spell CROSS	Repeat SEVEN
Copy TRIANGLE	Repeat/Explain HE SHOUTED THE WARNING.
Name TRIANGLE	Write HE SHOUTED THE WARNING.
Spell TRIANGLE	Compute 85 − 27 =
Name BABY	Compute 17 X 3 =
Write CLOCK	Name KEY
Name FORK	Demonstrate use of KEY
Read 7 SIX 2	Draw KEY
Read MGW	Read PLACE LEFT HAND TO RIGHT EAR.
Reading I	Place LEFT HAND TO RIGHT EAR Left hand to left ear, then self-corrected.
Reading II	Place LEFT HAND TO LEFT ELBOW

REITAN-KLØVE SENSORY-PERCEPTUAL EXAMINATION

(Instance indicated where stimulus was not perceived or was incorrectly perceived.)

TACTILE:

RH					LH					Both: RH					LH				
RH					LF					Both: RH					LF				
LH					RF					LH					RF				

AUDITORY:

RE					LE					Both: RE		X		X	LE				

VISUAL:

RV					LV					Both: RV					LV					– (Above eye level)
																			– (Eye level)
																			– (Below eye level)

TACTILE FINGER RECOGNITION:

	1				2				3				4				5				
Right:	1				2				3				4				5				0/ 20
Left:	1				2				3				4				5				0/ 20

COMMENTS:

FINGER-TIP NUMBER WRITING PERCEPTION:

	4	6	3	5	3	5	4	6	6	5	4	3	5	4	6	3	6	3	5	4	
Right:		8	8												3						3/ 20
Left:				3			3														2/ 20

COMMENTS:

VISUAL FIELDS: 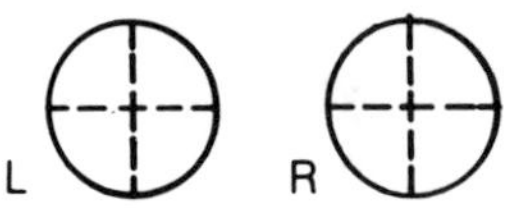 FULL

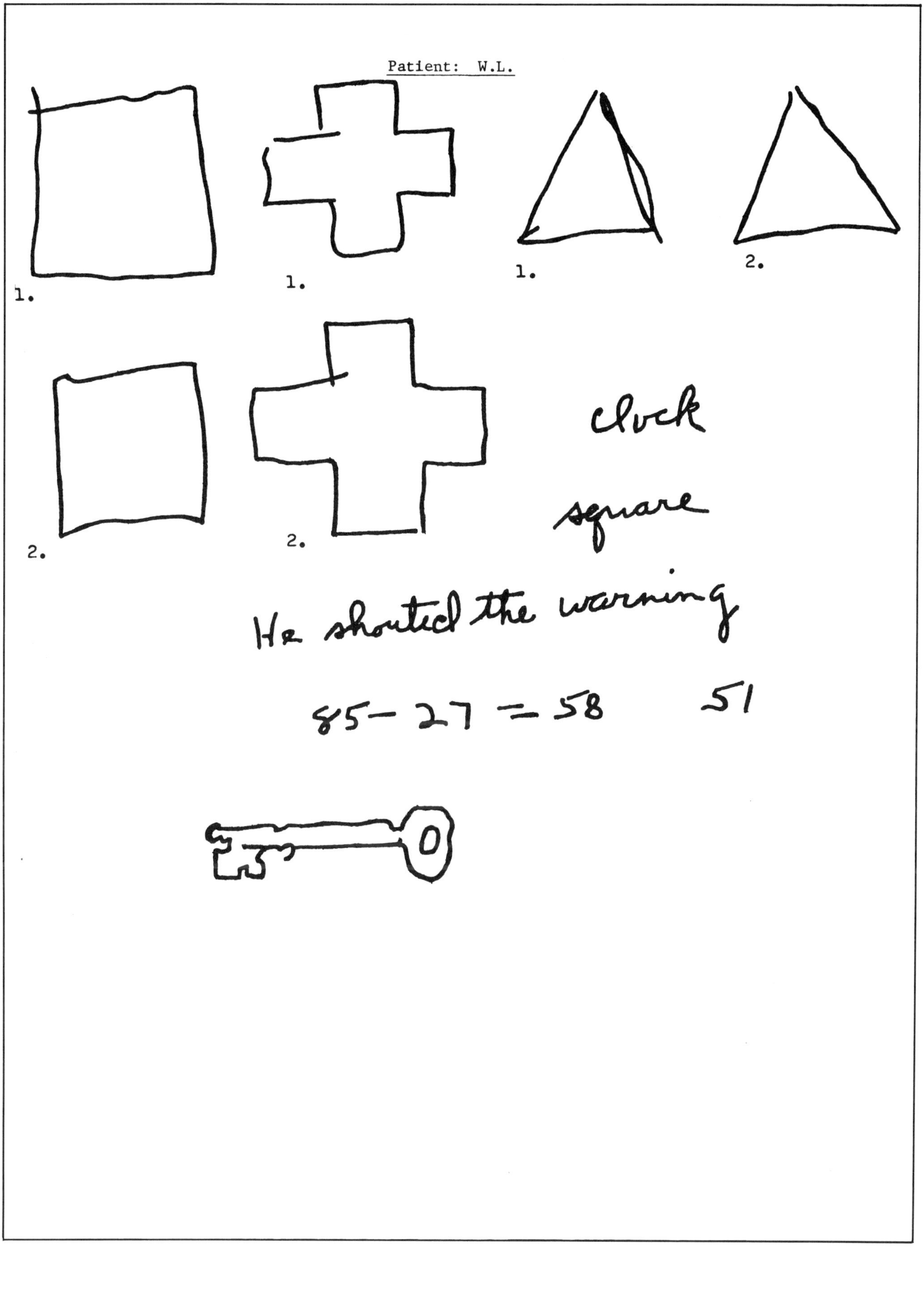
Patient: W.L.
1.
1.
1.
2.
2.
2.
clock
square
He shouted the warning
85 − 27 = 58
51

W.L. – A 41-year-old right-handed male bank officer with a college education.

Identification of brain-related deficits:

The Aphasia test form indicates that this man had relatively little difficulty with most of the items. When asked to put his left hand to his right ear he showed evidence of mild right-left confusion, but he corrected himself. His writing and drawings, however, showed evidence of some difficulties. He had no difficulties with the language or arithmetic items, but did show some mild but definitely pathological difficulties in his attempts to draw figures. His first cross duplicated the figure fairly well, but the extension of the upper horizontal line on the left side probably represents something of a problem in dealing with spatial relationships. This man did not show any definite evidence of problems in motor control, so the extension of the line cannot be attributed to this factor. In fact, when he drew the figure again, he made a similiar kind of mistake. If the drawings of the cross were considered by themselves, these errors might not be a sufficient basis to be confident of cerebral damage. The patient's difficulties in drawing the key, however, make his deficits much more obvious. First, he failed to show mirror images of the notches on the stem close to the handle. Secondly, he definitely deviated from symmetry in drawing the teeth of the key. The third error related to difficulty in completing the "nose" of the key. The final error, which probably is the most definitely pathological in significance, concerns the curved line extending from the bottom part of the stem, near the teeth. The patient seemed to be drawing this curve in the wrong direction; no part of the figure extended in this direction. This kind of error would not be at all likely to occur among control subjects. Thus, although the figures were drawn relatively well, they definitely deviated from the normal range.

The Sensory-perceptual Examination showed only a few deficits. The patient had a distinct tendency to fail to perceive an auditory stimulus to his right ear when stimuli were given bilaterally. He made no other mistakes on tests of double simultaneous stimulation. He also was entirely accurate on all 40 trials in tactile finger recognition. However, he made three mistakes with his right hand and two mistakes with his left hand in finger-tip number writing perception. It should be noted that errors with the right hand all represented instances of confusion involving curved stimulus figures and his answers also consisted of numbers made up of curves. In this sense, the errors were not particularly gross. Considering their nature, the two errors on the left hand may have been more significant than the three errors on the right hand.

Interpretation of the results:

There would be no way that one could definitely draw a conclusion of the presence of multiple sclerosis from these test results. Nevertheless, the complete neuropsychological test battery did provide evidence that permitted such a conclusion. Again, the importance of a complete neuropsychological evaluation is clearly suggested.

The patient did demonstrate scattered deficits of various types. His difficulty in the drawings shows evidence of a mild constructional dyspraxia and he also probably had mild right-left confusion. These findings would point toward involvement of both cerebral hemispheres, although the single instance of mild right-left confusion might not be sufficient by itself to implicate the left cerebral hemisphere.

The Sensory-perceptual Examination provided additional important information. While instances of sensory imperception are usually associated with serious and destructive lesions, the overall results in this case do not point toward such a condition. Nevertheless, the auditory imperception involving the right ear almost certainly would suggest some degree of left cerebral dysfunction. Finally, finger-tip number writing errors round out the picture of relatively mild and scattered losses that point toward involvement of both cerebral hemispheres. This set of results is rather typical for a person with mild deficits resulting from multiple sclerosis.

W.L.

NEUROLOGICAL SUMMARY

Symptoms:

Twelve years before hospitalization the patient first noted weakness of the left leg and foot. This condition progressed gradually and variably, finally involving both lower extremities and, more recently, the upper extremities also.

Signs:

Bitemporal pallor of the eye grounds.
Nystagmus.
Weakness of the left upper extremity and foot drop on earlier examinations which had progressed to spastic paraparesis.
Positive Babinski response and hyperactive reflexes on the left.
Dysdiachokinesis, left more than right.
Mild ataxia, left upper extremity.

Diagnosis:

Multiple sclerosis.

REITAN-INDIANA APHASIA SCREENING TEST

PATIENT: C.C.

Copy SQUARE	Repeat TRIANGLE "Ti-triang-o"
Name SQUARE	Repeat MASSACHUSETTS Correct but slurred.
Spell SQUARE "S-Q-U-A-I-R"	Repeat METHODIST EPISCOPAL Slurred.
Copy CROSS	Write SQUARE
Name CROSS "Plus." Could not think of another name.	Read SEVEN
Spell CROSS	Repeat SEVEN
Copy TRIANGLE	Repeat/Explain HE SHOUTED THE WARNING.
Name TRIANGLE	Write HE SHOUTED THE WARNING. Patient wrote then said, "I misspelled warning."
Spell TRIANGLE	Compute 85 – 27 =
Name BABY	Compute 17 X 3 =
Write CLOCK	Name KEY
Name FORK	Demonstrate use of KEY
Read 7 SIX 2	Draw KEY
Read MGW	Read PLACE LEFT HAND TO RIGHT EAR.
Reading I	Place LEFT HAND TO RIGHT EAR
Reading II "He is friendly animal, a famous winner of dog shows."	Place LEFT HAND TO LEFT ELBOW

REITAN-KLØVE SENSORY-PERCEPTUAL EXAMINATION

(Instance indicated where stimulus was not perceived or was incorrectly perceived.)

TACTILE:

RH					LH					Both: RH					LH			
RH					LF					Both: RH				X	LF			
LH					RF					LH					RF			

AUDITORY:

RE					LE					Both: RE					LE			

VISUAL:

																			– (Above eye level)
RV					LV					Both: RV					LV				– (Eye level)
																			– (Below eye level)

TACTILE FINGER RECOGNITION:

Right:	1			X		2					3					4					5	X		X	X	4/20
Left:	1					2					3					4					5					0/20

COMMENTS:

FINGER-TIP NUMBER WRITING PERCEPTION:

	4	6	3	5	3	5	4	6	6	5	4	3	5	4	6	3	6	3	5	4	
Right:	X		X	X	X	X						X	X	X							8/20
Left:												X									1/20

COMMENTS:

VISUAL FIELDS: 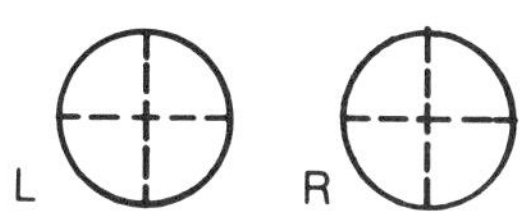 FULL

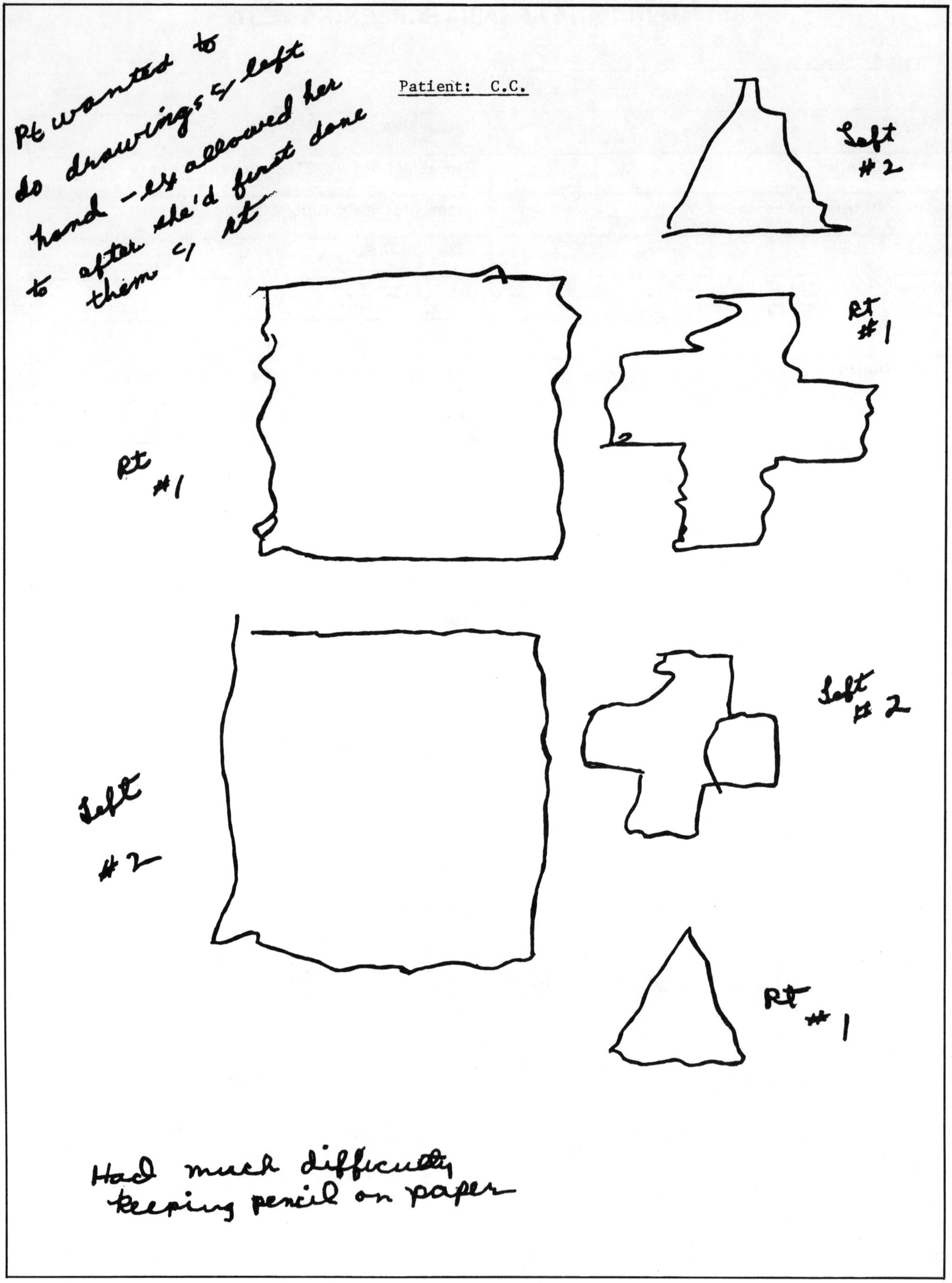
Pt wanted to
do drawings c̄ left
hand - so allowed her
to after she'd first done
them c̄ Rt
Patient: C.C.
Left
#2
Rt
#1
Rt
#1
Left
#2
Left
#2
Rt
#1
Had much difficulty
keeping pencil on paper

Patient: C.C.

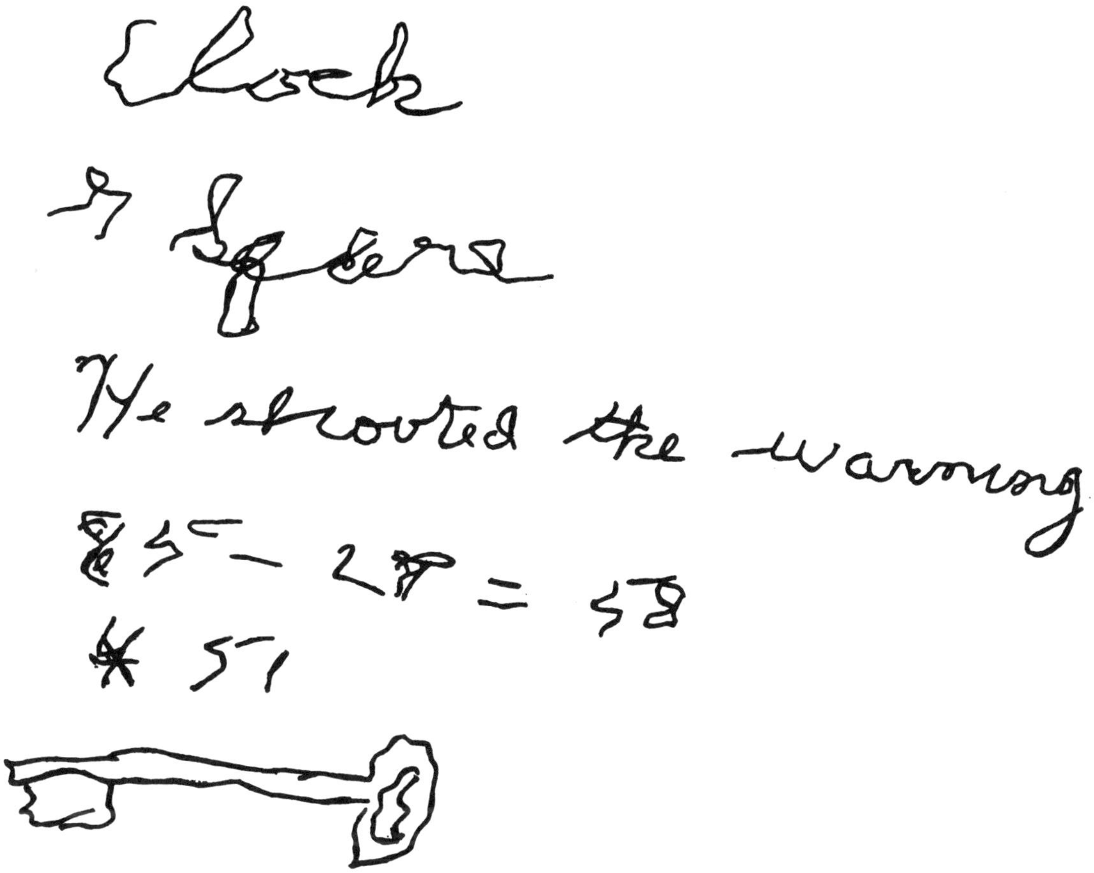

C.C. – A 52-year-old right-handed female homemaker with an eleventh grade education.

Identification of brain-related deficits:

The form for the Aphasia Test indicates that this woman had a few minor difficulties, but she was able to perform most of the verbal items fairly well. She did have a significant problem with motor control as will be noted below.

The first error was in spelling SQUARE, spelling the word S-Q-U-A-I-R. As has been previously noted, omission of the E with the rest of the word correctly spelled is not unusual for persons with somewhat limited educational experience. In this instance, however, the patient inserted an "i" and this is somewhat suspicious with regard to possible brain-related spelling difficulty. When she was shown the picture of the cross and asked to name it, the only name she could give was "plus." Even though she was encouraged by the examiner, she could not think of another possible name. She made no further mistakes until the second reading item, but her only problem in this instance was omission of the word "a." This mistake is probably of no significance. She had a little difficulty in enunciation, but principally it was a matter of slurring the sounds involved. However, on TRIANGLE, she began incorrectly, omitting the R, and this kind of mistake is sometimes suggestive of left cerebral damage.

The patient had a great deal of difficulty with the drawings and writing, but this principally was a manifestation of problems in motor control. She wanted to do the drawings with her left hand, even though she was right-handed, but the examiner had her do them first with her right hand and then with her left hand. Inspection of the drawings suggests that the patient did not have any fundamental problem with the shapes, but that her difficulties related to motor control. The patient had a great deal of difficulty actually keeping her pencil in contact with the paper as well as in drawing straight lines. Probably the principal error of possible significance occurred on the drawing of the second cross, using the left hand. the patient drew a line, involving the right lateral extremity, that went in the wrong direction. This could, however, have been nothing more than a slip of the pencil, considering the motor problems that the patient had.

The writing attempts must be studied carefully in order to differentiate between possible motor control problems and difficulties in dealing with the symbolic language aspects. The major problem occurred when the patient attempted to write the word SQUARE. Her first attempt at writing a capital S may have represented some language difficulty because it looks a little more like an attempt to write a G rather than an S. However, this might again have been a problem with motor control. Omission of the "u" was another matter, especially when the printed letters were directly in front of the patient. This mistake probably does represent a problem of left cerebral functioning. It is difficult to judge the "a" because the patient may have had some problems in getting the pencil to move just where she wanted it to go. Interestingly, the patient commented that she had misspelled WARNING on the next writing item. A careful inspection of her efforts indicates that this was not the case, but her concern, in its own right, revealed a degree of uncertainty in her ability to deal with language symbols. The 7 in the first arithmetic problem definitely was not clear, but the overall effort was correct and the difficulty probably was only due to a problem in controlling the pencil. However, the patient first wrote a 4 when she was attempting to give the answer to 17×3. Although an error of this kind may well be due to the patient's educational background, the corrected mistake may also suggest a little weakness in arithmetical computation. Finally, the drawing of the key was within normal limits, considering the woman's motor problems.

C.C. had some definite difficulties on the Sensory-perceptual Examination that go beyond expected limits for persons with normal brain functions. First, she had just a little difficulty perceiving a tactile stimulus to her right hand when it was given simultaneously with a stimulus to the left face. This single error on tests of double simultaneous sensory stimulation cannot, by itself, be considered a significant finding. However, results on tests for tactile finger recognition were clearly significant. The patient made a total of four mistakes on her right hand and no mistakes on her left hand. This difference is of significance particularly because the patient demonstrated, when her left hand was tested, that she had the basic attentional and discriminational capabilities to be able to do this kind of task correctly. Results on the test of finger-tip number writing perception were even more pronounced. The patient made a total of eight mistakes in 20 trials on her right hand but only one mistake on her left hand. Thus, these findings considered together definitely deviate from normal expectancy and point toward involvement of the left cerebral hemisphere.

Interpretation of the test results:

Although none of the mistakes made by this woman were absolutely of unequivocal significance with respect to cerebral damage, the aggregate probably was sufficient to suggest that she had significant difficulties over and beyond her problems of motor control. We would question whether technical terms should be used in describing the patient's difficulty because her mistakes hardly qualify as definite indications of aphasia. Nevertheless, the original misspelling of SQUARE, followed by omission of the "u" when attempting to write SQUARE, together with an inability to give the correct name for the cross, omission of the sound of the "r" in the first attempt to repeat TRIANGLE and a suggestion of just a little difficulty in confident expression of verbal communication (suggested by the patient's mistaken belief that she had misspelled WARNING) all suggest that this woman does not have quite the ability in dealing with language symbols for communicational purposes that is characteristic of a normal brain. These types of difficulties, in addition, suggest that this was not merely a matter of failure of prior acquisition through educational training. The types of mistakes, considered in total, suggest that the patient has lost some ability that was previously acquired.

It is clear from these findings that this woman did not show any striking deficiencies of an aphasic nature. We also would conclude that her drawings of figures were within normal limits except for the problems of motor control. Questions as to whether the difficulties on the Aphasia test were related to brain dysfunction or due to other factors such as limited educational experience were answered rather definitely by the results on the Sensory-perceptual Examination. C.C. made absolutely no mistakes on the left side of the body except in one instance when she failed to recognize a number written on the third finger-tip. She had relatively little difficulty on tests of double simultaneous sensory stimulation, but did make one error on the right hand when a stimulus was simultaneously given to the left face. The results on testing for tactile finger recognition and finger-tip number writing perception were distinctly more revealing, with errors occurring almost exclusively on the right side of the body. These findings were definitely of lateralizing significance and implicated the left cerebral hemisphere. Given results of this kind, with findings from the Sensory-perceptual Examination pointing toward left cerebral damage and errors on the aphasia examination being of somewhat equivocal significance, it is entirely likely that the difficulties on the aphasia examination represented some involvement of the left cerebral hemisphere. The fact that the mild language difficulties were not more pronounced, in turn, would argue against a recent destructive lesion of the left cerebral hemisphere and would be more compatible with a slowly progressive or relatively long-standing condition. Thus, results from the Sensory-perceptual Examination clearly pointed toward cerebral damage as being present in this patient and the relatively mild language deficits modified this conclusion in the direction of a relatively chronic type of disorder. Considering the obvious movement disorders, the findings are rather typical for two conditions – Parkinson's disease and multiple sclerosis. Considering the patient's age as a variable, one might be inclined to interpret the test results as suggesting the presence of Parkinson's disease rather than multiple sclerosis. However, the clinical diagnosis, based upon the history and neurological evaluation, was multiple sclerosis.

C.C.

NEUROLOGICAL SUMMARY

Symptoms:

Developed a stiff neck three years before current evaluation, went to a chiropractor, and his manipulation of her spinal cord and neck brought on nystagmus, dizziness, partial paralysis of her right side, and a tingling sensation over her entire body. Ten minutes after cessation of this treatment she suddenly lost her speech. The tingling sensation stopped in two days and the patient felt the other symptoms had completely subsided in three months. Two months later, however, she began to notice numbness on both sides of her body, followed in about three months by impairment of balance and occasional falls. Neurological evaluation, eight months after the chiropractic treatment, resulted in a diagnosis of multiple sclerosis, with current symptoms probably not intrinsically related to the chiropractic treatment.

Signs:

Complete neurological studies were done eight months after the chiropractic treatment (31 months before the current neuropsychological evaluation) including EEG, x-rays of the skull and cervical spine, radioactive brain scan, and a pneumoencephalogram. These were all normal and no evidence of a space-occupying lesion was found.

Clinical Diagnosis:

Multiple sclerosis.

REITAN-INDIANA APHASIA SCREENING TEST

Form for Adults and Older Children

Name: W.R.C. Age: 51 Date: ______ Examiner: ______

Copy SQUARE	Repeat TRIANGLE
Name SQUARE	Repeat MASSACHUSETTS "Massachusess"
Spell SQUARE	Repeat METHODIST EPISCOPAL "Methodis" "Espestica." Examiner had to give words individually to get the patient to respond.
Copy CROSS	Write SQUARE
Name CROSS "Kind of a cross."	Read SEVEN
Spell CROSS	Repeat SEVEN
Copy TRIANGLE	Repeat/Explain HE SHOUTED THE WARNING. Repeated correctly after examiner said it twice. Explained, "Afraid." Could not elaborate.
Name TRIANGLE "Kind of a triangle."	Write HE SHOUTED THE WARNING.
Spell TRIANGLE "T-R-Y (pause)." Could not finish.	Compute 85 - 27 = At first tried to add. Examiner questioned him, but he did not understand the minus sign. Examiner told him to subtract.
Name BABY	Compute 17 X 3 = Couldn't do. Examiner gave other problems and patient still had difficulty (see).
Write CLOCK Verbalized "clock", then wrote.	Name KEY
Name FORK	Demonstrate use of KEY Could not do even with props, but examiner noted he could stir his coffee when this occurred naturally.
Read 7 SIX 2 Responded slowly, but correctly.	Draw KEY
Read MGW	Read PLACE LEFT HAND TO RIGHT EAR.
Reading I	Place LEFT HAND TO RIGHT EAR Left hand to left ear.
Reading II "He's a friendly animal of famous winners of dog shows."	Place LEFT HAND TO LEFT ELBOW Crossed arms at wrists and said, "It just won't stay there."

REITAN-KLØVE SENSORY-PERCEPTUAL EXAMINATION

(Instance indicated where stimulus was not perceived or was incorrectly perceived.)

TACTILE:

RH					LH					Both: RH	X			X	LH			X	
RH					LF					Both: RH					LF		X		X
LH					RF					LH	X				RF			X	

AUDITORY:

RE					LE					Both: RE					LE	X		X	

VISUAL:

																				– (Above eye level)
RV					LV					Both: RV					LV					– (Eye level)
																				– (Below eye level)

TACTILE FINGER RECOGNITION:

Right:	1					2					3					4					5				0 / 20
Left:	1					2					3					4					5				0 / 20

COMMENTS:

FINGER-TIP NUMBER WRITING PERCEPTION:

	4	6	3	5	3	5	4	6	6	5	4	3	5	4	6	3	6	3	5	4	
Right:	X	X		X		X		X	X	X	X	X			X			X	X	X	13/ 20
Left:	X	X	X			X	X				X		X		X	X			X		10/ 20

COMMENTS:

VISUAL FIELDS:

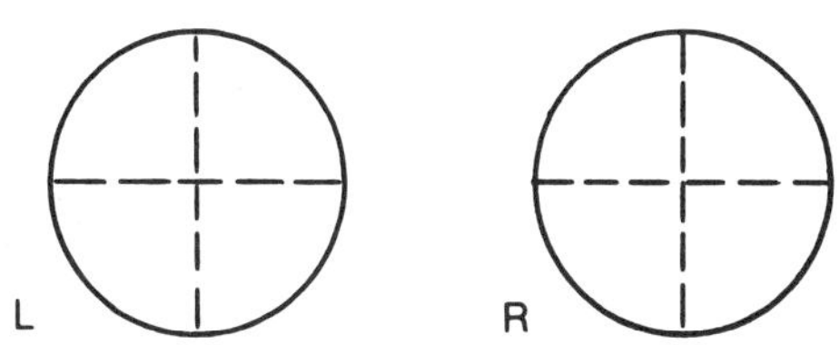

FULL

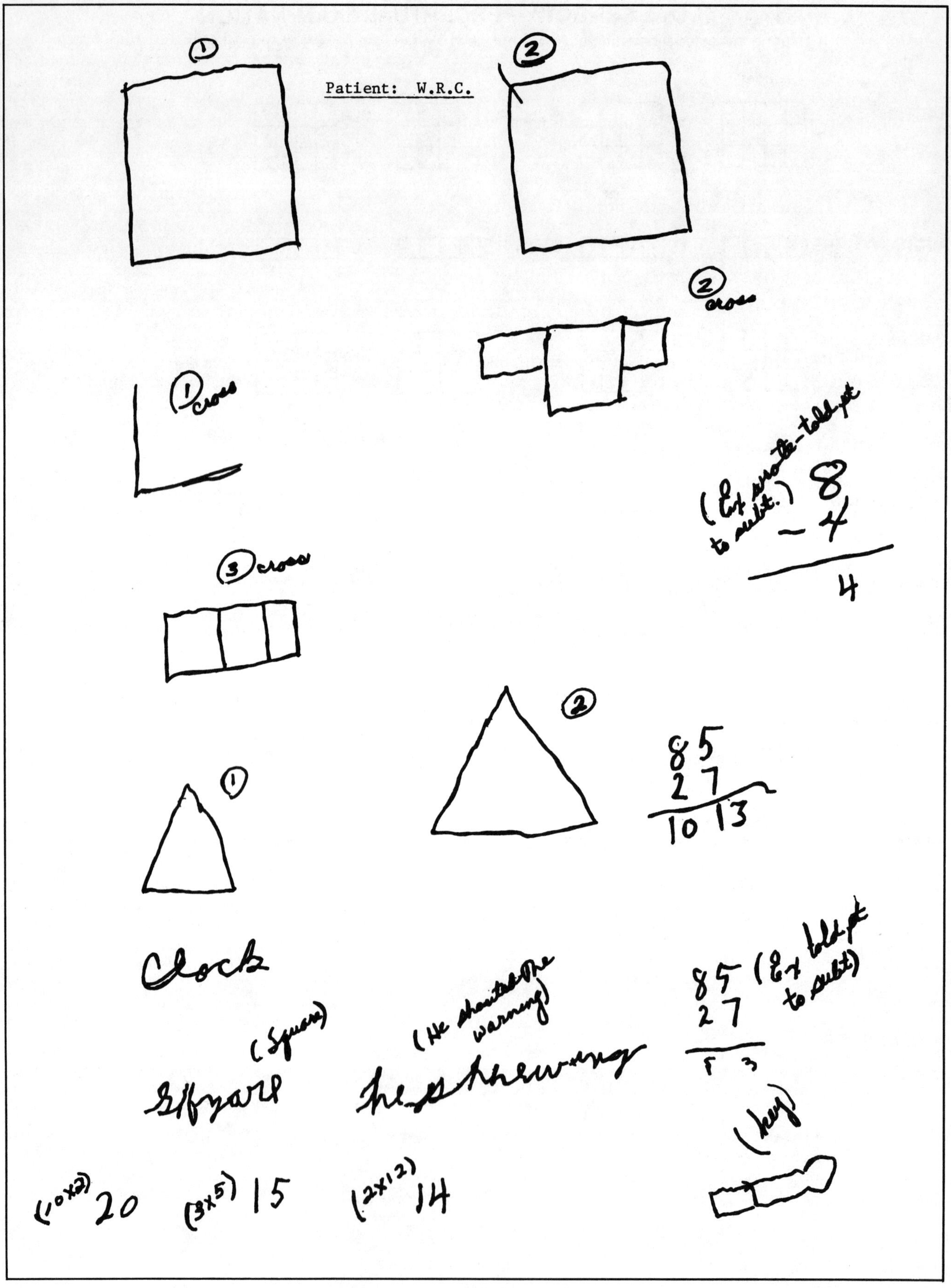
Patient: W.R.C.
cross
Clock
(key)

W.R.C. – A 51-year-old right-handed male janitor with a fifth grade education.

Identification of brain-related deficits:

This patient appeared to be rather limited in his capabilities, but he was able to perform many of the items on the Aphasia test. Spelling TRIANGLE was beyond his capability. It is not unusual for persons with limited educational backgrounds to substitute a "y" for an "i" but this man could not finish the word beyond the "y."

On the second reading item he substituted "of" for "a," but this may also be related to the patient's limited educational background. The first definite pathological manifestation occurred when the patient attempted to say METHODIST EPISCOPAL. The patient said the sounds of EPISCOPAL in the wrong sequence, demonstrating central dysarthria. The next deficit occurred when the subject was asked to explain the sentence HE SHOUTED THE WARNING. It is possible that this man was sufficiently impaired, in a general sense, that he just did not have an intellectual understanding of what the sentence might mean. Thus, his inability to give an explanation of the sentence, or its significance, might be due to general impairment rather than to a more specific deficit (auditory verbal dysgnosia). On the next item, however, the patient attempted to add 85 − 27, failing to understand the meaning of the minus sign. This is a clear indication of dyscalculia. He was able to do simple multiplication procedures, probably by rote memory, even though more complex problems were beyond him.

The patient also demonstrated evidence of ideokinetic dyspraxia. He was unable to demonstrate how he would use a key, even when using a prop such as a pencil. However, he could do things that occurred under natural circumstances, such as stirring his coffee after sugar had been added. The patient demonstrated some degree of right-left confusion when asked to place his left hand to his right ear. He showed general confusion when asked to place his left hand to his left elbow. He crossed his arms at the wrists and said, "It just won't stay there." It is difficult to interpret this response in a specific sense. Possibly the patient was again demonstrating an element of right-left confusion, but more likely he was so generally confused that he could not grasp the fact that the task was impossible.

The patient's writing and drawings demonstrated many deficits. He was able to copy the simple shape of a square but became entirely confused by the more complex shape of the cross. His three attempts, as may be noted, were grossly defective. Returning to a simpler figure such as the triangle, however, re-entered the realm of limited ability shown by this subject and he was able to perform fairly well. The patient had difficulty with the key, obviously drawing a very limited version. While he was able to write certain words, such as "clock," he became confused in attempting to write a "q" in the word "square" and he made little progress in his attempt to write "He shouted the warning." He was able to do very simple arithmetic, but needed to be told by the examiner whether to add, subtract, or multiply.

It is apparent from these findings that this man had limited abilities, although, rather than demonstrating specific deficits in the area of language and verbal functions, he principally performed only at a very low level. Thus, one might ask a question as to whether his deficits were related to his low level of education (having finished only the fifth grade) or to cerebral damage. Some of the deficits in dealing with language symbols probably could be explained in terms of the low educational level. However, other findings, including his failure to recognize the meaning of arithmetical signs and his extremely limited writing, together with his poor drawing of the cross and key, certainly reflect cerebral damage.

The Sensory-perceptual Examination yielded certain positive and certain negative findings. The patient showed a tendency toward imperception of tactile stimuli on both the right and left sides. Although he responded correctly to unilateral stimulation, he showed a definite tendency toward failure to perceive an auditory stimulus to his left ear when it was given simultaneously with a stimulus to the right ear. However, with visual stimulation he responded correctly in every instance. The patient was also able to identify fingers that were touched, although a verbal response system was somewhat beyond his capabilities. In performing the examination we had the patient use his other hand to identify the finger that had been touched by the examiner, and he was able to go through all 40 trials (20 on each hand) without error. However, the patient made many errors on the more difficult task involving finger-tip number writing perception.

Interpretation of the results:

This man demonstrated a tendency toward naming deficits (dysnomia), spelling dyspraxia, dyslexia, central dysarthria, auditory verbal dysgnosia, dyscalculia, dysgraphia, and right-left confusion (all implicating the left cerebral hemisphere) and definite constructional dyspraxia (reflecting right cerebral damage). On the Sensory-perceptual Examination the patient made errors on both sides in responding to double simultaneous tactile and auditory stimuli as well as in finger-tip number writing perception. Thus, the Aphasia examination pointed toward dysfunction of both cerebral hemispheres, the tests of double simultaneous tactile stimulation pointed toward involvement of both cerebral hemispheres, and finger-tip number writing errors did also. It is not surprising that there was not a preponderance of errors on one side or the other considering the fact that primary neuronal degenerative disease would be relatively diffuse in its distribution. Further, although the cognitive requirements of the usual response mode in the test for tactile finger recognition were beyond this man, he was able to recognize the fingers that were touched. This is an example of the resiliency of this test in the face of diffuse or generalized involvement, even when the patient's general competence has been severely compromised. When finger localization difficulties are clearly present the deficit is likely to relate to specific, focal, structural damage.

Even though the findings clearly point toward impairment of both left and right cerebral functions, it would be important to recognize that the results are suggestive of a serious overall deterioration of abilities and a loss in basic understanding. In one sense, the more complex the task became, the more difficulty the patient had. It seemed that he could do relatively simple things, at least within certain areas, fairly well but when the task became at all complex in terms of its cognitive requirements the patient's ability was not sufficient for the task.

This man complained of episodes of memory loss that had been present for about eight months. A pneumoencephalogram showed evidence of some degree of cerebral atrophy. A brain biopsy was done which resulted in a definite diagnosis of Alzheimer's disease. The results of the Aphasia test and the Sensory-perceptual Examination are fairly typical of relatively advanced Alzheimer's disease. However, identification of the full extent of the deficits would require a complete neuropsychological examination.

W.R.C.

NEUROLOGICAL SUMMARY

Symptoms:

Bilateral frontal headaches for about three years, occurring about twice weekly.
Memory loss, particularly involving recent events, for about eight months.
Difficulty in verbal expression, particularly in word finding, for about eight months.
Had gradually become less sociable, did not care to talk with others, and would sometimes just sit in a chair and say nothing to others for rather extended periods.
No indications of irritability or decline in personal hygiene.
Mild head injuries three years and again two years before admission.

Signs:

One neurologist felt that patient was a pleasant person with an apologetic air who did not waste words.
Another neurologist felt that the patient was confused, partially disoriented in space, location and time, and very forgetful. Both neurologists failed to elicit positive objective deficits on the neurological examination.
EEG: Mild generalized dysrhythmia, Grade I, and Delta waves, Grade I, left Sylvian area. Possible neoplastic disease could not be ruled out.
Pneumoencephalogram: Slight symmetrical dilatation of the lateral ventricles, suggesting a generalized degenerative disease.
Brain biopsy: Taken from right superior temporal gyrus. Findings typical of Alzheimer's disease.

Final Diagnosis:

Alzheimer's disease.

REITAN-INDIANA APHASIA SCREENING TEST

PATIENT: V.C.

Copy SQUARE	Repeat TRIANGLE
Name SQUARE	Repeat MASSACHUSETTS "Massachusess"
Spell SQUARE	Repeat METHODIST EPISCOPAL "Methodst Epis--" Could not complete.
Copy CROSS	Write SQUARE
Name CROSS	Read SEVEN
Spell CROSS	Repeat SEVEN
Copy TRIANGLE	Repeat/Explain HE SHOUTED THE WARNING.
Name TRIANGLE	Write HE SHOUTED THE WARNING.
Spell TRIANGLE	Compute 85 – 27 =
Name BABY	Compute 17 X 3 =
Write CLOCK	Name KEY
Name FORK	Demonstrate use of KEY
Read 7 SIX 2	Draw KEY
Read MGW	Read PLACE LEFT HAND TO RIGHT EAR.
Reading I	Place LEFT HAND TO RIGHT EAR
Reading II	Place LEFT HAND TO LEFT ELBOW

REITAN-KLØVE SENSORY-PERCEPTUAL EXAMINATION

(Instance indicated where stimulus was not perceived or was incorrectly perceived.)

TACTILE:	RH		LH		Both:	RH		LH		
	RH		LF		Both:	RH		LF		
	LH		RF			LH		RF	X X	
AUDITORY:	RE		LE		Both:	RE	X	LE		
VISUAL:	RV		LV		Both:	RV		LV		– (Above eye level) – (Eye level) – (Below eye level)

TACTILE FINGER RECOGNITION:

	1	2	3	4	5	
Right:						0 / 20
Left:						0 / 20

COMMENTS:

FINGER-TIP NUMBER WRITING PERCEPTION:

	4	6	3	5	3	5	4	6	6	5	4	3	5	4	6	3	6	3	5	4	
Right:																					0 / 20
Left:	X		X																		2 / 20

COMMENTS:

VISUAL FIELDS:

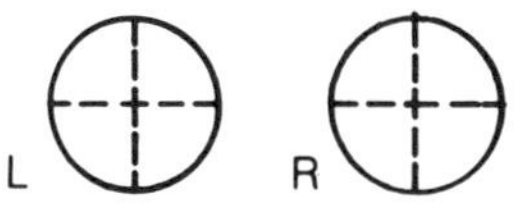

FULL

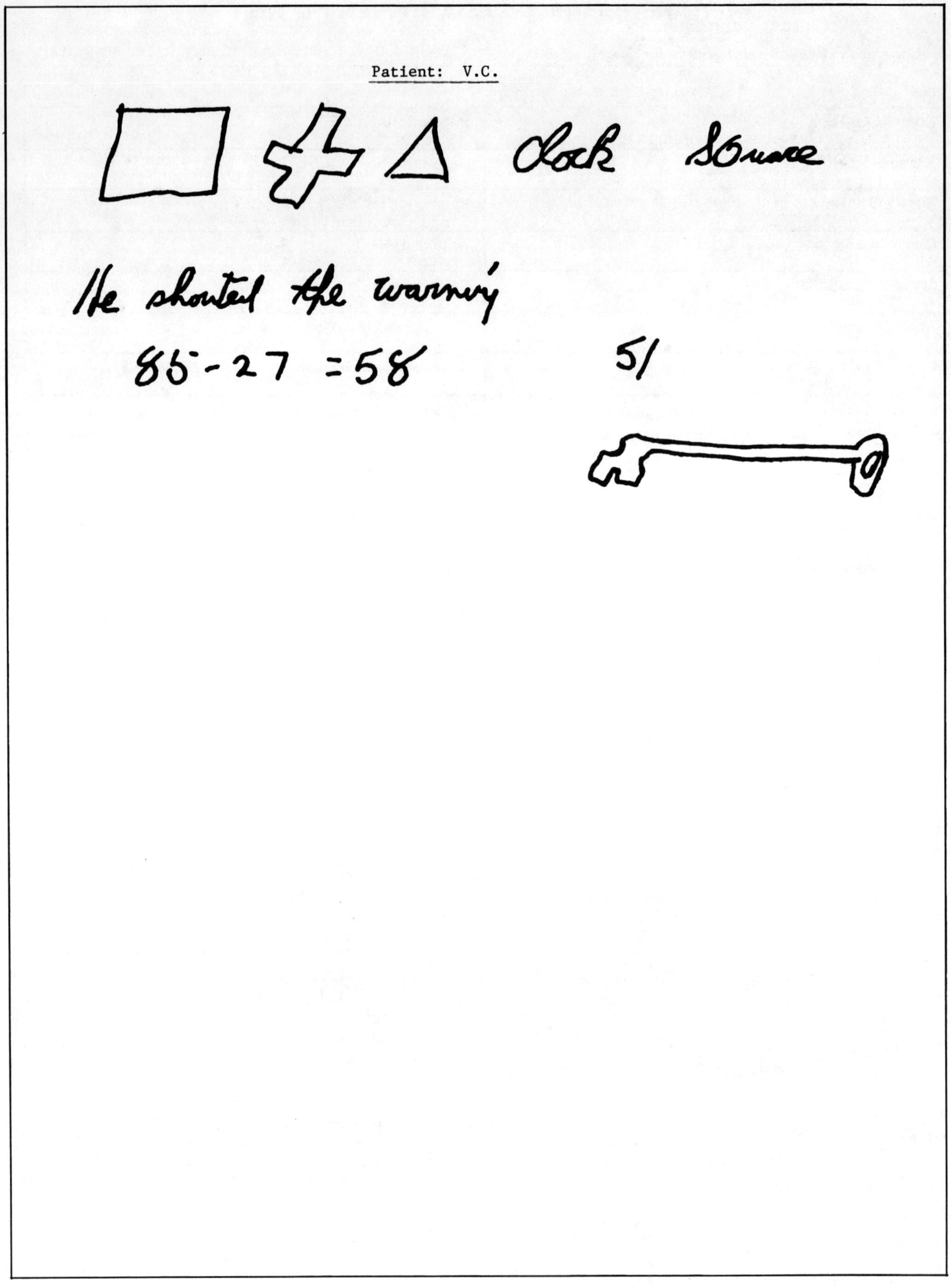
Patient: V.C.
Clock
He shouted the warning
85-27 =58
51

V.C. – A 56-year-old right-handed salesman with a twelfth grade education.

Identification of brain-related deficits:

As was true for the prior patient, this man also had a diagnosis of Alzheimer's disease, although the diagnosis was based upon clinical rather than histological evidence. The form for the Aphasia examination indicates that this man was able to do all of the verbal items correctly except for enunciating the word EPISCOPAL. The patient just was not able to say this word completely. He had a little difficulty in copying certain of the spatial configurations. He tended to tilt the cross and also had some difficulty with the symmetry of the teeth of the key. The loss of symmetry of the key may have some significance for impairment of brain functions, but it would be difficult from these points of information alone to be sure that the patient had a significant cerebral lesion. Tilting of the figures, especially to the right, occurs with a number of non-brain-damaged subjects and cannot be considered, by itself, as a pathognomonic sign. The patient also had difficulty writing the word "square," but some persons, especially ones with limited educational backgrounds, have difficulty writing a "q." Thus, this man did not show any striking evidence of serious losses in the simple tasks included in this test.

The Sensory-perceptual Examination showed evidence of certain deviant responses. For example, the patient had a definite tendency to fail to perceive a tactile stimulus to the right face when it was given simultaneously with a stimulus to the left hand. The patient also had a mild tendency toward imperception of a stimulus to the right ear with double simultaneous auditory stimulation. He had no difficulty in tactile finger recognition on either hand and performed quite well in finger-tip number writing perception. However, on the latter task he did make two mistakes on his left thumb.

More complete neuropsychological examination showed that this man had very striking impairment on higher-level tasks even though his IQ values were relatively intact. This is not uncommon in persons with Alzheimer's disease. This man was not able to perform the Category Test at all well and made relatively little progress with the Tactual Performance Test. Thus, in spite of evidence of severe higher-level impairment, he still had the abilities to do the simple tasks included in the Aphasia test and the Sensory-perceptual Examination. Almost certainly these residual abilities were a reflection of previous skills and the pronounced higher-level deficits reflected impairment in immediate problem-solving capabilities.

V.C.

NEUROLOGICAL SUMMARY

Symptoms:

Patient admitted to hospital because of angina pectoris. Neurosurgical consultation obtained because of history of a fall one month prior to admission. Following this fall he had developed difficulty with memory and slowness of thought.

Signs:

Patient depressed and slightly obtunded.
Neurological examination otherwise negative.

Diagnostic Tests:

Lumbar puncture: Pressure, 175; Protein, 65 and 45.
EEG: Dysrhythmia Grade I, generalized; Delta Grade I, left Sylvian.
X-rays: Skull films negative.
Ventriculogram: Negative.

Diagnostic Impression:

Alzheimer's disease.

REITAN-INDIANA APHASIA SCREENING TEST

Form for Adults and Older Children

Name: R.H. Age: 28 Date: ______ Examiner: ______

Copy SQUARE	Repeat TRIANGLE
Name SQUARE	Repeat MASSACHUSETTS
Spell SQUARE	Repeat METHODIST EPISCOPAL "Methodist Epistopal"
Copy CROSS	Write SQUARE
Name CROSS	Read SEVEN
Spell CROSS	Repeat SEVEN
Copy TRIANGLE	Repeat/Explain HE SHOUTED THE WARNING.
Name TRIANGLE "Diamond." Could not think of another name.	Write HE SHOUTED THE WARNING.
Spell TRIANGLE "T-R-I-G-A-N-G-L-E"	Compute 85 – 27 =
Name BABY	Compute 17 X 3 = Wrote "42". Examiner then gave other problems; made additional errors (see).
Write CLOCK	Name KEY
Name FORK	Demonstrate use of KEY
Read 7 SIX 2	Draw KEY
Read MGW	Read PLACE LEFT HAND TO RIGHT EAR.
Reading I	Place LEFT HAND TO RIGHT EAR
Reading II	Place LEFT HAND TO LEFT ELBOW

REITAN-KLØVE SENSORY-PERCEPTUAL EXAMINATION

(Instance indicated where stimulus was not perceived or was incorrectly perceived.)

TACTILE:

RH					LH					Both: RH					LH				
RH					LF					Both: RH					LF				
LH					RF					LH					RF				

AUDITORY:

RE					LE					Both: RE					LE				

VISUAL:

																				– (Above eye level)
RV					LV					Both: RV					LV					– (Eye level)
																				– (Below eye level)

TACTILE FINGER RECOGNITION:

Right:	1					2					3					4	X		X		5					2 / 20
Left:	1					2					3					4					5					0 / 20

COMMENTS:

FINGER-TIP NUMBER WRITING PERCEPTION:

	4	6	3	5	3	5	4	6	6	5	4	3	5	4	6	3	6	3	5	4	
Right:		X		X										X		X		X		X	6 / 20
Left:			X								X										2 / 20

COMMENTS:

VISUAL FIELDS:

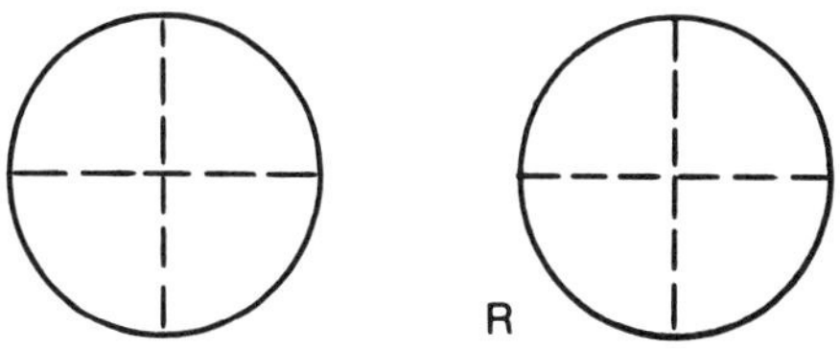

L R

FULL

Patient: R.H.

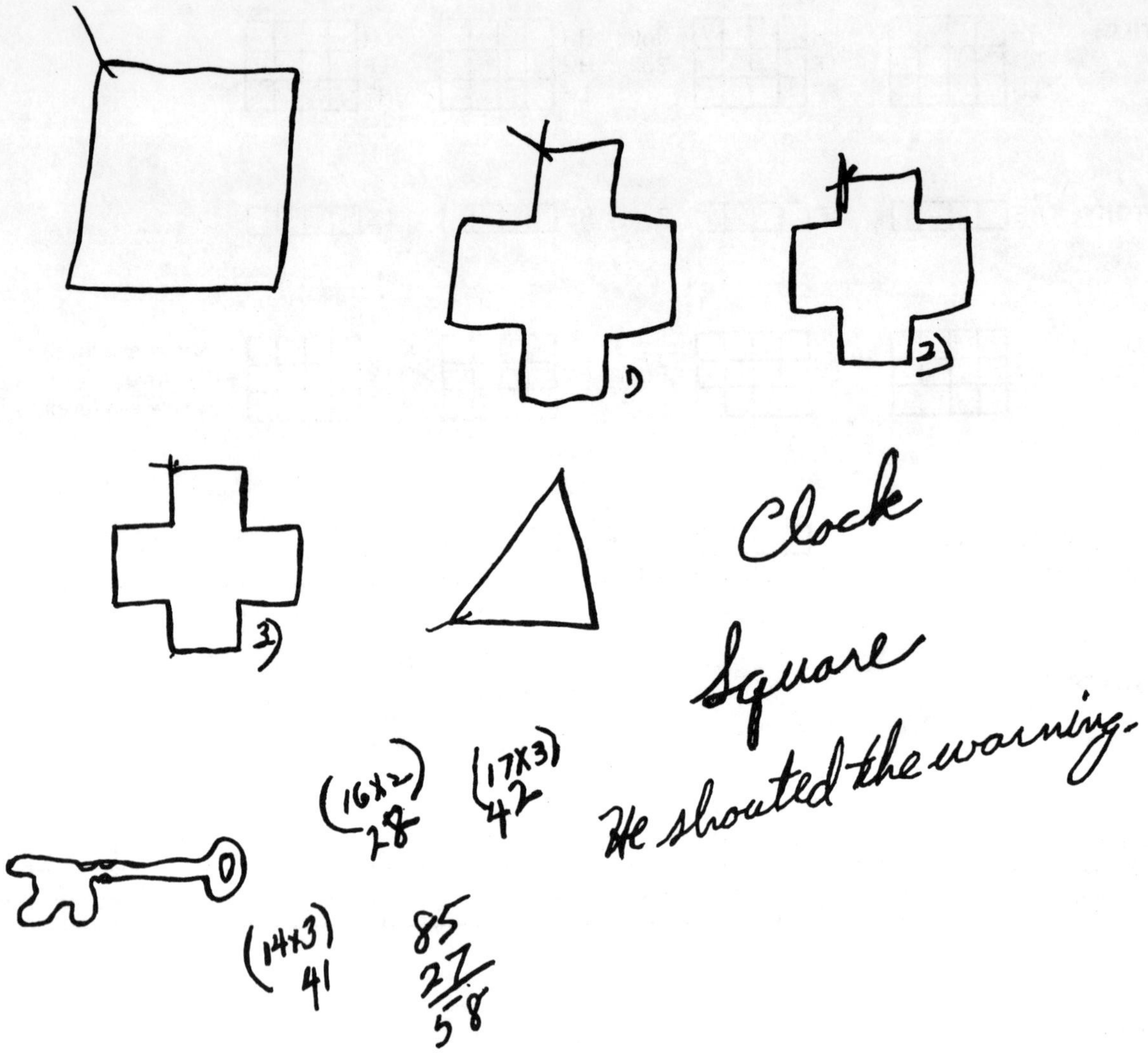
Clock
Square
He shouted the warning.
(16x2)
28
(17x3)
42
(14x3)
41
85
27
58

R.H. – A 28-year-old right-handed male security guard with a twelfth grade education.

Identification of brain-related deficits:

Patients who have had encephalitis may show a wide range of deficits depending upon the severity of the cerebral damage. This man is probably fairly typical, showing some deficits even though they are not very profound.

The form for the Aphasia test shows the presence of a few deficits. The patient probably does have a naming problem (mild dysnomia) as judged from his inability to give the correct name for the triangle. Further, he has a mild spelling problem as demonstrated by his spelling of TRIANGLE. We would not judge that his enunciation of EPISCOPAL was indicative of cerebral damage nor can we be sure that the errors in arithmetic computations are unequivocal indicators of cerebral damage. The patient did make suspicious mistakes in multiplication, especially in his "correction" of 16 × 2. He undoubtedly has some weakness in dealing with numerical relationships, but errors of this kind also occur among control subjects. Thus, the naming of the triangle and spelling of the word represent deviations from normal expectancy but the other difficulties are not definite indications of brain damage.

The patient's writing and drawings were nearly within normal limits. The writing shows no deficits. The drawing of the square, cross, and triangle were also probably within normal limits. However, the notches on the key, close to the teeth, suggest that the patient did have something of a problem with the spatial configuration. The lack of symmetry of the teeth also gives such a suggestion. We would not label these performances as showing evidence of constructional dyspraxia but they probably do reflect mild right cerebral dysfunction.

The patient showed no evidence of errors in tests of double simultaneous sensory stimulation. He had a little difficulty on the fourth finger of his right hand in tactile finger recognition and a little difficulty on both hands in finger-tip number writing perception. These findings would point toward a very mild degree of generalized cerebral dysfunction, with the left cerebral hemisphere perhaps a little more dysfunctional than the right. The findings from the Sensory-perceptual Examination, coupled with the evidence of very mild deficits on the Aphasia test, are probably sufficient to postulate that this man did have a mild degree of generalized cerebral damage. Again, it is important to note that a much more extensive neuropsychological examination would be needed in order to understand the overall adaptive abilities of this man as they related to the status of his brain.

R.H.

NEUROLOGICAL SUMMARY

Symptoms:

Patient developed an acute illness 1½ months before neuropsychological examination characterized by posterior headaches and neck pain, anorexia, lethargy, depression, and acute anxiety and feelings of tension. Psychiatric evaluation noted diminished emotional responsiveness, acute anxiety, paranoid feelings, and a preoccupation with religious matters. A diagnosis was made of schizophrenic reaction, acute undifferentiated type. The patient's emotional problems improved during the next few weeks, but episodes of nausea with projectile vomiting occurred frequently and the patient developed a severe pain and blurring of vision in his right eye. Examination revealed a probable retrobulbar neuritis and this led to referral for hospitalization.

Signs:

Reduced visual acuity of right eye.
Right optic disc was small in size and elevated about three diopters. Disc capillaries were dilated.
Tangent screen examination revealed an enlarged blind spot in right visual field.
No other significant findings on physical and neurological examinations.
EEG, CSF studies, bilateral cervical angiograms all normal.

Course:

Eight days after admission the patient developed a small hemorrhage at the margin of the right optic disc and nausea and vomiting continued.
Eleven days after admission patient began gradually to improve.
Eighteen days after admission the patient was feeling well and all signs and symptoms were gone except for signs of some secondary optic atrophy that was beginning.
Psychiatric evaluation suggested that the patient had a schizoid personality but no diagnosis was made.

Clinical Impression:

Acute encephalitis.

LISTING OF NEUROLOGICAL DIAGNOSES FOR INDIVIDUAL PATIENTS

Patient		*Page*
J.A.	Glioblastoma multiforme – left temporal lobe	48
V.S.	Glioblastoma multiforme – left parietal area	57
J.B.	Ependymoma – left occipital-temporal-parietal area	63
P.H.	Astrocytoma Grade III – right parietal-temporal-occipital area	67
C.B.	Large oligodendroglioma – right	71
V.N.	Glioma – right frontal	77
W.P.	Glioblastoma multiforme – primarily right temporal	81
C.L.	Cystosarcoma phyllodes with metastases to lung and cerebrum – temporal lobes bilaterally	87
A.C.	Metastatic bronchogenic carcinoma – left fronto-parietal	92
W.M.	Probable metastatic melanoma – right posterior parietal-occipital	98
W.F.	Cerebral infarction – distribution of left posterior and middle cerebral arteries	104
C.S.	Cerebral thrombosis – right middle cerebral artery	110
J.B.	Arteriovenous malformation – right fronto-temporal-parietal	114
W.E.	Essential hypertension	118
R.S.	Intracerebral hematoma – left frontal	121
F.C.	Cortical atrophy, with convulsions due to irritation of the left motor area	126
G.P.	Gunshot wound of left eye and head; post-traumatic epilepsy	130
L.P.	Post-encephalitic Parkinson's disease	134
G.D.	Parkinson's disease, probably post-encephalitic	137
W.V.	Retrobulbar neuritis – right; multiple sclerosis suspected	142
W.L.	Multiple sclerosis	146
C.C.	Multiple sclerosis	149
W.R.C.	Alzheimer's disease	154
V.C.	Alzheimer's disease	159
R.H.	Acute encephalitis	162

CHAPTER 8

Conclusions

This book has essentially ignored the many types or categories of aphasia that have been proposed by aphasiologists, taking seriously the observation by almost every student in the field that the individual patient rarely fits any of these categories and, in fact, especially among persons with recent or biologically disruptive cerebral lesions, frequently shows intra-individual variability in the manifestation of specific deficits. Instead, the principal purpose of this volume has been to instruct the reader in conducting a series of simple but standardized tests that deal with language, non-language, and sensory-perceptual functions (using the *Reitan-Indiana Aphasia Screening Test* and the *Reitan-Kløve Sensory-perceptual Examination*) to identify specific brain-related deficits in performance, and to relate these deficits to pathological aspects of the brain. To facilitate this aim a selective review was presented of the area of aphasia as well as the rather extensive research results based upon our particular testing procedures.

No attempt will be made at this point to summarize all of the conclusions, supported by the literature generally, that might be stated regarding aphasia. Instead, we shall cover certain summarical statements that are based upon our own experiments using the Aphasia Screening Test and Sensory-perceptual Examination.

1. Aphasia represents a condition of language deficit, based on impaired brain functions, that is rather specific in nature. This observation is consistent with nature's attribution of only about one-sixth of the cerebral cortex to language and verbal abilities. If one presumes that the entire cerebral cortex subserves other abilities, a corollary of the above conclusion is that other areas of function, in total, constitute a more significant aspect of the human ability structure than do language functions. A second implication is that a complete neuropsychological examination must include far more than an assessment of language functions alone.

2. Research findings have demonstrated that the presence of aphasia is demonstrable with the use of tests that explicitly require expressive and/or receptive language abilities, but that aphasia carries with it no additional consequences (beyond the effects of cerebral damage without aphasia) for the additional major higher-level neuropsychological areas of abstraction, reasoning and logical analysis, or visuo-spatial and manipulatory skills (Reitan, 1960). An implication of this finding is that the left cerebral hemisphere, contrary to popular reports, appears to have no specific or special role in logical analysis and deductive thinking unless language content is involved (Doehring & Reitan, 1962). While certain publications would contest this conclusion, we believe that variables such as early cerebral damage (which leads to alterations in the organization of brain-behavior relationships), the use of abstraction tests that include language content, or imperfect control of pathophysiological status in comparison groups have been responsible for conflicting findings.

3. A methodological approach that employs both intra- and inter-individual comparative data greatly facilitates identification and interpretation of aphasic manifestations in the individual subject.

4. Various aphasic symptoms occur with markedly differing frequency, suggesting that certain deficits are readily produced by even relatively mild cerebral damage whereas other types of deficits that appear to represent "core" aspects of language structure, are much less susceptible to impairment and occur much less frequently. This finding suggests the possibility of an approach to analysis of aphasic manifestations that might relate dissolution of language functions to the acquisition of language functions.

5. Intercorrelations of aphasic and related symptoms show a broadly ranging magnitude, although symptoms of right cerebral damage generally correlate negatively with left cerebral deficits. This finding suggests a methodological approach for the eventual rigorous evaluation and further understanding of language acquisition and language dissolution. A limiting factor in implementation of such an analysis might be the inadequacy and inability of statistical methods and models to simulate the organizational complexity of human brain-behavior relationships.

6. Study of intercorrelations of aphasic and sensory-perceptual deficits indicates a high correlation between the presence of expressive and receptive language deficits, a differential relationship of right vs. left sensory-perceptual deficits to language and aphasic deficits, rather high correlations between symptoms within a single sensory modality but lower correlations between sensory modalities and, in general, a sufficiently complex and diversified situation to recommend caution in any attempt to postulate refined and separate categories of aphasic disorders.

7. That high rates of accuracy are possible in classifying individual subjects to control, right, left, or

generalized cerebral damage groups on the basis of results obtained in individual examinations (Wheeler & Reitan, 1962).

8. Analysis of data from the Aphasia and Sensory-perceptual tests, as compared with data representing 23 major variables from the Halstead-Reitan Battery (Wheeler, Burke & Reitan, 1963; Wheeler & Reitan, 1963), suggests that the Aphasia and Sensory-perceptual tests permit correct classification to groups with right, left, generalized or no brain damage with an accuracy rate approaching that of data based on the 23-variable matrix (Wheeler, 1963). This finding suggests that the tests presented in this volume have a broadly ranging relevance to cerebral functions generally. The limitation implicit in evaluation and interpretation of the findings, however, is a function of the competence and experience of the rater.

Certain additional conclusions can be drawn that pertain more specifically to Aphasia Screening Test and the Sensory-perceptual Examination.

1) These measures include a broadly ranging set of performances that test the adequacy of both left and right cerebral functions, requiring only a short time for administration.

2) They can be administered at bedside and require minimal equipment.

3) They may serve as an initial type of evaluation, with due recognition being given to the likelihood of producing false-negatives when using a sign approach. Positive findings, however, may serve to recommend more complete neurological and neuropsychological evaluation.

4) They have the advantage of an extensive research base for interpretation of results for individual patients.

5) They combine inter-individual and intra-individual inferential approaches as well as verbal and non-verbal (drawings and sensory-perceptual functions) tasks, exploiting their complementary value for individual interpretation.

6) They are oriented toward eliciting specific deficits or abnormalities in performance, as contrasted with the growing tendency of many aphasia tests to assess verbal abilities (verbal intelligence?) on a continuous distribution.

7) We must also note, however, that the Aphasia and Sensory-perceptual tests are not detailed, are not organized according to any specific or selected theory of aphasia and related disorders, and are principally supported by empirically validated findings rather than by formal theoretical positions.

References

Albert, M.L., Goodglass, H., Helm, N.A., Rubens, A.B., and Alexander, M.P. 1981. *Clinical Aspects of Dysphasia.* New York: Springer-Verlag.

Beck, S.J. 1944. *Rorschach's test: I. Basic Processes.* New York: Grune and Stratton. 1945. *Rorschach's test: II. A Variety of Personality Pictures.* New York: Grune and Stratton.

Benson, D.F. 1967. Fluency in aphasia: Correlation with radioactive scan localization. *Cortex, 3,* 373-394.

Benton, A.L. 1964. Contributions to aphasia before Broca. *Cortex, 1,* 314-327.

Benton, A.L. 1965. J.A.P. Gesner on aphasia. *Medical History, 9,* 54-60.

Benton, A.L. 1967. Problems of test construction in the field of aphasia. *Cortex, 3,* 32-58.

Benton, A.L. 1976. Historical development of the concept of hemispheric cerebral dominance. In S.F. Spicker and H.T. Engelhardt, Jr. (Eds.), *Philosophic Dimensions of the Neuromedical Sciences.* Dordrecht, Holland: Reidel.

Benton, A.L. 1977. The interplay of experimental and clinical approaches in brain lesion research. In S. Finger (Ed.), *Recovery from Brain Damage: Research and Theory.* New York: Plenum.

Benton, A.L. 1981. Aphasia: Historical perspectives. In Sarno, M.T. (Ed.), *Acquired Aphasia.* New York: Academic Press, Inc., Pp. 1-25.

Benton, A.L. and Joynt, R.J. 1960. Early descriptions of aphasia. *Archives of Neurology, 3,* 205-221.

Bouillaud, J.P. 1825. Recherches cliniques propres a. demontrer. que la prete de la parloe correspond a la lesion des lobulas anterieurs de cervau. *Journal on Archives Generales de Medecine, 8,* 25-45.

Broman, S.H., Nichols, P.L., and Kennedy, W.A. 1975. *Preschool I.Q.: Prenatal and Early Development Correlates.* Hillside: Lawrence Erlbaum Associates.

Brookshire, R.H. 1978. *An Introduction to Aphasia.* Minneapolis: BRK Publishers.

Brown, J.W. 1972. *Aphasia, Apraxia and Agnosia: Clinical and Theoretical Aspects.* Springfield, Illinois: Charles C. Thomas, publisher, x + 309.

Conrad, K. 1954. New problems of aphasia. *Brain, 77,* 491-509.

Courville, C.B. 1942. Coup-contrecoup mechanism of craniocerebral injuries: Some observations. *Archives of Surgery, 45,* 19-43.

Damasio, A. 1981. Cerebral localization of the aphasias. In Sarno, M.T. (Ed.), *Acquired Aphasia.* New York: Academic Press.

Damasio, A. 1981. The nature of aphasia: Signs and syndromes. In Sarno, M.T. (Ed.), *Acquired Aphasia,* New York: Academic Press.

Darley, F.L. (Ed.). 1967. *Brain Mechanisms Underlying Speech and Language.* New York: Grune and Stratton.

Darley, F.L. and Spriestersbach, D.C. 1978. *Diagnostic Methods in Speech Pathology.* New York: Harper and Row, xvii + 574.

Davis, L.J., Jr. and Reitan, R.M. 1967. Dysphasia and constructional dyspraxia items, and Wechsler verbal and performance IQ's in retardates. *American Journal of Mental Deficits, 71,* No. 4.

DeRenzi, E. 1980. The Token Test and the Reporter's Test: A measure of verbal input and a measure of verbal output. In Sarno, M.T. and Hook, O. (Eds.), *Aphasia: Assessment and Treatment.* New York: Masson Publishers.

DeRenzi, E. and Ferrari, C.1979. The Reporter's Test: A sensitive test to detect expressive disturbances in aphasics. *Cortex, 15,* 279-291.

DeRenzi, E. and Vignolo, L.A. 1962. The Token Test: A sensitive test to detect receptive disturbances in aphasics. *Brain, 85,* 665-678.

Dunn, L. 1965. *Peabody Picture Vocabulary Test, Manual.* Circle Pines, Minnesota: American Guidance Service.

Eisenson, J. 1973. *Adult Aphasia Assessment and Treatment.* New York: Appleton-Century-Crofts.

Emerick, L.L. 1971. *The Appraisal of Language Disturbance, Manual.* Marquette: Northern Michigan University.

Goldstein, K. 1942. *After Effects of Brain Injuries in War.* New York: Grune and Stratton.

Goldstein, K. 1948. *Language and Language Disturbances.* New York: Grune and Stratton.

Goodglass, H. and Blumstein, S. 1973. *Psycholinguistics and Aphasia.* Baltimore: Johns Hopkins Press.

Goodglass, H. and Kaplan, E.1972. *The Assessment of Aphasia and Related Disorders.* Philadelphia: Lea and Febiger.

Halstead, W.C. 1947. *Brain and Intelligence.* Chicago: University of Chicago Press.

Halstead, W.C. and Wepman, J.M. 1949. The Halstead-Wepman aphasia screening test. *Journal of Speech and Hearing Disorders, 14,* 9-15.

Head, H. 1926. *Aphasia and Kindred Disorders of Speech.* Cambridge, England: The University Press, Volume 1.

Head, H. 1951. Hughlings Jackson on aphasia and kindred affections of speech. *Brain,* 38:1.

Hécaen, H. 1979. Aphasias. In Gassaniga, M.S. (Ed.), *Handbook of Behavioral Neurobiology,* Vol. 2. *Neuropsychology,* New York: Plenum Press, Pp 239-292.

Hécaen, H. and Albert, M.L. 1978. *Human Neuropsychology.* New York: John Wiley and Sons, xix + 509.

Heilman, K.M., Rothi, L.J., and Valenstein, E. 1982. Two forms of ideomotor apraxia. *Neurology, 32,* 342-346.

Heimburger, R.F. and Reitan, R.M. 1961. Easily administered written test for lateralizing brain lesions. *Journal of Neurosurgery, 18,* 301-312.

Holland, A.L. 1980. *Commnicative Abilities in Daily Living: Manual.* Baltimore: University Park Press.

Howes, D. and Geschwind, N. 1964. Quantitative studies of aphasic language. In Rioch, D.M. and Weinstein, E.A. (Eds.), *Disorders of Communication.* Baltimore: Williams and Wilkins.

Jackson, J.H. 1932. *Selected Writings.* Edited by James Taylor, London: Hodder and Stoughton, Vol. 2, Pp. 3-237.

Keenan, J.S. and Brassell, E.G. 1975. *Aphasia Language Performance Scales.* Murfreesboro, Tennessee: Pinnacle Press.

Kennedy, F. and Wolf, A. 1936. The relationship of intellect to speech defect in aphasic patients. *Journal of Nervous and Mental Disorders,* 84:125 and 293.

Kertesz, A. 1979. *Aphasia and Associated Disorders: Taxonomy, Localization, and Recovery.* New York: Grune and Stratton.

Kertesz, A. 1980. *Western Aphasia Battery.* London, Ont.: University of Western Ontario.

Kertesz, A., Lesk, D., and McCabe, P. 1977. Isotope localization of infarcts in aphasia. *Archives of Neurology, 34,* 590-601.

Kimble, G.A. 1956. *Principles of General Psychology.* New York: Ronald Press.

Klopfer, B. and Kelley, D.M. 1942. *The Rorschach Technique.* New York: World book, Pp. 436.

Lendau, W.M., Goldstein, R., and Kleffner, F.R. 1960. Congenital aphasia: A clinicopathologic study. *Neurology, 10,* 915-921.

Lenneberg, E. 1967. *Biological Foundations of Language.* New York: Wiley.

Marie, P. 1906. La troisième circonvolution frontale gauche ne joue aucun rôle special dans la function du langage. *Semaine Médicale,* May 23rd, reprinted in P. Marie, 1926, *Travaux et Memoires,* Tome I, Paris: Masson, pp. 3-30. For translation, see M.F. Cole and M. Cole, 1971, *Pierre Marie's papers on speech disorders,* New York: Hafner.

Marin, O.S.M., Schwartz, M.F., and Saffran, E.M. 1979. Origins and distribution of language. In Gassaniga, M.S. (Ed.), *Handbook of Behavioral Neurobiology,* Vol. 2, *Neuropsychology,* New York: Plenum Press, Pp. 179-213.

Meyers, R. 1947. The relationship between "thinking" and language: An experimental approach using dysphasic patients. *Transcripts of the American Neurological Association,* Pp. 65-69.

Meyers, R. 1948. Relation of "thinking" and language: An experimental approach using dysphasic patients. *Archives of Neurology and Psychiatry, 60,* 119-139.

Mohr, J.P. 1978. Broca aphasia: Pathological and clinical. *Neurology, 28,* No. 4, 311.

Munn, N.L. 1951. *Psychology* (Second Ed.). New York: Houghton Mifflin Company.

Ojemann, G.A. (Ed.) 1975. Language and the thalamus: Object naming and recall during and after thalamic stimulation. *Brain and Language, 2,* 101-120.

Oppenheimer, P.R. 1976. Diseases of the basal ganglia, cerebellum, and motor neurons. In W. Blackwood and J.N. Corsellis (Eds.), *Greenfield's Neuropathology.* London: Arnold.

Penfield, W. and Roberts, L. 1959. *Speech and Brain-Mechanisms.* Princeton, N.J.: Princeton University Press, xiii + 286.

Piotrowski, Z. 1937. On the Rorschach method and its application in organic disturbances of the central nervous system. *Rorschach Res. Exch.,* 1:23; 1937. The Rorschac ink-blot method in organic disturbances of the central nervous system. *Journal of Nervous and Mental Disorders,* 86:525.

Porch, B.E. 1967. *Porch Index of Communicative Ability: Theory and Development,* Vol. 1. Palo Alto, California: Consulting Psychologists Press.

Porch, B.E. 1973. *Porch Index of Communicative Ability: Administration, scoring and interpretation.* Vol. 2, Palo Alto, California: Consulting Psychologists Press.

Reitan, R.M., 1953. Intellectual functions in aphasic and non-aphasic brain injured subjects. *Neurology,* 3 (3).

Reitan, R.M. 1954. The performance of aphasic, non-aphasic, and control subjects on the Rorschach Test. *The Journal of General Psychology, 51,* 199-212.

Reitan, R.M. 1954. Intelligence and language functions in dysphasic patients. *Diseases of the Nervous System, 15,* 1-8.

Reitan, R.M. 1955. The relation of the Trail Making Test to organic brain damage. *Journal of Consulting Psychology, 19,* 393-394.

Reitan, R.M. 1958. Validity of the Trail Making Test as an indicator of organic brain damage. *Perceptual and Motor Skills, 8,* 271-276.

Reitan, R.M. 1960. The significance of dysphasia for intelligence and adaptive abilities. *Journal of Psychology, 50,* 355-376.

Reitan, R.M. 1962. Problems in evaluating the psychological effects of brain lesions. Spl. supplement, *A.P.A. Div. 22, Newsletter.*

Sarno, M.T. 1969. *The Functional Communication Profile: Manual of Directions.* New York: New York University Medical Center – The Institute of Rehabilitation Medicine.

Sarno, M.T. (Ed.) 1981. *Acquired Aphasia.* New York Academic Press.

Schuell, H. 1965. *Differential Diagnosis of Aphasia with the Minnesota Test.* Minneapolis: University of Minnesota Press.

Schuell, H. 1973. *Differential Diagnosis of Aphasia with the Minnesota Test* (Second Edition). Minneapolis: University of Minnesota Press.

Schuell, H.M., Jenkins, J.J., and Jimenez-Pabon, E. 1964. *Aphasia in Adults: Diagnosis, Prognosis, and Treatment.* New York: Hoeber.

Shewan, C.M. 1980. *Auditory Comprehension Test for Sentences.* Chicago: Biolinguistics Clinical Institute.

Sinnott, E.W. 1950. *Cell and Psyche.* Chapel Hill: University of North Carolina Press, Pp. 20.

Sklar, M. 1973. *Sklar Aphasia Scale* (Revised Edition). Los Angeles: Western Psychological Services.

Spreen, O. and Benton, A.L. 1977. *Neurosensory Center Comprehensive Examination for Aphasia* (1977 Revision). Victoria, B.C.: Neuropsychology Laboratory, University of Victoria.

Spreen, O. and Risser, A. 1981. Assessment of Aphasia. In Sarno, M.T. (Ed.), *Acquired Aphasia,* New York: Academic Press, Pp. 67-127.

Spreen, O. and Wachal, R.S. 1973. Psycholinguistic analysis of aphasic language: Theoretical formulations and procedures. *Language and Speech, 16,* 130-146.

Watson, J.B. 1924. *Behaviorism.* New York: People's Institute.

Weisenburg, T.H. and McBride, K.E. 1935. *Aphasia.* New York: Commonwealth Fund.

Wepman, J.M. and Jones, L.V. 1964. Five aphasias: A commentary on aphasia as a regressive linguistic phenomenon. In Rioch, D.M. and Weinstein, E.A. (Eds.), *Disorders of Communication.* Baltimore: Williams and Wilkins.

Wepman, J.M. 1951. *Recovery from Aphasia.* New York: Ronald.

Wertz, R.T. 1979. Word fluency measure. In Darley, F.L. (Ed.), *Evaluation of Appraisal Techniques in Speech and Language Pathology.* Reading, Mass.: Addison-Wesley.

Wheeler, L. 1963. Predictions of brain damage from an aphasia screening test; an application of discriminant functions and a comparison with a non-linear method of analysis. *Perceptual and Motor Skills, 17,* 63-80.

Wheeler, L., Burke, C.H., and Reitan, R.M. 1963. An application of discriminant functions to the problem of predicting brain damage using behavioral variables. *Perceptual and Motor Skills, 16,* 417-440 (Monograph Supplement).

Wheeler, L. and Reitan, R.M. 1962. The presence and laterality of brain damage predicted from responses to a short aphasia screening test. *Perceptual and Motor Skills, 15,* 783-799.

Wheeler, L. and Reitan, R.M. 1963. Discriminant functions applied to the problem of predicting cerebral damage from behavior tests: A cross validation study. *Perceptual and Motor Skills, 16,* 681-701.

Whitaker, H. and Whitaker, H.A. (Eds.) 1977. *Studies in Neurolinguisitics.* New York: Academic Press, xiv + 322.

Wilson, E.B. 1925. *The Cell in Development and Heredity* (Third Ed.). New York: Macmillan.

Index

Agnosia, 3, 4, 32, 34
  apperceptive visual, 4
  associated visual, 4
  color, 4
  musical, 4
  sound, 4
  visual spatial, 4
Agraphia, 2, 3
Alexia, 2, 3, 4
  with agraphia, 5
Amnesia verbalis, 2
Anomia, 4, 5
Anosognosia, 4
Aphasia, v, 3-4, 32, 37, 39, 167
  amnestic, 15
  anomic, 15
  auditory, 3
  brain lesions and, 1, 2, 4-5
  Broca's, 4, 6, 10, 13
  categories of, v, 1
  classification of, 32ff, 167-168
    (problems in), 2-3, 4, 5, 6
  clinical tests for (see *Tests for Aphasia*)
  conduction, 4, 5
  definition of, v, 1, 4, 5, 9, 19
  fluent, 1-2, 5, 10
  global, 5, 10
  historical considerations, 1-2, 6, 15ff
  identification of, 1-2, 2ff
    (problems in), 2
  intelligence (and), 6, 14ff, 35
  interindividual variability, 1, 2-3, 5, 6, 8
  nominal, 3
  non-fluent, 1, 5, 10
  semantic, 3, 4
  syntactical, 3
  transcortical motor, 5
  transcortical sensory, 5
  verbal, 3
  Wernicke's, 4, 5, 10
Apraxia, 3, 5, 32, 34
  bimanual, 4
  dressing, 4
  facial, 4
  ideational, 4
  ideo-motor, 4
  limb-kinetic, 4
  truncal, 4
Army General Classification Test, 16-17
Auditory-verbal dysgnosia, 26, 34
Autopagnosia, 4, 5
Body dysgnosia, 29, 34
Brain (see also *Cerebral hemispheres*)
  lesions, 46
  localization, 1, 5-6, 13
  neuropsychological function (and), 35
Central dysarthria, 34
Cerebral hemispheres
  electrical stimulation, 6-7
  lobes of (and functions), 6, 7
  localization, 5ff
Computational dyspraxia, 34
Constructional dyspraxia, 33, 34, 37, 40
Developmental deficits, 4
Dyscalculia, 34
Dysgnosia, 26
Dysnomia, 26, 33-34
Dysgraphia, 34
Dyslexia, 33-34, 36-37
Dyspraxia, 26
Halstead-Reitan Neuropsychological Test Battery, 22, 23, 24
Hypesthesia, 30
Ideo-kinetic dyspraxia, 34
Jargonagraphia, 5
Neuropsychological assessment, 8, 23, 24, 26, 35, 46, 167
  Methods of Inferential Approach,
    – level of performance, 11, 22
    – differential scores, 22
    – pathognomonic "sign", 4, 21, 22-23, 24, 27
    – comparison of right-left body sides, 22, 24-25
Pallilalia, 4
Paraphasia, 15
Paroxysmal speech disorders, 4
Pathognomonic "sign" (see *Neuropsychological assessment*)
Prosopagnosia, 4
Psychometric tests, 8, 12, 17-18
Receptive amusia, 4
Reitan-Indiana Aphasia Screening Test, 18, 21, 26ff
  aging (and), 47
  approach to, v, 21-22, 26-27, 33, 167
  content, 21-22, 32, 33
  deficits
    – expressive vs. receptive, 26, 33, 39-40, 167
    – frequency of, 35-36, 167
    – intercorrelations of, 36-40, 167

– lateralizing implications, 35, 39, 40-45, 167-168
instructions for Administering, 26ff
– recording responses (on), 27, 46-47
interpretation and "scoring", 23, 33, 47
purpose of, 21-22, 26
research results, 35ff, 167-168
results on individual patients, 46ff
validity of (see research results)
Reitan-Kløve Sensory-perceptual Examination, 23, 29ff
cerebral lateralization (and), 24
classification of deficits, 32, 34
comparison of right and left body sides (see *Neuropsychological assessment*)
content of, 23-24
deficits
– frequency of, 35-36, 167
– intercorrelations of, 36-38
– lateralizing implications, 35, 39-40, 44
double simultaneous stimulation, 24-25, 29, 30, 34
– auditory, 29
– tactile, 25, 29, 30
– visual, 29-30
finger agnosia (see tactile finger localization)
finger-tip number writing perception, 24, 30, 31
instructions for administration, 29ff
lateralization (and) 29-30
purpose of, 24, 29
right-left confusion (and), 29
research results, 35ff
results for individual patients, 46ff
"sign" approach (see *Neuropsychological assessment*)
tactile finger localization, 24, 30, 31
tactile form recognition, 31
unilateral stimulation, 24-25, 29-30, 31
validity (see research results)
visual fields, 29-30, 31
Right-left confusion, 34, 39
Rorschach Test, 16-17, 18
Spelling dyspraxia, 33
Tests for Aphasia
Aphasia Language Performance Scales, 10
Appraisal of Language Disturbance, 11
Auditory Comprehension Test for Sentences (ACTS), 9
Boston Diagnostic Aphasia Examination, 7, 11
Communicative Abilities in Daily Living, 10
Functional Communication Profile, 10
Halstead-Wepman Aphasia Screening Test, 10, 21
Minnesota Test for Differential Diagnosis of Aphasia, 11-12
Multilingual Aphasia Examination, 11
Neurosensory Center Comprehensive Examination for Aphasia (NCCEA), 11, 12
Peabody Picture Vocabulary Test, 11
Porch Index of Communicative Ability, 11, 12
Reporters Test, 9
Sklar Aphasia Scale, 10
Token Test, 9
Western Aphasia Battery, 11, 12
Visual form dysgnosia, 26, 33
Visual letter dysgnosia, 33, 34, 36-37
Visual number dysgnosia, 33
Visual word dysgnosia, 33, 34
Wechsler-Bellevue Scale, 18
Wechsler Bellevue Scale of Adult Intelligence, 16, 17
Wechsler Mental Ability Scale, 16, 18